HEALTH LITERACY IN PRIMARY CARE

ABOUT THE AUTHORS

GLORIA G. MAYER, RN, EdD, FAAN, is president and CEO of the Institute for Healthcare Advancement (IHA), a nonprofit organization whose mission is, "Empowering people to better health." IHA is a leader in health literacy, producing educational materials aimed at providing those with limited reading skills the health information they need.

Dr. Mayer has spoken and written extensively on a number of clinical and management topics. Her most recent publications include three of the five books in IHA's "What To Do For Health" series: *What To Do When Your Child Gets Sick* (2000), *What To Do For Teen Health* (2000), and *What To Do When You're Having a Baby* (2001). Books in the series are written at a third- to fifth-grade reading level so that the 90 million American adults who cannot read above a fifth-grade level can have access to this much needed health information.

Dr. Mayer received her BS degree from the University of Miami, an MS degree from the University of Maryland, and her masters and doctorate in education from Columbia University in New York City. Dr. Mayer consults nationally on health literacy and other health care topics.

MICHAEL VILLAIRE, MSLM, is Director of Programs and Operations for IHA. His background includes 20 years in various editor roles in health care publishing, including work on peer-reviewed journals in nursing, hospital publications, physician news magazines, and an online health care portal experiment. He has helped redesign and launch several medical and nursing journals and managed the development of a multimedia, interactive curriculum in critical care.

Mr. Villaire has been key in designing and launching annual medical symposia, including an annual conference in the complementary and alternative medicine field and, in his current position, IHA's annual Health Literacy Conference. He has written numerous articles on various aspects of health literacy and lectures on how to design and print health education materials for a low-literacy audience.

Mr. Villaire earned BA degrees in English and in communications from Western Michigan University in Kalamazoo, MI. He also earned a Masters of Science in Leadership and Management degree from the University of La Verne in La Verne, CA.

HEALTH LITERACY IN PRIMARY CARE

A CLINICIAN'S GUIDE

Gloria G. Mayer, RN, EdD, FAAN,
and
Michael Villaire, MSLM

With a Foreword by Albert E. Barnett, MD

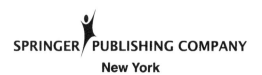

SPRINGER PUBLISHING COMPANY

New York

Springer Publishing Company, LLC.
11 West 42nd Street
New York, NY 10036
www.springerpub.com

Acquisitions Editor: Sally J. Barhydt
Production Editor: Shana Meyer
Cover design: Mimi Flow
Composition: Aptara, Inc.

08 09 10/ 5 4 3 2

_____

Library of Congress Cataloging-in-Publication Data

Mayer, Gloria G.
    Health literacy in primary care : a clinician's guide / Gloria G. Mayer and Michael Villaire ; with a foreword by Albert E. Barnett.
        p.   cm.
        Includes bibliographical references and index.
        ISBN-13: 978-0-8261-0229-4 (pbk.)
        ISBN-10: 0-8261-0229-8 (pbk.)
    1. Health education.   2. Patient education.   3. Communication in medicine.
4. Primary care (Medicine)   I. Villaire, Michael.   II. Title.
[DNLM: 1. Patient Education.   2. Communication Barriers.   3. Educational Status.
4. Professional-Patient Relations.
WA 590 M468h 2007]

RA440.5.M42   2007
613—dc22

                                                                    2006101856

_____

Printed in the United States of America by Bang Printing.

CONTENTS

PREFACE

The emergence of health literacy as a clinical issue should come as no surprise to health care providers. Patients with low literacy skills have always been a part of their practice. A persistent challenge, however, has been to understand low health literacy and to put a face on those affected in order to develop clear, straightforward strategies for overcoming the problem.

Health Literacy in Primary Care: A Clinician's Guide offers an excellent starting point to answer such a challenge. Written for the primary care practitioner, the text provides an in-depth view of the issue of health literacy, including definitions of low health literacy, a review of much current research, and efforts to quantify the problem.

The authors systematically address numerous aspects of the intersection of practice and health literacy, from creating a patient-friendly environment in the office and hospital setting to health literacy assessment; from understanding and avoiding medical errors to dealing with the interface between culture and health literacy; from improving patient–provider communication to writing and designing effective patient education materials; and from exploring alternative forms of patient communication to incorporating the use of foreign-language interpreters and translators in the clinical encounter.

With its broad view of literacy-related topics, however, *Health Literacy in Primary Care* needn't be read in sequence from chapter 1 to chapter 10; readers are encouraged to find entrée into the book at virtually any point. For example, those readers interested in designing easy-to-read patient education materials may want to skip right to chapters 7, 8, and 9, which are designed to simplify and improve that critical task. Those interested in sharpening their communication skills might look first to chapters 1 and 6, which focus on optimizing the clarity of patient–provider encounters. Those who serve a number of non-English-speaking patients may want to begin at the end, with chapter 10, which deals with the challenge of finding and evaluating qualified interpreters and underscores their role in providing effective care to patients at all literacy levels.

Low health literacy is a costly problem, both in terms of dollars and in terms of human suffering. But health care providers can play a crucial role in mitigating the effects of low health literacy if they attempt to educate themselves about the issue. By doing so, providers can work more effectively with this segment of the population and improve the health care such patients receive. Low health literacy is a much more pervasive problem than some people think, and the consequences of this ignorance—on the part of the practitioner as well as the patient—can be devastating.

Health Literacy in Primary Care is a valuable resource that raises awareness of the problem and provides hands-on tools for working with patients to dispel their shame, increase their understanding, and ultimately strengthen the bond of trust between patient and provider. These goals are the basis for an effective clinical partnership.

The text's authors are from the Institute for Healthcare Advancement (IHA), a nonprofit health care organization with a mission of empowering people to better health. Health literacy has been a primary focus at IHA since 1999. This book represents one more effort to *increase understanding* of this widespread phenomenon and to work toward *solving the problem* of low health literacy. Awareness and effective strategies are key for diminishing the impact of low health literacy on patients, even if this persistent problem remains part of clinical practice many years into the future.

Valuable though it is, this book is only one of many tools in the health care provider's arsenal. Additional resources are listed throughout the text, and readers are encouraged to do further research on their own. To help raise awareness and provide the easy-to-read materials so many patients need so desperately, IHA offers an annual health literacy conference and publishes a series of self-help books for consumers as well as caregivers. The "What To Do for Health" series is written at a third- to fifth-grade reading level, making the books easy to use and understand for the roughly 90 million adults who lack the functional literacy skills needed to navigate the U.S. health care system. Visit the IHA Web site at http://www.iha4health.org to learn more about these and other tools.

Gloria G. Mayer and Michael Villaire

ACKNOWLEDGMENTS

The authors wish to acknowledge the contributions of Michael Muscat and Lynne Pantano for their research efforts in gathering materials for this book, as well as Judith Connell, DrPH, for her contributions during the planning phase. They also wish to thank the Institute for Healthcare Advancement for its commitment to health literacy and its support during the writing of this book.

FOREWORD

Not so many years ago, the language of medicine was Latin. I remember, as a child, looking through my father's old medical tomes and seeing all the diseases described in Latin. I prepared myself for medical school by taking 4 years of Latin in high school, confident that this regimen would enable me to understand and communicate with my fellow physicians.

Few of us in those days thought very much about communicating with patients. Wasn't Latin and the rest of our medical jargon our private language? It was as if it were primarily designed to confound patients. After all, "good patients" were not expected or advised to question a physician's evaluation or proposed treatment. One of my best-remembered medical school professors made clear, on more than one occasion, that to be a great physician requires only "an accurate diagnosis and appropriate treatment." Patients were treated like small children. The patient's sole role in the health care equation was to be the uncomplaining object of the physician's ministrations. Health care illiteracy on the part of the public was not a problem, but actually a desired condition.

Today, the situation is profoundly altered. The only vestiges of Latin still existing are in some disease nomenclatures and prescription notations. But it seems that low health literacy is even more problematic now than in the days of medical Latin. For one thing, largely ineffective and inadequate treatments of past decades mostly have been displaced. Present-day therapies and procedures are not only far more effective but also are more complicated and in many ways more dangerous.

Disease prevention and efforts at screening for medical problems have made dramatic strides, but they also require a large dollop of patient cooperation and acceptance. The importance of diet and lifestyle to a patient's well-being has been firmly established. Patients are now required to participate in their own health care in order to maximize the benefits of modern treatments. Poor health literacy skills put patients at a severe disadvantage in the present health care system. And weak communication skills on the part of providers greatly reduce and can even obliterate otherwise successful therapeutic choices.

Health literacy actually is assuming even greater relevance as more and more of the cost of health care is borne by the individual patient, rather than by a corporate entity. How can patients select the appropriate medical management of their problem from countless television ads and Web sites? How can patients understand the priorities and nuances of their health problems? What measures can they take to ensure effective value for their health dollar? How can they avoid unnecessary and often dangerous overuse of health care resources? What can they do at home? When do they call the doctor? When is it an emergency?

Individuals with low health literacy have a difficult task in answering these and other questions when they attempt to take accountability for their own and their family's well-being. The so-called digital divide only serves to aggravate the problem further because a significant threshold of literacy is required just to use the Internet for information. As a society, it is difficult for us to embrace an existential belief in individual responsibility when the literacy playing field is so uneven.

Much research has been done on ways to diminish the real and potential harm that may afflict individuals with low health literacy. Dedicated and able workers across the country have made useful and exciting strides in dealing with the problem. In *Health Literacy in Primary Care: A Clinician's Guide,* Gloria Mayer and Michael Villaire have brought together in a single volume the major issues in health literacy from the standpoint of the patient, as well as the challenges facing health care providers. Importantly, this text encompasses and distills some specific methodologies that have been demonstrably effective in communicating with low-literate patients. Dr. Mayer has used her extensive literacy experience and teaching techniques to craft a compelling introduction to the topic in the opening chapters. Then, clearly and succinctly, the authors go on to define the various issues and offer pathways for effectively dealing with patients with weak literacy skills.

One might ask if this is a textbook for a course that does not exist. In a sense, that is true. We know of no academic discipline at an American university specifically in health literacy. Schools of public health deal, among other things, with pure food and water, safety, and environmental issues. Because of our vast knowledge base, medical school and public health school curricula already are crammed with courses of great importance. But, as the authors state so ably in chapter 1, health literacy is an extremely pervasive and costly issue, both financially and in terms of human suffering.

Perhaps the time is not far off when health literacy will be recognized as a problem worthy of inclusion in formal university curricula.

Albert E. Barnett, MD
Chairman and Medical Director
Institute for Healthcare Advancement
Clinical Professor, Public Health and Preventative Medicine
Loma Linda University School of Medicine

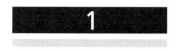

UNDERSTANDING HEALTH LITERACY

Imagine you are an exclusively English-speaking American and you find yourself very far from home. Maybe you're on the west coast of Karnataka, in a largely rural area miles from Mangalore City, India, where the Kannada, Konkani, and Tulu languages are widely spoken, but English is rare. Sitting outside a small village eatery overlooking part of the Arabian Sea, you suddenly feel sick to your stomach. Glancing around, you see dozens of locals filing past, beasts of burden in tow, but only the occasional sign in a language you cannot read.

You realize your phrase book is back in your hotel room and you begin to panic; it's late and there isn't a hospital in sight. You grip your abdomen, praying the nausea will pass. Maybe it was the *uppittu* or *rava dosa* you ate this morning, or maybe you're having a reaction to the digestive pills the chemist recommended when you were in Bengalooru. Weak in the knees, your head spinning, you stand up, brace yourself against a nearby wall, and hope you can explain to someone—to *anyone*—that you need medical attention urgently.

But it's hopeless. Though the village is buzzing with activity, most of its inhabitants are Coorgis and nomadic Lambanis who don't speak a word of English. Maybe you can signal your distress using hand gestures? Unfortunately, the locals just stare at you puzzled or smile and nod: your clothes are strange and your customs are unfamiliar. Were you to make it to a hospital, how would you explain your plight to the clinical staff? If you were lucky enough to get to a local pharmacy for medicine, what would you do if the instructions on the bottle were written entirely in Tulu or in some other language? You'd be at the mercy of a translator or interpreter. Would you understand what you were being told? Questions like these race through your mind, making you feel sicker.

Sounds desperate, doesn't it? Imagine feeling so utterly lost and isolated when you are ill. Imagine being confused by or unfamiliar with your surroundings when you are desperately in need of help. Imagine receiving medical instructions you could not possibly follow, no matter how much you wanted to. Imagine not knowing what you should do next.

* * *

Unfortunately, for roughly 90 million Americans—and possibly even more—this extraordinary circumstance is not difficult to imagine. And it's not because these Americans cannot speak the native language (though surely some of them can't). Nor is it because these millions of people are necessarily world travelers, though for some Karnataka is neither exotic nor distant. It's not even because all 90 million know what it's like to be taken ill in a public place. (Then again, how many of us have never had *that* unpleasant experience?) No, the reason so many millions of Americans can sympathize with the unsettling experience of the nauseated tourist in Karnataka is that they struggle with low literacy. And the vast majority of these individuals—perhaps all of them—also have low *health* literacy. It means they've been there. They know the feeling.

However, low health literacy is not about what language you speak or how well educated you are. It is not limited to immigrants, the poor, or the elderly, though each of these groups is affected disproportionately. And perhaps most important, it is by no means something that health care providers can afford to ignore. *Health literacy is about access to care.* Specifically, it is about who has the ability to use the health care system available to them in a way that is appropriate for their circumstances. It is about power and about effective patient–provider communication. In fact, it is about the very nature of the relationship between patients and their providers. And low health literacy is around us all the time—in every clinic, in every community, in every county, and in every state.

But how specifically are the day-to-day experiences of those with low health literacy similar to the desperate circumstances of the sick tourist in Karnataka? Simple: those with low health literacy skills feel similarly isolated and alone when they encounter health-related information phrased in language they cannot effectively "translate." They feel equally lost and overwhelmed when dealing with prescription labels or when they attempt to understand what's said to them by health care providers, many of whom use highly specialized jargon yet rarely make sure their patients can understand the message. Often low-literate patients cannot use the densely written health materials they're given because they lack the literacy skills necessary to decipher them, just as an exclusively English speaker would have little use for medical instructions written entirely in Tulu.

HEALTH LITERACY DEFINED

So far we seem to be using the terms *literacy* and *health literacy* interchangeably. There is considerable overlap between the two concepts, so this practice is actually quite common, even in the medical literature. (Occasionally you may even notice the two terms substituted for one another throughout the chapters of this book.) Still, important distinctions exist between the terms. Literacy refers to the ability to read, write, and understand one's native language in both written and spoken forms. What, then, is *health literacy?* Can we distinguish it from other kinds of literacy, such as media or computer literacy, that call for skills in specific and sometimes technical contexts?

Yes, we can, but health literacy is not much different from these other kinds of literacy; it simply refers to how well one applies a broad range of literacy skills *in the context of health care.* Functional media literacy may call for an understanding of the way music and special effects heighten the drama in a movie or television program, for example. By contrast, computer literacy skills may require familiarity with CD-ROMs, word-processing programs, and the ins and outs of the World Wide Web.

The proper context for health literacy, however, is health care. If you have difficulty understanding terms your doctor uses in an office visit, it's not necessarily because you are low literate: chances are you simply haven't reached a sufficient *health literacy* level to translate the jargon you hear into standard English that makes sense to you. Likewise, if the abbreviations on a chart or prescription bottle trip you up, it may be due to your *health* literacy level, not your *general* literacy skills. Even if you're an excellent reader, in other words, you may have a hard time understanding texts dealing with a specific health concept, disease, or condition.

An example might help illustrate the point. Witness this startling confession from Gloria G. Mayer, RN, EdD, president and CEO of the Institute for Healthcare Advancement (IHA), and coauthor of *Health Literacy in Primary Care: A Clinician's Guide:*

> I am a nurse with advanced degrees. I read on a college level. Yet, I am a total health illiterate. How can this be? Well, I've been diagnosed with an unusual type of autoimmune disease that has extended into several other diseases, one of which— lymphoma—might be fatal. Yet, despite my health care background, my ability to understand the written word at a high grade level, and the many resources at my immediate disposal, I still don't understand everything I need to know about my condition (Mayer, 2003, p. 2).

Obviously, then, based on the comments above, health literacy involves more than one's ability to read texts.

Yet so does *general* literacy, assuming we rely on the definition of literacy offered by the National Literacy Act of 1991: "an individual's ability to read, write, and speak English, *and compute and solve problems* [emphasis added] at levels of proficiency necessary to function on the job and in society, to achieve one's goals, and develop one's knowledge and potential" (National Institute for Literacy, 1991). Based on this definition, literacy encompasses more than just reading; *numeracy,* or competence in math skills needed in everyday life, is equally important for *functional literacy,* itself defined as the literacy level needed to perform specific tasks (Institute of Medicine, 2004, p. 37).

In this respect, literacy is actually quite similar to health literacy. After all, the skills required to navigate the health care system are essentially functional skills; that is, they serve a specific purpose, allowing patients to function in everyday life. Simple computations are necessary for following the instructions on a prescription bottle, for example, as is some facility with calculating times based on those instructions. If you are asked to take a pill every 4 to 6 hours and it's 10 a.m. now, you must be able to calculate that your next dose should fall between 2 p.m. and 4 p.m. We're not born knowing how to use a clock; at some point we all must *learn* how to do so.

What distinguishes literacy from health literacy is context, as Barry D. Weiss, MD, explains: "Health literacy differs from general literacy, which refers to the basic ability to read, write, and compute, without regard to the context in which the reading and writing occur" (Weiss, 2005, p. 17). According to the American Medical Association (AMA), health literacy calls for "a constellation of skills, including the ability to perform basic reading and numerical tasks required to function in the health care environment" (Ad Hoc Committee, 1999). The word *constellation* is appropriate here. Although these abilities seem scattered and independent from one another, when properly aligned—that is, when the patient can translate information using his or her literacy skills—they bring a much larger picture into focus. The stars align; the patient suddenly understands.

Functional health literacy is critically important during the typical patient–provider encounter, during a pharmacy visit when patients are reading the label on a prescription bottle for the first time, at home when they're opening a book to learn about their child's illness, and in many other situations. It's not enough simply to *understand* the information, however; we also must *act* on it. That's why *Healthy People 2010* and the Institute of Medicine (IOM) define health literacy as "the degree to which individuals have the capacity to obtain, process, and understand basic health information and services needed to make appropriate health decisions" (Ratzan & Parker, 2000). We must use the information we encounter to make decisions that affect our health and well-being. In fact, one could argue that the most useful health information is presented in a problem-solving or behavioral context (i.e., the how-to approach). As the IOM's Committee on Health Literacy notes:

> While general facts about cancer, nutrition, or care-giving are helpful, unless the health information is cast within a problem-solving context, it is often lost. . . . For example, instructions provided to an elderly man with diabetes on the importance of foot care would be more effective if the information is presented within the context of how to achieve the necessary care. . . . In other words, "getting the message out" does not mean that people will act on the information (IOM, 2004, pp. 155–156).

LITERACY SURVEYS IN THE UNITED STATES: INTRODUCING THE "AVERAGE" AMERICAN

Much of what we know about literacy in the United States we owe to the National Adult Literacy Survey (NALS) of 1992 and the National Assessment of Adult Literacy (NAAL) of 2003, the most recent nationally representative surveys of literacy skills among adults. The 1992 NALS did not specifically test knowledge of health-related concepts; such instruments as the Rapid Estimate of Adult Literacy in Medicine (REALM) and the Test of Functional Health Literacy in Adults (TOFHLA), which we discuss later in this book, have been used on individuals expressly for that purpose.

However, because the more recent NAAL, a follow-up study to the 1992 NALS, expanded the number of background questions about health and included health-related tasks as part of its item pool, it provides considerably more insight into the relationship between health and literacy than did its predecessor (Comings & Kirsch, 2005).

The NALS and the NAAL present participants with everyday tasks, such as totaling the entries on a bank deposit slip, identifying a piece of information in a news article, determining the difference in price between two items, locating an intersection on a street map, and other tasks that involve the use of written documents varying from relatively simple to complex. Sixty-five of the 152 tasks on the NAAL were taken from the earlier NALS in order to measure changes in literacy that took place between 1992 and 2003 (National Center for Education Statistics, 2005). Recognizing that functional literacy requires a broad spectrum of skills, the researchers who developed these surveys designed them to assess abilities along three literacy scales: prose literacy, document literacy, and quantitative literacy. A short newspaper article might be used to test *prose* skills, *documents* tend to be charts and forms the participant reads and deciphers, and *quantitative* skills usually involve mathematical computations.

Although the NALS of 1992 categorized respondents into five different levels (from level 1, the lowest, associated with the most basic tasks and the lowest literacy levels, to level 5, the highest, associated with the most complicated tasks and the highest literacy levels), the 2003 NAAL recognized only four: *proficient,* indicating that the survey respondent possessed skills necessary for performing complex and challenging literacy activities; *intermediate,* meaning that he or she had the skills necessary to perform moderately challenging activities; *basic,* signaling a respondent who had the skills necessary for performing simple, everyday tasks; and *below basic,* the lowest level, signifying a respondent with no more than the most simple and concrete literacy skills. These four levels were based on recommendations from a committee of the National Research Council's Board on Testing and Assessment (BOTA). A full description of BOTA's methodology in determining the four levels for the 2003 NAAL is available at http://books.nap.edu/catalog/11267.html.

The NALS of 1992 originally surveyed nearly 13,600 individuals aged 16 years and older, plus 1,000 adults in each of 12 states to provide state-level results comparable to the national data. More than 26,000 adults were surveyed in all, and each participant was asked to spend about an hour responding to a series of tasks and questions asking about demographic characteristics, education, reading practices, and other topics related to literacy (Kirsch, Jungeblut, Jenkins, & Kolstad, 1993, p. xv). The more recent NAAL, by contrast, surveyed more than 19,000 adults aged 16 years or older, roughly 18,000 of whom lived in households and more than 1,000 of whom lived in prisons, yielding a statistically valid representation of the total adult population of about 222 million people, based on U.S. Census Bureau and Bureau of Justice statistics for 2003 (White & Dillow, 2005).

Figure 1.1 shows the percentage of adults in each literacy level in 1992 and 2003. Fourteen percent of adult respondents in the 2003 NAAL fell into the below basic category in prose literacy, 12% in document literacy, and 22% in quantitative literacy. Twenty-nine percent were categorized as basic in prose

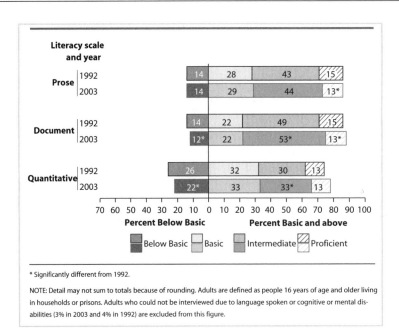

FIGURE 1.1 Percentage of U.S. adults in each literacy level: 1992 and 2003. *Source:* U.S. Department of Education, Institute of Education Sciences, National Center for Education Statistics, 1992 National Adult Literacy Survey, and 2003 National Assessment of Adult Literacy.

literacy, 22% in document literacy, and 33% in quantitative literacy. Those at the basic level were unable to perform such tasks as consulting reference materials to determine which foods contain a particular vitamin, identifying a specific location on a map, or calculating the cost of ordering specific office supplies from a catalog—tasks that could be performed by those scoring at the intermediate level (NCES, 2005).

Thirteen percent of respondents were labeled proficient, meaning they could read and understand lengthy, complex prose texts, synthesizing information and making complex inferences; integrate, synthesize, and analyze multiple pieces of information in complex documents; and use abstract quantitative information to solve multistep problems when the mathematical operations were not easily inferred and the problems were complex (NCES, 2005).

What does the 2003 NAAL tell us about functional literacy? It's true that some of those categorized at the lowest level, below basic, could be described as nonliterate; others, however, were able to perform simple tasks, such as locating easily identifiable information and following written instructions in simple documents, signing a form, and adding the amounts on a bank deposit slip. Still, we might see such individuals as functionally illiterate because they could not perform the described tasks reliably. (Note, however, that those with limited literacy skills cross all ethnic and educational boundaries.) If those who fell into the below basic category could be called marginally or functionally illiterate, what broader term describes those participants in the basic category?

What if we assumed that those scoring in the basic category could function well in the context of everyday literacy tasks? After all, the NAAL defines a basic reader as one who has "the skills necessary for performing simple, everyday tasks" (NCES, 2005). Because prose, document, and quantitative skills all are necessary for functional literacy, we would be justified in considering the largest group in the below basic category as functionally literate, which in this case would be those who scored below basic in quantitative tasks. (Considerably more respondents tested below basic in quantitative skills than in prose [14%] or document [12%] skills.) In this case we would arrive at a figure of at least 48.8 million people who cannot perform the literacy tasks necessary to function in everyday life. (Twenty-two percent of NAAL respondents scored below basic in quantitative skills; 22% of 222 million people is roughly 48.8 million.)

We must qualify such a figure, however. Bear in mind that, within each category, participants demonstrated a range of abilities, just not enough to qualify for the next level. Those categorized as below basic scored anywhere from 0 to 234 on the quantitative scale, 0 to 209 on the prose scale, and 0 to 204 on the document scale. To achieve basic categorization, however, a test-taker had to score between 235 and 289 on the quantitative scale, 210 and 264 on the prose scale, and 205 and 249 on the document scale. Someone scoring 235 in quantitative literacy would not be as proficient as someone scoring 289, even though both would be categorized as basic. In addition, someone who scored below basic on prose literacy yet intermediate on quantitative literacy would have a difficult time performing tasks that call for more advanced prose skills. Basically, those scoring below basic in any of the three categories—regardless of how they scored in the other two—would have considerable trouble understanding certain pieces of information they encounter every day.

In other words, many in the basic category, in addition to all those in the below basic category, would have a hard time dealing with clinical information, which tends to be fairly complicated. Results from both the NALS and the NAAL suggest as much about readers at the lowest levels. More than a decade ago, 21% to 23% of respondents on the NALS, roughly 40 million to 44 million adults, scored in the lowest of the five levels, level 1, qualifying them as functionally illiterate. Twenty-five to 28% or 50 million adults, demonstrated literacy skills in the next highest level, level 2, which corresponded with "marginal" literacy skills. Add 40 million to 50 million, and that brings us to the figure of 90 million Americans who have poor or marginal literacy skills.

On the more recent NAAL, 43% of adults were found to be either basic or below basic in prose literacy, 34% fell into these two categories in document literacy, and 55% were at these levels in quantitative literacy. Across the three categories of prose, document, and quantitative literacy, then, an average of 44% of U.S. adults surveyed scored in the lowest two of four levels on the NAAL. Extrapolating these percentages to an adult population of roughly 222 million (as of 2003), this means that close to 98 million Americans may struggle with or be unable to perform everyday tasks, such as adding the amounts on a bank deposit slip, using a television guide to find out what programs are on, or comparing ticket prices for two events.

Again, based on the 1992 NALS, the IOM estimated that roughly 90 million Americans (the figure we cited in the opening paragraphs of this chapter), or as many as 94 million, lack sufficient literacy skills to function in the health care system (IOM, 2004). Our calculations here suggest that the 2003 NAAL recorded a similar statistic, arriving at the higher number because of 11 additional years of population growth.

Forty-eight million, 90 million, 94 million, 98 million: whatever the exact figure, the sheer numbers of Americans affected by this problem make it worthy of our attention. Scores of millions of average Americans—that's right, *average* Americans, not exceptions to the rule, not statistical outliers—live in fear and anxiety because they are poorly equipped to navigate our increasingly complex health care system. And it's because they lack the literacy skills they need to make sense of health information. This is one take-home lesson of surveys like the NALS and the NAAL. Full summaries of NALS and NAAL data are available in several references listed at the end of this chapter (Kirsch et al., 1993; NCES, 2005; White & Dillow, 2005).

But these are just surveys, you may be thinking; they aren't real. In real life, people can get by when they have to. They can ask for help, or they have relatives who can help them.

Don't be so sure. Research suggests that those with limited literacy skills report poorer overall health, are less likely to make use of medical screenings, seek medical care after they have reached later stages of disease, are more likely to be hospitalized, have poorer understanding of their treatments, and have lower adherence to medical regimens (Berkman et al., 2004; Rudd, 2002). Many are getting no help at all.

ALL AROUND US

Evidence of the adverse effects of low health literacy is all around us—just pick up a newspaper or turn on your television. Even ads suggest there's a problem. Advertisers, one might argue, have a vested interest in recognizing trends and needs in the marketplace, especially those advertisers doing public relations for multimillion-dollar health benefits companies.

A recent advertisement from Blue Cross Blue Shield, for example, features a blue and white bookmark with a collegiate-looking tassel hanging down one side. The text on the bookmark begins, "We Could Save Billions in Healthcare Costs if We Could Just Get Kids to Read," and then touts a mentoring program that the organization sponsors with the Department of Health Care Policy at Harvard Medical School. The program "uses health related children's books to raise health awareness," and the ad explains that "[s]ome consumers aren't able to read basic health information . . . [which] compromises the quality of healthcare and adds billions to America's annual health care cost." It's no exaggeration:

research by Friedland and colleagues suggests that low health literacy increases U.S. health expenditures by roughly $73 billion per year (National Academy on an Aging Society, 1998).

The Blue Cross Blue Shield ad appeared not only in such newspapers and magazines as the *New York Times, U.S. News and World Report,* the *Wall Street Journal, USA Today,* the *Washington Post,* the *New Republic,* and the *Atlantic Monthly* but also in employee trade publications circulated by human resources departments. Many of these publications are geared toward a general readership; others, however, such as the *Atlantic Monthly* (with a circulation of about 500,000) and the *Wall Street Journal* (which reaches roughly 2 million readers), are read by some of the highest-paid Americans, among whom one would find health policy elites and other business decision makers.

On average, readers of the *Atlantic Monthly* earn $82,983 per year (Project for Excellence in Journalism, 2004). One-third of *Wall Street Journal* readers are in top management, one-fifth are in mid-management, and more than a quarter are either professional or technical (2000 Beta Travel Study, 2000). In other words, ads such as these not only share information with general readers about the activities of a major health plan but also target high-end stakeholders with a vested interest in improving efficiency in the delivery of health care services. These professionals know that such efforts as the Blue Cross Blue Shield/Harvard University cosponsored mentoring program can save health care costs in the long run, preventing the unnecessary use of emergency services, for example.

Business interests are certainly catching on to the importance of low health literacy as a national issue. Although Blue Cross Blue Shield has not developed a campaign specifically around health literacy, notes Joe Bogardus, executive director of brand marketing communications for the Blue Cross Blue Shield Association, the company is concerned with demonstrating how its plans across the country are working to identify programs that enhance quality of care and work to keep health care costs more affordable (J. Bogardus, personal communication, February 2006). Pilot research programs sponsored by Blue Cross are examining employer–employee communication with an eye toward what works to improve employee health habits. Can posters in the break room cause a measurable increase in the use of generic drugs, for example? Could a video- or Web-based employer education program encourage employees to exercise more?

That patient education can improve health outcomes and save costs is one premise of Blue Cross's *Walking Works* initiative, which it sponsors with the President's Council on Physical Fitness and Sports. The campaign seeks to help Americans live healthier lives by helping them set and achieve personal walking goals. Although some believe that money spent by managed care organizations on health literacy efforts would be better spent on efforts to help health care providers improve the clarity of their communications with patients (Kantor, 2005), what matters is that stakeholders in health-related fields have taken notice of the health literacy problem and are seeking organized solutions.

Literature reviews reveal increasing awareness among researchers as well. In January 2000, for example, Rudd and colleagues from the National Center for the Study of Adult Learning and Literacy (NCSALL) published an annotated bibliography of medical and public health literature addressing literacy issues that appeared between 1990 and 1999 (Rudd, Colton, & Schacht, 2000). Their review suggests a growing recognition of literacy issues and communication barriers within the health fields. Follow-up reviews were published for the years 2000 (Greenberg, 2001) and 2001 (Zobel, 2002). In their 2003 bibliography of health literacy research published between January and December 2002, Zobel, Rowe, and Gomez-Mandic note,

> The most significant difference in [2002's] bibliography is that there has been a marked increase in the body of literature addressing the issues of literacy and health. The number of articles published in public health and medical journals has almost doubled from . . . [2001]. Specifically, there has been an increase in the area of computer literacy and health education in the information age. This issue emerged [in 2002] for the first time, but there is now much more attention being paid not only to issues concerning readability of Internet materials but also to the differences between print and computer based health education materials.

Much of this new research is undertaken at institutions of higher learning. And whereas few official requirements or curricula address health literacy in schools of medicine, public health, nursing, dentistry, or pharmacy, efforts to expose students to the subject are on the rise. Courses and curricula touching on health literacy have been offered at the Harvard School of Public Health, the University of Colorado Medical School, and the University of Virginia School of Medicine (IOM, 2004). As our understanding of the relationship between literacy and health improves, such offerings will likely spread to other schools in the future.

Still, one needn't subscribe to the *Journal of the American Medical Association (JAMA)* or have clinical training to come to the conclusion that we have a nationwide low literacy problem with significant implications for health care. In 1998, in fact, President Clinton sent a memo to the heads of all executive departments and agencies in the federal government directing them to use plain language in "all new documents, other than regulations, that explain how to obtain a benefit or service or how to comply with a requirement you administer or enforce. For example, these documents may include letters, forms, notices, and instructions" ("President Clinton's memorandum," 1998).

Among these executive departments and agencies is the U.S. Department of Health and Human Services (HHS), which houses the Agency for Healthcare Research and Quality (AHRQ), the Centers for Disease Control and Prevention (CDC), the Food and Drug Administration (FDA), the National Institutes of Health (NIH), and other agencies charged with safeguarding the health of all Americans. Indirectly, then, President Clinton's directive recognized the need for easy-to-read materials that communicate health-related information between government entities and the lay public. After all, limited access to public health information not only decreases knowledge and awareness, but also hampers action and civic involvement (Rudd, Kaphingst, Colton, Gregoire, & Hyde, 2004).

More recently, in July 2005, the AMA and the Blue Cross Blue Shield Association cosponsored the Official White House Conference on Aging (WHCoA), the purpose of which was to provide recommendations that the WHCoA policy committee could incorporate into final policy recommendations for the president and Congress (AMA Foundation, 2005). It remains to be seen what actions the White House or Congress will take based on the committee's advice, but the committee did raise many of the issues and cite many of the studies that are featured in subsequent chapters of this book. (To read the full proceedings from the conference, visit the AMA Web site at http://www.ama-assn.org/ama/pub/category/7639.html.)

SEEING THE SYSTEM THROUGH THE PATIENT'S EYES

By now it's easy to see that there is a significant problem with respect to literacy and health literacy skills in the United States. Awareness is growing, but judging by the $73 billion figure cited earlier, the health literacy problem remains exorbitantly expensive. Nevertheless, data and statistics can be cold and abstract. How does low health literacy manifest in a patient's everyday life?

One way to put yourself in the shoes of the low-health-literate patient is to think carefully about the range of literacy-related skills needed just to make a visit to the doctor, even for something fairly routine. First the patient must use a calendar or some other means for remembering the date and time of the appointment—a basic skill, yes, but one we should not take for granted. (As noted earlier, numeracy skills such as using a calendar must be learned.) Then the patient must secure transportation to the appointment. This could mean planning around bus schedules, with all the logistical savvy such a task entails. If the patient is driving, he or she may be faced with dozens of road signs along the way, some signaling one-way streets, others explaining detours and road construction complete with dates and phone numbers for further information, and perhaps other signs obscured by trees.

Once the patient arrives at the destination, he or she will probably be asked to interpret signage at the hospital or clinic, including parking signs, building identification signs, and directories. Hospitals often have multiple entrances that go by various names: "admitting," "receiving," "ambulatory care," or "emergency entrance" (Rudd, Renzulli, Pereira, & Daltroy, 2005, p. 74).

Inside the waiting room the patient may be asked to fill out patient information and consent forms and to read and acknowledge receipt of a Notice of Privacy Practices as required by the Health Insurance Portability and Accountability Act (HIPAA) of 1996, no doubt written several grade levels above his or her actual reading ability and in a miniscule type size that makes reading the document far too burdensome. (Using several software programs, Hochhauser [2003] analyzed more than 30 HIPAA privacy notices and found that their reading level averaged grade 14.5, or the second or third year of college.) With a waiting room full of sick and weary patients and the potential for embarrassment if he or she seems confused, the patient may decide that the path of least resistance is simply to pretend to understand everything he or she is told. After all, the patient's just there to see the doctor.

Once inside the examination room, the patient will likely be interviewed by a nurse practitioner, which means having to articulate something about his or her symptoms and probably establishing a reason for the visit. A patient who does not speak English may have the option of communicating through an interpreter, which adds another layer of complexity to the clinical encounter. (For more about the role of interpreters in health care, see chapter 10, Interpreters and Their Role in the Health Care Setting.) In any event, those mysterious charts, containers, needle depositories, and drawers full of equipment can be intimidating, raising the patient's stress level and discouraging open communication. Use of jargon, even in posters on the wall, already has set in motion a process of bewilderment.

Virtually all of these activities, from the simplest to the most complex, require some degree of reading proficiency, facility with language, and effective communication skills. Each calls for informed decision making as well. Most assume a level of ease with technical terms or vocabulary that could be unfamiliar to the average American. Many of these are the very skills tested on the NALS and the NAAL, which found that almost half of all Americans (43% in prose literacy, 34% in document literacy, and 55% in quantitative literacy, for an average of approximately 44%) scored in the lowest two literacy levels.

The bottom line is this: in addition to all the other concerns that health care providers have about their patients—from whether their outcomes and quality of life will improve to whether they will experience drug interactions; from whether they will comply with a physician's orders to whether they will receive quality care even after being discharged—low health literacy adds yet another layer of complexity to the already dense tissue of interrelationships that comprise good care and effective patient–provider communication. Can health care providers be sure that their low-literate patients understand their chronic diseases and how to treat them? Are low-literate patients clear about the directions they are given concerning new medications? Do their nods signal genuine understanding, or is that just a defense mechanism to avoid appearing ignorant? Will low-health-literate patients take advantage of all the medical resources they are offered?

Answering such questions is the task of health care providers themselves. Patients who have difficulty completing a job application or reading tables and charts are unlikely to fare very well in our demanding health care system, in which information is sometimes presented in multipage formats and with strangely la-beled graphs featuring masses of vertical bars and other mysterious abbreviations, such as mm Hg, EKG, and °F. Health care providers need to understand problems caused by low literacy. Those with poor literacy skills are like the sick tourist in Karnataka, who must find help despite her lack of understanding of native customs or dialects. The best time for a crash course is not when you are sick.

Some researchers know that all too well because they have quite liter-ally walked in their patients' footsteps. Along with a group of research assis-tants, Rudd (2004) conducted an examination of hospital navigation issues to gain insight into the literacy environment that helps and hinders patients as they seek care. Interviewers and informants—including graduate students, re-search staff, adult education teachers, and students enrolled in adult education programs—walked around the public areas of 10 municipal hospitals. The investigators found that "when people need assistance, they currently rely more heavily on other people than they do on signs and maps." This preliminary study also confirmed that "a dense and demanding literacy environment can be intimidating, that most people find complex signs difficult to read, and that a person with average literacy skills is not familiar with many of the medical terms used on signs and in forms" (Rudd, 2004, p. 23).

TEXTS AND CONTEXTS: BROADENING OUR PERSPECTIVE

Earlier we mentioned that literacy differs from health literacy only with respect to the context in which each takes place. Difficulty reading a poem or a novel, following cooking instructions, or calculating a 15% gratuity, for example, suggests that an individual may have a literacy problem. The context of such tasks is everyday life, but they are not necessarily encountered in the process of seeking health care. Difficulty complying with a doctor's orders because you don't understand them or in deciding what to do if your child sprains his or her ankle, however, suggests a health literacy problem. The context of these challenges is health care.

Next we asked that you put yourself in the patient's shoes by considering the constellation of skills that are required to make a simple doctor visit. Now let's take the process of empathizing with patients a step further.

All of us are literate and illiterate only within a specific context, as Dr. Rima Rudd, primary investigator in the navigation study discussed above, reminds us. "I'm a highly literate person," she explains, "but if you gave me a textbook in neuroscience or car mechanics, you would find that I have low functional literacy with these texts" (*Law of averages*, 2003). All specialized languages can give us pause. We saw poignant evidence for such selective literacy in the confession from this book's coauthor, Gloria Mayer—a nurse with advanced degrees—who is unable to understand everything she needs to know about her autoimmune disorder. To demonstrate further, however, let's try an experiment. Imagine you are confronted with the following paragraph by Homi K. Bhabha, professor of English and African American studies at Harvard University, in your everyday reading:

> From the subaltern perspective, are we demanding that Foucault should historicize "imperialism" as the origin of modernity, so that he may "complete" the argument? Definitely not.... [T]he colonial and postcolonial is, metaleptically, partially present in the text, in a spirit of subaltern resistance that will turn it toward other things.... By disavowing "the colonial moment" as enunciative, transferential discursive relation, Foucault can say nothing of the power and knowledge that constitutes the position of the Western ratio, in its moment of modernity, as a dialogic "colonial" relation (Bhabha, 1992, p. 64).

Did reading Bhabha's words make you feel at least mildly illiterate? (And to think: they were written in English, not Tulu.) If not, then congratulations: you are functioning at or above the 16th-grade reading level, easily two or three times that of the average American adult. For most readers, however, the passage would be seriously confusing, especially to those unfamiliar with multisyllabic, esoteric terms, such as *subaltern, metaleptically, transferential, enunciative,* and *dialogic.* The material also would leave even highly educated readers nonplussed who had little or no prior knowledge of French philosopher and social critic Michel Foucault's work or the assumptions of postcolonial theory.

Similarly, how would the nonspecialist make sense of Professor T. W. Anderson's explanation for why we ought to study normal multivariate distributions in statistics:

> One of the reasons the study of normal multivariate distributions is worthwhile is that marginal distributions and conditional distributions derived from multivariate normal distributions are also normal distributions. Moreover, linear combinations of normal variates are again normally distributed. First we shall show that if we make a nonsingular linear transformation of a vector whose components have a joint distribution with a normal density we obtain a vector whose components are jointly distributed with a normal density (Anderson, 1958, p. 19).

Even if Anderson's point is not entirely clear, let us hope that ours is: we must think twice before making assumptions about or judging those who have low health literacy or low literacy in general. Despite our privileges of higher education or of specialized training, we too can be low literate in certain situations. Often it simply depends on the text and context in which we encounter information.

DISPELLING MYTHS ABOUT LOW HEALTH LITERACY

Myths about low health literacy persist among health care professionals and the lay public. Identifying these misconceptions affords us the opportunity to discuss factors that really do affect health literacy, such as age, income, education, language, and country of origin. Some populations are more vulnerable to the effects of this problem than are others. Should we assume that a patient who is poor has low health literacy, whereas a patient who is affluent functions at a higher level? On average that may be safe to assume, but making such assumptions is generally unwise. Much like those with limited literacy skills, those with low health literacy come from a variety of backgrounds.

"Some adults who displayed limited skills [in the 1992 NALS] reported working in professional or managerial jobs," note Kirsch and colleagues (1993, p. xxi), "earning high wages, and participating in various aspects of our society . . . while others who demonstrated high levels of proficiency reported being unemployed or out of the labor force. Thus, having advanced literacy skills does not necessarily guarantee individual opportunities."

A few stereotypes about the low literate contain a kernel of truth, but they are unreliable, based on hasty generalizations. According to a 2004 report by the Educational Testing Service, U.S. adults with low literacy skills typically have not completed high school or obtained a GED, have health-related limitations on their ability to go to school or work, are members of minority groups, and are immigrants to the United States (Rudd, Kirsch, & Yamamoto, 2004, p. 41). We should be cautious about jumping to conclusions, however. "An important and as yet unanswered question," note the authors of a January 2004 Agency for Healthcare Research and Quality (AHRQ) evidence report, "is whether literacy is a mediator of adverse outcomes or whether it is merely a marker for other associated factors, such as poverty, lack of access to care, or lack of health insurance, that actually lead to poorer health outcomes" (Berkman et al., 2004, p. 6).

It is not entirely clear, in other words, whether limited literacy skills should be seen as a cause or an effect—whether, for example, low literacy forces people into poverty or afflicts them with poorer health outcomes or whether being poor and suffering ill health simply makes it less likely that consumers will gain access to a quality education or to the best our health care system has to offer. The same goes for those with low health literacy, so this might be a good time to separate a few facts about low health literacy from several common myths.

Myth #1: If I Give Patients Easy-to-Read Materials, They'll Be Offended Because I'm "Dumbing Down" to Them

This simply isn't true. When a patient feels condescended to or disrespected, it probably has more to do with the caregiver's tone of voice, body language, and mistaken cultural assumptions, stated or implied, than with the reading level of materials the patient receives. In a study of Chinese- and Vietnamese-speaking patients with limited English proficiency, for example, Ngo-Metzger and colleagues (2003) found that Asian-American patients perceived their Western doctors as critical of or suspicious about traditional medical practices, such as coining and cupping, which led to a level of distrust and misunderstanding. When a language barrier is present, patients with limited English proficiency value providers and staff who express nonverbal emotional support and seek to establish a trusting relationship. Presumably those with low health literacy feel similarly, whatever language they speak.

There is a clear mismatch between the reading level of typical health information (e.g., handouts, brochures, forms) and the reading level of the average patient. Although most health material is written at a 10th-grade level, in fact, the average American adult cannot read above the 8th-grade level (Schwartzberg, VanGeest, & Wang, 2005). And normally a person's reading level is actually several grades below the last grade he or she finished. In other words, if a patient has completed the 12th grade, chances are that he or she reads at a 9th- or 10th-grade level at best. More than 300 studies have established the disconnect between patient reading levels and patient education materials (Doak, Doak, Friedell, & Meade, 1998; Dollahite, Thompson, & McNew, 1996; Hearth-Holmes et al., 1997).

To close the gap, either the reading level of materials must be brought down, the reading level of patients must be raised, or both. It falls naturally within the purview of the U.S. educational system to improve student reading and literacy levels, though some researchers have argued that consistent, cross-grade health curricula—including efforts to teach the teachers—could go a long way toward improving health literacy levels among Americans. Studies suggest that inadequate attention to teacher health literacy impedes student health literacy (IOM, 2004, p. 143). And reports by the National Research Council and the National Institute of Child Health and Human Development address the failure of schools to produce adults with sufficient literacy skills to participate in an increasingly information-driven and competitive economy (IOM, 2004; National Reading Panel, 2000; Snow, Burns, & Griffen, 1998). Legislative efforts such as the No Child Left Behind Act have been undertaken to correct this failure (IOM, 2004), but the provision of adequate health and science education continues to elude us.

As the IOM's Committee on Health Literacy suggests, there is some justification for embedding health literacy instruction into existing literacy instruction for children and adults because learners retain and apply information best in contexts similar to those in which they first encountered the information (IOM, 2004, p. 149). Reading and writing skills must be learned in the context of texts and literacy purposes that readers find in their everyday lives, which may be one reason the 2003 NAAL incorporated more health-related texts to determine the relationship between general literacy and functional health literacy.

Studies examining the outcomes of introducing more expository texts into primary-grade instruction have found that students whose teachers diversify their materials learn as much as those who do not (IOM, 2004, p. 150). In other words, there's no need to wait until middle or high school to teach students about the different text types that are commonly used to convey health information. Increasing young people's exposure to such materials early in their education increases the odds that they will have more facility with such texts later in life.

Implementing higher standards for health education in elementary and secondary schools, adult education programs, college courses, and continuing education programs for health care providers is one way to improve health literacy among Americans of all age groups. However, several barriers that may hinder the implementation of school health programs at the local, state, national, and international levels have been described by the World Health Organization (WHO, 1996). Therefore, striving to simplify patient education materials seems like a logical and reliable approach for now. After all, unlike patient education levels, reading levels of handouts and other clinical materials are within the direct control of health care providers. It may take time before students exposed to improved health literacy education reap the benefits as independent health care consumers, but health materials can be improved and made easier to read right now.

Such improvements stand to benefit all health care consumers, regardless of their background. Studies have shown that even highly literate patients are not offended simply because they are offered easy-to-read materials by their health care providers (Ad Hoc Committee on Health Literacy, 1999; Braddock, Fihn,

Levinson, Jonsen, & Pearlman, 1997; Plimpton & Root, 1994; Winslow, 2001). Across the board, in fact, simpler just seems to work better for all patients, no matter what reading level they have achieved. If the goal of health care providers is to improve patient outcomes and quality of life—and undoubtedly it is—then anything that helps meet that goal should be a top priority. Caregivers may not be able to make better readers out of their patients, but they can treat them and make them feel better. Simplifying the language of written and oral instructions is one way to do that.

Myth #2: Patients With Low Health Literacy Are Dumb or Don't Know How to Read

We've already established the difference between literacy and health literacy. By definition, those with low health literacy are not necessarily unable to read; they simply have difficulty understanding and using information that pertains to health. Only about 10% of participants in the 1992 NALS could be seen as illiterate in the sense that they failed even at the earliest stages of learning to read. (In 2003, about 3% of adults in the NAAL study sample took an alternative assessment because they were unable to complete a minimum number of simple literacy screening questions [NCES, 2005].) Three times as many individuals, or 30% of the total sample size in the NALS study, demonstrated an ability to read most everyday print items and could fill out simple forms, even if they approached fairly simple texts in a slow and unreliable fashion. Low-literate readers may avoid reading because of their limited skills, but generally they are able to read (Strucker & Davidson, 2005).

Research suggests an imperfect correlation between education and literacy, though the correlation between fewer years of formal education and lower health outcomes is well established. In other words, those with high school diplomas and even several college credits may lack literacy skills, just as someone with adequate literacy (as measured by certain instruments) may never have completed high school. As Weiss notes, "education level measures only the number of years an individual attended school, not how much the individual learned in school" (Davis, Kennen, Gazmararian, & Williams, 2005, p. 158). As one might expect, however, more than 80% of those who never finished high school ranked in the lowest two levels of the 1992 NALS (Kirsch et al., 1993), suggesting that their educational background, although not necessarily predictive of literacy, is correlated with it. In 2003, literacy was lowest across the three scales for adults who did not complete high school; they accounted for the largest group with below basic skills on the NAAL (NCES, 2005).

Even if the NALS and the NAAL revealed broad trends in literacy, exceptions to the rule remain critically important for us to consider. Along these lines, we must be careful to distinguish between low health literacy and low intelligence. Patients who need more time to absorb information are not "dumb." Even physicians from one specialty of medicine may believe they are reading a foreign language when they encounter studies by those in other specialties. And it's certainly possible to achieve a high level of academic or professional success in society despite having few or no literacy skills. One instructive example is the experience of John Corcoran, the 48-year-old high school teacher who sought help for his hidden illiteracy and eventually overcame it. His story is told in the book *The Teacher Who Couldn't Read* (Corcoran & Carson, 1994). Simply put, different people learn differently, regardless of their level of education or their literacy skills. We must understand that how information is presented can do more to muddy an intended message than to clarify it.

Myth #3: If I Just Explain It Slowly and Clearly, the Patient Will Understand

The benefits of speaking slowly and clearly to patients cannot be overestimated. Nevertheless, it's not the speed of the message that matters, but its content, how it is presented, and the amount of information it conveys. Studies have shown that patients remember and understand as little as half of what they are told by their physicians. According to Doak and colleagues, the essential condition required to activate a patient's understanding and memory system is "the existence of a reasonable match between the logic, language, and experience in the information and the patient's logic, language, and experience" (Doak, Doak, & Root, 1996; Youmans & Ngoh, 2005). In other words, caregivers should be mindful of an individual patient's abilities before attempting to communicate; health-related messages should be evenly matched with the intended audience.

In fact, the more information a patient is asked to remember, the less likely he or she will be to actually recall it. "At present," note Schillinger and Davis (2005, p. 190), "clinicians do not have the means to determine how patients learn best, nor the tools to more effectively engage patients who do not appear to be maximally benefiting from clinical interactions."

What's more, there is considerable embarrassment and shame associated with limited literacy, as Parikh, Parker, Nurss, Baker, and Williams (1996, pp. 33–39) found in a study of low-income African American patients; 40% admitted feeling shame about their reading skills. Complicating matters is the fact that many patients are not forthright about their abilities or judge their skills to be higher than they are. Many people are adept at hiding low literacy skills, using excuses or coping strategies such as "I forgot my glasses" or offering to read handouts at home. During a medical emergency, such evasions could jeopardize a patient's life, so many patients are forced to abandon them, sometimes with disturbing results. (Consider the patient who grants informed consent for a life-threatening procedure he or she cannot fully understand.) Health care providers cannot assume patients understand what they are told or what they are signing just because they nod or claim to understand.

Why not simply screen patients for literacy? That way we could target our efforts only to those who would benefit most from them. According to Davis and colleagues (2005, p. 175), there is no evidence that literacy testing results in improved delivery of health care or improved health outcomes. For this and other reasons, there is considerable controversy about whether patients should be screened at all. For one, we risk stigmatizing people when we seek to label them. Most people with low literacy are embarrassed about it, refusing to admit it even to loved ones. Some don't realize they have limited literacy skills, which means that categorizing them could change their behavior in potentially negative ways.

The most commonly used health literacy assessment tools, two of which are briefly mentioned in this chapter, are the REALM, the TOFHLA, and the Wide Range Achievement Test (WRAT). Each has benefits as well as drawbacks. The REALM, for example, does not discriminate above a ninth-grade reading level (Davis et al., 2005, p. 165). (For a more detailed discussion of literacy screening tools, see chapter 3, Assessing Patients' Literacy Levels.) At this point, suffice it to say that widespread literacy screening is an imperfect solution for a multifaceted problem and that even the best assessment tools are not without their flaws.

One of the most reliable means for determining whether patients understand is the teach-back method. Health care providers simply ask patients to explain back to them, in their own words, what they feel they learned from the exchange (as opposed to asking "Do you understand?" which rarely elicits an honest "no" response or further questions). The provider may ask something like, "If you were asked by your spouse all the things you need to do to care for your condition, what would you tell him or her about it?"

Teach-back is potentially very effective. A study by Schillinger and colleagues (2002) showed that patients whose doctors used this method to ensure understanding treated their diabetes more effectively. The study also revealed, however, that teach-back is used in only 20% of patient–physician encounters. This is but one glaring example of a potential solution that simply begs for implementation by more health care providers.

Myth #4: Only Patients Who Come From Foreign Countries and Don't Speak English Are Low Literate; That's Not My Patient Population

There is no question that a considerable number of immigrants have low literacy skills in English. According to the 1992 NALS, more than half of immigrants who entered the United States after childhood scored in the lowest literacy level (Kirsch et al., 1993). Bear in mind, though, that the NALS and the NAAL tested only English-language literacy; adult immigrants from non-English-speaking nations may very well be highly literate in their own languages, even if research suggests otherwise (Weiss, 2005). Although minority groups and immigrant populations have disproportionately higher rates of limited literacy, because of their lower numbers they represent a smaller percentage of Americans with limited literacy skills. Most Americans with limited literacy skills are White, native-born Americans. Therefore, even health professionals who serve largely White and English-speaking populations are likely to encounter low-literate patients throughout their day.

What about the elderly? Because older Americans, regardless of socioeconomic status, tend to have a higher rate of limited health literacy than do those

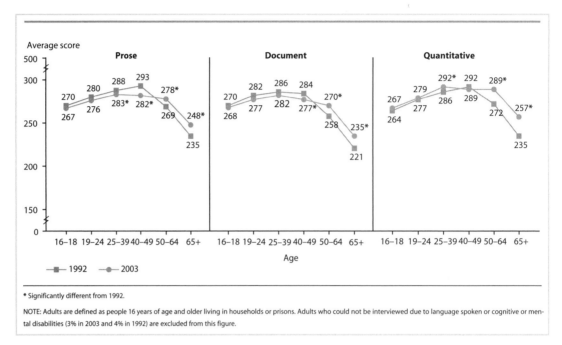

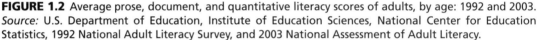

FIGURE 1.2 Average prose, document, and quantitative literacy scores of adults, by age: 1992 and 2003. *Source:* U.S. Department of Education, Institute of Education Sciences, National Center for Education Statistics, 1992 National Adult Literacy Survey, and 2003 National Assessment of Adult Literacy.

in other age groups (based on studies using literacy screens, such as the English- and Spanish-language TOFHLA), any practice that treats older patients also will have a statistically higher likelihood of encountering the problem of low health literacy (Gazmararian et al., 1999; Weiss, Reed, & Kligman, 1995). In the NALS of 1992, roughly half of those aged 65 years and older scored at level 1, the "functionally illiterate" level, with another third scoring at level 2, the "marginally literate" level (Kirsch et al., 1993). Only one of five respondents over 65 scored higher than level 2 (Weiss, 2005). The line graphs in Figure 1.2 show the average prose, document, and quantitative literacy scores by age in 1992 and 2003. Notice how each line dips down as the NAAL or NALS respondent ages.

There were similar findings for patients from different racial and ethnic groups: 1992 NALS data revealed that 41% of Whites scored in the two lowest literacy levels, as did 64% of American Indians and Alaskan natives, 60% of Asians and Pacific Islanders, 77% of Blacks, and 78% of Hispanics (Weiss, 2005). Average prose and document literacy scores increased among Blacks and Asians/Pacific Islanders between 1992 and 2003. Averages among Hispanics, however, decreased during those years (NCES, 2005).

Finally, there's the question of socioeconomic status. After all, one unspoken corollary of the assumption that only foreigners have low health literacy is the belief that only those who are less affluent have limited literacy skills. Several studies suggest that low health and limited general literacy skills are common among low-income populations (Weiss, 2005). As with other factors affecting literacy, however, it's unclear whether limited literacy contributes to poverty or if those in lower income groups have limited literacy because of fewer educational opportunities (Weiss, 2005).

The truth, as an AMA educational video aimed at raising awareness about low health literacy suggests, is that "you can't tell by looking." The video features excerpts from interviews with people whose problems with low health literacy have interfered with their access to quality care. One segment features a physician talking to a senior citizen who clearly is confused by his diagnosis of hypertension. He thinks his condition may have something to do with being hyperactive, but he isn't sure (American Medical Association Foundation, 2005). What the video demonstrates is that low-literate patients may be young or old, rich or poor, White or non-White, male or female, well or casually dressed, frail or robust. We must take care not to stereotype.

WHY HEALTH LITERACY MATTERS: INCREASING PATIENT SAFETY

If it were determined that the design of automobile steering wheels were the primary cause of fatal highway accidents, industry engineers would set to work redesigning them. After they demanded changes, consumer advocates might caution drivers to use their steering wheels differently, at least until the new designs were widely available, but almost certainly the paramount concern would be driver safety. Why, then, does medical information continue to be written above the average comprehension level of its target audience?

After all, one of the most obvious dangers of low health literacy is the potential for misunderstanding medical instructions—something that could lead to hazardous dosing errors. (For a discussion of the relationship between medical errors and low health literacy, see chapter 4, Understanding and Avoiding Medical Errors.) Studies have found medical dosing errors in patients asked to follow directions for preparing oral rehydration solution for children with diarrhea, among those charged with determining the correct dosage from a label of children's cough medicine, among parents administering albuterol inhalers to their asthmatic children, and in diabetes patients asked to dose and administer insulin shots (Weiss, 2005). Just as some parents might bring their children to the hospital emergency department for nonurgent conditions, such as a slightly higher-than-normal temperature of 99°F (Herman & Mayer, 2004), others may fail to seek care for potentially fatal conditions, such as dental cellulitis, all because they lack easily acquired knowledge.

And it isn't just medical information that could be misconstrued, thereby endangering some of the most vulnerable members of society. A study by Wegner and Girasek (2003) found that the readability of child safety seat installation instructions measured from the 7th- to the 12th-grade level, far exceeding the abilities of average Americans. According to the National Safe Kids Campaign, roughly four out of five car safety seats are used incorrectly, with an average of three mistakes per seat (Karp, 1998).

SPREADING THE WORD, CLOSING THE GAP

Luckily, awareness about low health literacy continues to grow every year. Thanks to the initial wake-up call of the 1992 NALS, the prevalence of the problem has attracted the attention of numerous segments of society, from public to private entities, the government, universities, clinics, nonprofit groups, and individual health care providers. Some landmarks in public awareness include the publication of the AMA report on health literacy in the *Journal of the American Medical Association* (Ad Hoc Committee, 1999) and the publications of the IOM report *(Health Literacy: A Prescription to End Confusion),* the AHRQ's evidence report/technology assessment *(Literacy and Health Outcomes),* and the AMA's textbook *(Understanding Health Literacy: Implications for Medicine and Public Health)* in 2004.

Organizations dealing with health literacy continue to proliferate. Founded in 2002 with initial funding from Pfizer Inc., the Partnership for Clear Health Communication is one such example. This coalition of national organizations is committed to offering free and low-cost resources and programs to deliver patient information, medical education, and practice management tools to health care providers. Among its most prominent resources is the Ask Me 3 program, which encourages patients to understand the answers to three questions: (1) What is my main problem? (2) What do I need to do? and (3) Why is it important for me to do this? Visit http://www.askme3.org to learn more. In 2003, the AMA Foundation developed its Health Literacy Educational Kit, which includes a CD-ROM, a manual for clinicians, the video documentary mentioned earlier, and other resources aimed at teaching physicians, health care professionals, and patients' advocates about health literacy (IOM, 2004, p. 160).

Professional conferences and symposia sponsored by such organizations as the AMA, Pfizer Inc., Kaiser Permanente, the Institute for Healthcare Advancement, and the H. Lee Moffitt Cancer Center & Research Institute have become increasingly common; numerous private efforts, such as Pfizer's Health Literacy Initiative and the Blue Cross Blue Shield Association's *Walking Works* initiative, offer innovative self-care solutions; and educational programs in hospitals and other health service organizations continue to expand. Government-sponsored, private, and public–private health initiatives, such as *Healthy People 2010* (whose objective 11–2 seeks to "improve the health literacy of persons with inadequate or marginal literacy skills"; U.S. Department of Health and Human Services, 2000), the California Health Literacy Initiative, the Florida Health Literacy Study, and the New York City Health Literacy Initiative, increasingly spread the word to individuals and organizations, as do major universities through publicly and privately funded research.

New accreditation standards by the Joint Commission on the Accreditation of Health Organizations (JCAHO) and the National Committee for Quality Assurance (NCQA) help ensure that health care organizations and programs in the United States maximize their effectiveness by reaching out to those with limited health literacy. This is great news for health care providers because it translates into new sources of funding and helps raise awareness.

As awareness grows, those with the power to make changes to public policy increasingly take notice, sometimes engineering progress through new legislation or new programs. Examples include the Media Smart Youth program developed by the National Institute of Child Health and Human Development (NICHD) and the Curriculum Linking Science Education and Health Literacy program, funded by the National Center for Research Resources. The goal of the latter program is to "transform the food experiences of inner-city children, teachers and parents, and caregivers into an inquiry-based science program" (IOM, 2004, p. 153).

On the state level, California's "Health Framework for California's Public Schools, Kindergarten through Grade Twelve," Alaska's "Healthy Reading Kits" for grades 2 through 8, and New Jersey's core curriculum content standards for comprehensive health and physical educations programs (which include health literacy) all are designed to address health literacy in public schools (IOM, 2004).

With each passing year, we know more about the people who have low health literacy, more about the best means for correcting the problem, more about the effects of health literacy on a host of other factors (e.g., chronic disease, quality of life, income, and socioeconomic status), and more about how these various factors contribute to our patients' health and general literacy. We share much of this information in subsequent chapters of this book, sometimes through stories or advice from nurses and other health care professionals on the frontlines of patient care, but also through examination of a growing body of published literature that establishes a firm link between literacy and health.

HEALTH LITERACY: DON'T LEAVE HOME WITHOUT IT

One of the key messages of *Health Literacy in Primary Care: A Clinician's Guide* is that you needn't go far to find someone hobbling along in circumstances similar to those described in the opening paragraphs of this chapter—certainly not as far as Karnataka, India. The low health literate are your friends, your family members, your colleagues, and your patients. Many Americans in search of quality medical care really do find themselves adrift, desperately seeking to communicate what ails them and to understand how to treat their conditions despite their limited literacy skills.

Our titanic health care system makes extraordinary demands even on those with the privilege of higher education, not to mention those who may never have had formal schooling or for whom English is a second or third language. Think of the exclusively Spanish-speaking patient who encounters a label instructing him in English to take a certain medication "once" a day. Considering that the Spanish word *once* means "eleven" and not "one time," it seems that the potential for confusion—even a lethal overdose—in such a situation is particularly grave (IOM, 2004, p. 116; Weiss, 2005, p. 26).

Even those who speak English fluently and are comfortable with insurance forms or medical jargon may find themselves awash in conflicting information, especially in light of the ever-expanding information overload of the Internet, which for various reasons remains a text-intensive environment (Baur, 2005). Journalist Jan Hoffman refers to this information overload as part of the "blessing and the burden of being a modern patient." Writing in the *New York Times* on August 14, 2005, she notes,

> A generation ago patients argued for more information, more choice and more say about treatment. To a great extent, that is exactly what they have received: a superabundance of information, often several treatment options and the right to choose among them. As this new responsibility dawns on patients, some embrace it with a sense of pride and furious determination. But many find the job of being a modern patient, with its slog through medical uncertainty, to be lonely, frightening and overwhelming (Hoffman, 2005).

Navigating a "superabundance" of information can be lonely, frightening, and overwhelming for highly literate health care consumers, so just imagine trying to navigate that same complex system—encountering "several treatment options" and having "the right to choose among them"—if you didn't finish high school or if you have trouble focusing on dense, health-related material. How much more overwhelming is it for a 2003 NAAL basic or below basic reader?

As we've discussed, someone with highly specialized knowledge who is well educated and perfectly literate in his or her own field—say, automobile systems engineering or computer programming—may still feel lost when confronted by the arcane language of poststructuralist literary criticism or quantum physics. He or she is by no means illiterate, but neither is he or she a member of the elite club. Such a person is bathed in esoteric and unfamiliar language, required to navigate a puzzling new text as if learning English for the first time.

The idea of navigating a puzzling new text accurately describes the experience of low-health-literate patients, and it is the goal of this book to share stories and to educate caregivers about the needs of these patients. Metaphorically, at least, raising patients' health literacy skills to the functional level teaches them the Kannada, Konkani, and Tulu they need to survive that sudden bout of nausea in Karnataka we evoked earlier, regardless of what they eat or what new medications they take as they gaze out at the Arabian Sea.

REFERENCES

2000 Beta Travel Study—Business. (2000). Beta Research Corporation. *WSJ On-line*. Retrieved January 27, 2006, from http://advertising.wsj.com/Research/Cons/2000BetaTravelBusiness_h1.htm

Ad Hoc Committee on Health Literacy for the Council on Scientific Affairs. (1999). Health literacy: Report of the Council on Scientific Affairs. *Journal of the American Medical Association, 281*(6), 552–557.

American Medical Association. (2005). *Mini-conference on health literacy and health disparities.* Retrieved January 10, 2006, from http://www.ama-assn.org/ama/pub/category/15250.html

American Medical Association (AMA) Foundation. (2005). *Health literacy video.* Retrieved August 20, 2005, from http://www.ama-assn.org/ama/pub/category/8035.html

Anderson, T. W. (1958). *An introduction to multivariate statistical analysis.* New York: Wiley.

Baur, C. E. (2005). Using the Internet to move beyond the brochure and improve health literacy. In J. G. Schwartzberg, J. B. VanGeest, & C. C. Wang (Eds.), *Understanding health literacy: Implications for medicine and public health* (pp. 141–154). Chicago: American Medical Association Press.

Berkman, N. D., DeWalt, D. A., Pignone, M. P., Sheridan, S. L., Lohr, K. N., Lux, L., et al. (2004, January). *Literacy and health outcomes* (Evidence Report/Technology Assessment No. 87. AHRQ Publications No. 04-E007-2). Rockville, MD: Agency for Healthcare Research and Quality.

Bhabha, H. K. (1992). Postcolonial authority and postmodern guilt. In L. Grossberg, C. Nelson, & P. Treichler (Eds.), *Cultural studies* (pp. 56–68). New York: Routledge.

Braddock, C. H., Fihn, S. D., Levinson, W., Jonsen, A. R., & Pearlman, R. A. (1997). How doctors and patients discuss routine clinical decisions: Informed decision making in the outpatient setting [Abstract]. *Journal of General and Internal Medicine, 12,* 339–345.

Comings, J. P., & Kirsch, I. S. (2005). Literacy skills of US adults. In J. G. Schwartzberg, J. B. VanGeest, & C. C. Wang (Eds.), *Understanding health literacy: Implications for medicine and public health* (pp. 43–53). Chicago: American Medical Association Press.

Corcoran, J., & Carson, C. C. (1994). *The teacher who couldn't read: The true story of a high school instructor who triumphed over his illiteracy.* Colorado Springs, CO: Focus on the Family Publishing.

Davis, T., Kennen, E. M., Gazmararian, J. A., & Williams, M. V. (2005). Literacy testing in health care research. In J. G. Schwartzberg, J. B. VanGeest, & C. C. Wang (Eds.), *Understanding health literacy: Implications for medicine and public health* (pp. 157–179). Chicago: American Medical Association Press.

Doak, C. C., Doak, L. G., Friedell, G. H., & Meade, C. D. (1998). Improving comprehension for cancer patients with low literacy skills: Strategies for clinicians. *CA—A Cancer Journal for Clinicians, 48,* 151–162.

Doak, L. G., Doak, C. C., & Root, J. H. (1996). *Teaching patients with low literacy skills* (2nd ed.). Philadelphia: J.B. Lippincott.

Dollahite, J., Thompson, C., & McNew, R. (1996). Readability of printed sources of diet and health information. *Patient Education and Counseling, 27,* 123–134.

Gazmararian, J. A., Baker, D. W., Williams, M. V., Parker, R. M., Scott, T. L., Green, D. C., et al. (1999). Health literacy among Medicare enrollees in a managed care organization. *Journal of the American Medical Association, 281,* 545–551.

Greenberg, J. (2001). *An updated overview of medical and public health literature addressing literacy issues: An annotated bibliography of articles published in 2000.* Retrieved September 22, 2005, from the Harvard School of Public Health Web site: http://www.hsph.harvard.edu/healthliteracy/literature/lit_2000.html

Hearth-Holmes, M., Murphy, P. W., Davis, T. C., Nandy, I., Elder, C. G., Broadwell, L. H., et al. (1997). Literacy in patients with chronic disease: Systematic lupus erythematosus and the reading level of patient education materials. *Journal of Rheumatology, 24,* 2335–2339.

Herman, A. D., & Mayer, G. G. (2004). Reducing the use of emergency medical resources among Head Start families: A pilot study. *Journal of Community Health, 29*(3), 197–208.

Hochhauser, M. (2003). Why patients won't understand their HIPAA privacy notices. *Privacy Rights Clearinghouse.* Retrieved December 29, 2005, from http://www.privacyrights.org/ar/HIPAA-Readability.htm

Hoffman, J. (2005). Awash in information, patients face a lonely, uncertain road. *New York Times Online*. Retrieved August 14, 2005, from http://www.nytimes.com/2005/08/14/health/14patient.html?ex=1281672000&en=6ec6abca057820c9&ei=5088&partner=rssnyt&emc=rss

Institute of Medicine (IOM) of the National Academies Committee on Health Literacy, Board on Neuroscience and Behavioral Health. (2004). *Health literacy: A prescription to end confusion*. Washington, DC: National Academies Press.

Kantor, A. (2005). Can health literacy programs cut costs? *Managed Healthcare Executive*. Retrieved February 10, 2006, from http://www.managedhealthcareexecutive.com/mhe/article/articleDetail.jsp?id=170611

Karp, H. (1998, May 1). *Car seat safety check: 8 common mistakes you must avoid*. Retrieved September 1, 2005, from http://www.parents.com/parents/story.jhtml?storyid=/templatedata/parents/story/data/5198.xml

Kirsch, I., Jungeblut, A., Jenkins, L., & Kolstad, A. (1993). *Adult literacy in America: A first look at the findings of the National Adult Literacy Survey*. Washington, DC: National Center for Education Statistics, U.S. Department of Education.

Law of averages: Casting a wide net in health literacy efforts with Rima Rudd, ScD. 2001, Center for the Advancement of Health. (2003, March). *Facts of life: Issue briefings for health reporters, 8*(3). Retrieved August 27, 2005, from http://www.cfah.org/factsoflife/vol8no3.cfm

Mayer, G. G. (2003). Confessions of a health illiterate. *Healthcare Advances, 5*(2), 2.

National Academy on an Aging Society. (1998, October). *Understanding health literacy: New estimates of the costs of inadequate health literacy*. Paper presented at the Pfizer Conference on Health Literacy: Promoting Health Literacy: *A Call to Action*, Washington, DC.

National Center for Education Statistics (NCES). (2005). *A first look at the literacy of America's adults in the 21st century* (NCES 2006-470). Retrieved December 16, 2005, from http://nces.ed.gov/NAAL/PDF/2006470.PDF

National Institute for Literacy (NIFL). (1991). *Public Law 102–73, the National Literacy Act of 1991. H.R. 751. July 25, 1991*. Retrieved September 2, 2005, from http://www.nifl.gov/public-law.html

National Reading Panel. (2000). *Teaching children to read: An evidence-based assessment of the scientific research literature on reading and its implications for reading instruction*. Bethesda, MD: National Institute of Child Health and Human Development.

Ngo-Metzger, Q., Massagli, M. P., Clarridge, B. R., Manocchia, M., Davis, R. B., Iezzoni, L. I., et al. (2003). Linguistic and cultural barriers to care: Perspectives of Chinese and Vietnamese immigrants. *Journal of General and Internal Medicine, 18*, 44–52.

Parikh, N. S., Parker, R. M., Nurss, J. R., Baker, D. W., & Williams, M. V. (1996). Shame and health literacy: The unspoken connection. *Patient Education and Counseling, 27*, 33–39.

Plimpton, S., & Root, J. (1994). Materials and strategies that work in low literacy health communication. *Public Health Report, 109*(1), 86–92.

President Clinton's memorandum on Plain Language in Government Writing. (1998). Retrieved October 7, 2005, from http://www.plainlanguage.gov/whatisPL/govmandates/memo.cfm

Project for Excellence in Journalism. (2004). *State of the news media 2004: An annual report on American journalism*. Retrieved January 23, 2006, from http://www.stateofthenewsmedia.org/2004/narrative_magazines_audience.asp?media=7&cat=3

Ratzan, S. C., & Parker, R. M. (2000). Introduction. In C. R. Selden, M. Zorn, S. C. Ratzan, & R. M. Parker (Eds.), *National Library of Medicine current bibliographies in medicine:*

Health literacy (NLM Pub. No. CBM 2000–1). Bethesda, MD: National Institutes of Health.

Rudd, R. E. (2002). *Health literacy overview presentation.* Retrieved August 27, 2005, from the Harvard School of Public Health, Health Literacy Studies Web site: http://www.hsph.harvard.edu/healthliteracy

Rudd, R. E. (2004). Navigating hospitals. *Literacy Harvest, 11*(1),19–24. Retrieved January 30, 2006, from http://www.lacnyc.org/resources/publications/harvest/HarvestFall04. pdf#search='rima%20rudd%20navigation%20study%20hospital

Rudd, R. E., Colton, T., & Schacht, R. (2000). *An overview of medical and public health literature addressing literacy issues: An annotated bibliography* (National Center for the Study of Adult Learning and Literacy Report No. 14). Retrieved September 22, 2005, from the Harvard Graduate School of Education Web site: http://www.hsph. harvard.edu/healthliteracy/litreview.pdf

Rudd, R. E., Kaphingst, K., Colton, T., Gregoire, J., & Hyde, J. (2004). Rewriting public health information in plain language. *Journal of Health Communication, 9*(3), 195–206.

Rudd, R. E., Kirsch, I., & Yamamoto, K. (2004). *Literacy and health in America.* Princeton, NJ: Educational Testing Service.

Rudd, R. E., Renzulli, D., Pereira, A., & Daltroy, L. (2005). Literacy demands in health care settings: The patient perspective. In J. G. Schwartzberg, J. B. VanGeest, & C. C. Wang (Eds.), *Understanding health literacy: Implications for medicine and public health* (pp. 69–84). Chicago: American Medical Association Press.

Schillinger, D., & Davis, T. (2005). A conceptual framework for the relationship between health literacy and health care outcomes: The Chronic Disease Exemplar. In J. G. Schwartzberg, J. B. VanGeest, & C. C. Wang (Eds.), *Understanding health literacy: Implications for medicine and public health* (pp. 181–203). Chicago: American Medical Association Press.

Schillinger, D., Grumbach, K., Piette, J., Wang, F., Wilson, C., Daher, C., et al. (2002). Association of health literacy with diabetes outcomes. *Journal of the American Medical Association, 288*(4), 475–482.

Schwartzberg, J. G., VanGeest, J. B., & Wang, C. C. (Eds.). (2005). *Understanding health literacy: Implications for medicine and public health.* Chicago: American Medical Association Press.

Snow, C. E., Burns, M. S., & Griffen, P. (Eds.). (1998). *Preventing reading difficulties in young children.* Washington, DC: National Academy Press.

Strucker, J., & Davidson, R. (2005). What does low literacy mean? In J. G. Schwartzberg, J. B. VanGeest, & C. C. Wang (Eds.), *Understanding health literacy: Implications for medicine and public health* (pp. 55–68). Chicago: American Medical Association Press.

U.S. Department of Health and Human Services, Office of Disease Prevention and Health Promotion. (2000, January 25). *Healthy people 2010.* Retrieved September 16, 2005, from http://www.healthypeople.gov/lhi

Wegner, M. V., & Girasek, D. C. (2003). How readable are child safety seat installation instructions? *Pediatrics, 111*(3), 588–591.

Weiss, B. D. (2005). Epidemiology of low health literacy. In J. G. Schwartzberg, J. B. VanGeest, & C. C. Wang (Eds.), *Understanding health literacy: Implications for medicine and public health* (pp. 17–39). Chicago: American Medical Association Press.

Weiss, B. D., Reed, R. L., & Kligman, E. W. (1995). Literacy skills and communication methods of low-income older persons. *Patient Education and Counseling, 25,* 109–119.

White, S., & Dillow, S. (2005). *Key concepts and features of the 2003 National Assessment of Adult Literacy* (NCES 2006-471). Washington, DC: U.S. Department of Education, National Center for Education Statistics.

Winslow, E. H. (2001). Patient education materials: Can patients read them, or are they ending up in the trash? *American Journal of Nursing, 101*(10), 33–38.

World Health Organization (WHO). (1996). *Improving school health programs: Barriers and strategies.* Geneva, Switzerland: World Health Organization.

Youmans, S., & Ngoh, L. (2005, May). *Communicating medication instructions to patients: Cultural challenges and possible solutions.* Paper presented at Culture, Language, and Clinical Issues: Operational Solutions to Low Health Literacy, Institute for Healthcare Advancement Fourth Annual Health Literacy Conference, Anaheim, CA.

Zobel, E. (2002). *An updated overview of medical and public health literature addressing literacy issues: An annotated bibliography of articles published in 2001.* Retrieved September 22, 2005, from the Harvard School of Public Health Web site: http://www.hsph.harvard.edu/healthliteracy/literature/lit_2001.html

Zobel, E., Rowe, K., & Gomez-Mandic, C. (2003). *An updated overview of medical and public health literature addressing literacy issues: An annotated bibliography of articles published in 2002.* Retrieved September 23, 2005, from the Harvard School of Public Health Web site: http://www.hsph.harvard.edu/healthliteracy/literature/lit_2002.html

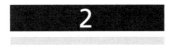

2

CREATING A PATIENT-FRIENDLY ENVIRONMENT

Mr. Martinez was born in the United States and has lived here his entire life. He is 46 years old, married with three children, and bilingual in English and Spanish; he does not speak with an accent. He is a construction worker in Hollywood, making movie sets there and in other cities and states as needed. He earns between $100,000 and $140,000 per year and has good health insurance. His wife does not work, and the couple lives in a very nice area in the Hollywood Hills. Mr. Martinez is also illiterate, but no one knows this fact—not even his children, who do well in school.

Mr. Martinez has not gone to a doctor in years. Lately, though, he has been having severe headaches that keep him home in bed and he feels that he must discover their cause. He makes an appointment with an internist in Beverly Hills and walks into the office by himself, approaching the receptionist first to give her his name. At this point, things become a bit tense.

First he is asked to sign in, to state the time he arrived, and to indicate the time of his appointment. Because Mr. Martinez cannot read or write, however, he doesn't know what the sheet is asking for. He can write his name and he does so, but he leaves the other areas on the sheet blank. He sits down, and before long the receptionist calls him back up to the desk and gives him three additional forms to complete, including a health history, a Health Insurance Portability and Accountability Act (HIPAA) of 1996 Notice of Privacy Practices, and an insurance form. Mr. Martinez cannot read any of them. He sits down with the clipboard and begins to struggle through the words, but he can't do it.

Although he wants to tell the receptionist that he can't read or write, there are many other people waiting around and Mr. Martinez feels embarrassed. So he decides just to sit there and do nothing. At last the receptionist asks him if he has finished, and he simply walks up and hands her the incomplete forms. She looks at them and Mr. Martinez whispers that he can't read. The receptionist has never dealt with a patient who could not read; she doesn't know quite what to do with this information or with him.

After thinking about the situation, the receptionist goes back and talks to the health care provider. The provider has some experience with this issue and tells the receptionist to take the patient to an exam room and fill out the questionnaire for him. Basically, the receptionist reads the questions to Mr. Martinez and writes the answers in the appropriate places. Now the patient feels much more at ease. And because the provider knows that Mr. Martinez cannot read or write, she works more closely with him, avoiding medical jargon and speaking to him in lay terms.

Of course, Mr. Martinez is neither dense nor stupid; he can understand what his provider is saying as long as she uses "living room" language. The provider writes a few directions clearly and simply and tells Mr. Martinez to have his wife read them to him and to call if there's anything he can't understand.

* * *

In the somewhat idealized story above, the patient's outcome was vastly improved because the provider did all the right things. Although Mr. Martinez had high blood pressure and was under a lot of stress, the patient–provider interaction was so positive that he decided to go to the doctor routinely after his initial visit. He was no longer fearful of the unknown. His health care provider, now realizing that patients with low health literacy have special needs, drafted new policies to guide her office staff in the future. She also provided her employees with continuing education on how to identify and treat patients with low health literacy.

Unfortunately, most patients find going to the doctor to be inconvenient and sometimes even frightening. People with special needs find it very difficult to make medical visits, and those who are illiterate or have low literacy skills have an even harder time doing so. One reason is that physicians' offices are not very user friendly. Often staff members do not recognize literacy problems in their patients, even though these patients must have basic literacy skills just to get past the reception area. Specialists, ancillary providers, and hospitals present additional challenges to the low-literate patient. Sometimes it is difficult for these patients to find the correct office or to get through the admission procedure in a hospital because of the signs and various written documents they must decipher (Rudd, 2004). After all, we live in a society in which reading is the expected norm. We generally assume that people know how to read.

Several areas must be addressed before we can achieve more patient-friendly offices and hospital environments. First of all, health care providers and support staff must know something about the principles of adult education. Too often patient education efforts are focused on providing sound clinical information even though the health care providers lack awareness of the most effective teaching methods for adult learners (Padberg & Padberg, 1990). In addition, providers ought to understand the reasons why their patients are literacy challenged. Such information affects the approach they take with such patients. Office staff, hospital staff, and providers must use technology, printed materials, and other patient educational materials that are well suited for the literacy challenged. Last, the office or hospital settings themselves must be conducive to dealing with patients with special literacy needs.

As we discuss our goal of creating a more patient-friendly environment for those with low health literacy, in this chapter we mention many issues and topics that are treated in depth in later parts of the book. In fact, each part of this book reflects the concern of the whole, which is to share information and advice that can help providers offer better and more humane care to their patients—especially to those patients who have difficulty understanding or using the written and spoken information they encounter in their attempts to navigate the health care system.

ADULT TEACHING AND LEARNING

Adults learn differently than children do. A child, for example, relies on other people to decide what is important to learn. Children accept information as it is presented, have little or no past experience to draw on, and understand that the information presented will be used in the future (Collins, 2004). A child also has a limited ability to serve as a resource to teachers or to other students in the learning environment.

An adult, however, is different. Adults can decide what is important to learn. They have past experience to verify or nullify information that is presented to them (Collins, 2004). Adults want information that is useful now, and they have a significant ability to serve as a resource to teachers and to other students.

Accepting the fact that adults and children learn differently means that a teacher must understand the characteristics of adult learners when attempting to educate them in health care. These characteristics must be recognized and incorporated into teaching strategies regardless of the patients' ability to read or write. One of the main goals of any teaching program is to effect behavior change in the student. Therefore, we should carefully evaluate the skills patients have learned in order to demonstrate that our teaching efforts have been effective.

Adults are autonomous and self-directed and must recognize the need for learning (Lieb, 1991). Our patients want to be an integral part of any learning activity and want to learn information about their health care. We must incorporate these adults into any learning activity and make sure they understand the need for the information we are presenting. In other words, if our patients feel that what they're hearing is just general knowledge, or that it somehow is not pertinent to them or to their family members, they will tune it out.

For this reason, it is the teacher's job to make his or her content relevant and to demonstrate how the information can be used to achieve better health. According to research, in order to remember and to use new information, adults must integrate the information into existing frameworks of understanding. They must participate in the learning process by linking the information to what they already know (Blackburn, 2005; Lieb, 1991).

Adults are interested in learning practical things rather than abstract theory (Collins, 2004). Again, health educators must demonstrate how new information applies to the patient personally. Not everyone is interested in knowledge for its own sake. Adults have accumulated a wealth of life experiences that can be used in the teaching/learning process. Even if someone cannot read, he or she has lived life, had many experiences, and come into contact with a wide variety of people. It is important to draw on an individual's past experiences to teach new ideas (Gamonal, 2003). If the teacher can show some relationship between a previous event and a current one, patients are more likely to see the connection and to make positive changes.

Therefore, hands-on learning rather than a straight lecture is preferable for adult learners. The more hands-on your educational program is, in fact, the more your adult students are likely to learn. It has been said that people retain roughly 15% to 25% of what they hear, 50% to 55% of what they see and hear, and 80% to 85% of what they hear, see, and do (Collins, 2004). Although these statistics vary from source to source, most educators agree that adults, adolescents, and children have three main learning styles—*visual, auditory,* and *kinesthetic*—that determine how much they will retain.

Visual learners learn more by looking and watching. Auditory learners, by contrast, learn more when they can listen, hear, and speak. And kinesthetic learners need to experience, move, and do to reinforce what they learn (Kolb, 1984; *Principles of Adult Learning*, n.d.). Videos, flip charts, and demonstrations appeal to visual learners. Group discussions or shared stories and examples are better for auditory learners. Kinesthetic learners remember more when they are engaged with role-playing, practice demonstrations, and similar activities. Everyone learns using all three styles, but usually one style is dominant (*Principles of Adult Learning*, n.d.).

Evaluating the learning styles of patients and focusing teaching strategies to meet those styles can increase patients' motivation and make education efforts more effective (Chase, 2001). Low-literate learners are less inclined to absorb information through written materials or by listening to long, dry lectures. A kinesthetic approach, then, is usually most effective with these patients. We must strive to have low-literate adults *do* the task, *make* the low-fat dessert, and *take* their own blood pressure. The more we allow our patients to do for themselves, in other words, the more likely they are truly to learn the tasks.

All learners need respect, and this is especially true of adult learners. Adult learners need an opportunity for input and discussion. The adults we teach should be seen as our peers and should be included in the decision-making process (Lieb, 1991). If we are teaching patients about their medications and when to take them, for example, we should ask the patients about their lifestyles. In fact, this information should help determine the time of day the patient takes medications. If a patient usually arises at 6 a.m., his or her morning pill ought to be taken at 6 a.m. If the patient arises at 9 a.m., however, clearly 9 a.m. would be a better time to take that morning pill.

Health professionals must adjust their teaching efforts to fit with a patient's lifestyle. Failure to do so will only lead to noncompliance and increased morbidity, which are exactly the kinds of results we're trying to avoid.

There are several barriers to the learning process that we must consider. Poor language and reading skills are a major obstacle. It is important for the provider or staff member to determine whether the patient is a poor reader or cannot read at all, and then to adapt his or her teaching style to meet this challenge.

There are many ways to address reading skills, many of which are presented in this book (see, for example, chapter 3, Assessing Patients' Literacy Levels, and chapter 8, Principles of Writing for Low Literacy). Ignoring the patient's reading skills or assuming that the patient can read does not help anyone meet his or her objectives. Whether or not the patient can read, we must understand that adults learn differently than do children and adapt our teaching methods to meet the needs of adults.

REASONS FOR LOW HEALTH LITERACY

There are many who believe that people with literacy challenges are dropouts or stupid or just don't try. This is far from the truth. There are several reasons why people have literacy problems, including limited education; language barriers; cognitive impairment caused by dementia, delirium, or medication effects; learning disorders; affective disorders; and illness. These circumstances are not the fault of the patient or the family. No one purposely chooses to be sick or to have dyslexia. If given the choice, everyone would like to be able to read and write. In fact, shame and embarrassment drive many patients to hide their low literacy (Baker et al., 1996; Parikh, Parker, Nurss, Baker, & Williams, 1996). As a result, it is harder for health care providers and clinical staff to know which patients have difficulty reading and which cannot read at all, but they must discover this information if they are to provide the additional help and devote the additional time that low-health-literate patients require.

Limited Education

Those people with limited or poor education may be able to enroll in adult reading classes. These classes are offered at many public schools in the evening or at local libraries and other locations. Some are taught by volunteers and have demonstrated positive results. According to the National Reporting System of the U.S. Department of Education's (DOE's) Office of Vocational and Adult Education, adult basic and literacy education programs steadily improved in effectiveness during 2000–2001, 2001–2002, and 2002–2003 (U.S. Department of Education, 2004). The DOE report, titled *Adult Education and Family Literacy Act: Program Year 2002–2003: Report to Congress on State Performance*, includes evaluative data from all 50 states. It is available at http://www.ed.gov/about/reports/annual/ovae/2003adulted.pdf.

Adult reading classes are usually either free or may charge a very low fee. They require a large time commitment from the student, however, so to succeed the student truly must be motivated to learn to read. Clinical office staff may be in a good position to recommend educational programs to patients. Even if the patient decides to enroll in a reading class, the health care provider and his or her staff still must be cognizant of the fact that the patient cannot read today. Such awareness affects whether and how well the patient takes his or her medications, understands preprocedure orders, reads directions, and fills out forms.

If members of a patient's family know about the patient's literacy problems and are able to read, it may be appropriate to include family members in the educational process. If this is the appropriate action, someone in the family should be identified as the patient's partner. The patient's partner needs to have permission from the patient to be included in the clinical and education process and should take responsibility for assisting the patient at home.

If, however, the family does not know about the patient's literacy problems or the patient does not have a family, office staff must realize that alternative options to the written word may be necessary. Examples of alternative resources are discussed in chapter 9, Using Alternative Forms of Patient Communication. Among these options are videotapes, audiotapes, *fotonovelas*, pictographs, and telephone callbacks.

Language Barriers

Language barriers are another obstacle to literacy. A literacy problem could exist if the patient's native tongue is, say, Spanish or Chinese and he or she has come to the United States, where virtually everything is written in English. Another issue is whether the patient is literate in his or her own language. In other words, is it a language or a literacy-plus-language problem? If the patient reads well in his or her native language, translation is an option. Bilingual staff members can do translations of English-language materials internally, but there is also the option of contracting with a business that uses certified translators to do translations. To locate translators in your area, you can visit the American Translators Association Web site at http://www.atanet.org.

Trained health care translators must be familiar with medical terms and jargon so that the translation conveys both the literal meaning and spirit of the original (Sobero & Giraldo, 2004). Once a text has been translated, one major hurdle has been overcome. However, the mere availability of translated materials does not mean that patients have been taught the information; it just means they can read the information if they choose to do so.

If the patient cannot read in his or her native language, then it is a problem both of translation and of low literacy. Sending the patient to a reading program may be appropriate if there is a program in that patient's native language. But more than 300 languages are spoken in the United States, so unless the language is fairly common, classes may be difficult to locate. In addition, in light of the patient's low literacy level, translations must be easy to read in the native language. Developing such translations is not a simple task. First, the clinician must find someone to translate the piece into the correct language. Then he or she must find someone else who can make the text low literate or easy to understand in the target language. After these steps have been taken, the text must be back-translated into English again, and the two pieces must be compared with each other. Comparing the back-translation with the original text can help identify trouble spots in the translation process (Yahya, 2002–2004).

Finally, those producing the materials may need to conduct a focus group with native speakers of the language to proof them again. After all, regions of the same country in which related languages are spoken often have their own geographical, cultural, and regional differences. Think of all the countries in which Spanish is spoken, for example. Would one Spanish translation meet everyone's needs? In spoken Chinese, slight variations in tone or the way words sound can make one dialect—from Mandarin to Gang to Cantonese—impossible to understand for speakers of another dialect. These variations become especially challenging in multiethnic regions, such as California or New York City, where so many cultures and languages coexist. (For more about the relationship between culture and low health literacy, see chapter 5, Factoring Culture Into the Care Process.)

As difficult as some translations are to make, many translations are produced successfully and used all over the United States. To translate texts into easy-to-read versions in a different language simply takes more time and work, but it is well worth the effort (Figure 2.1a, b, and c). Again, the availability of a translation will not necessarily solve the problem for those who cannot read, but easy-to-read translations certainly can help those with low-literacy skills.

Cognitive Impairment and Affective Disorders

Cognitive impairment may be caused by dementia, delirium, and medication effects. When patients have any of these diseases or symptoms, it can be impossible to teach them about their own self-care. For this reason, it is important to know whether the disease or symptom is temporary or permanent. For example, if medication effects are associated with some medicine that the patient will stop taking in the future, efforts to educate the patient will be more successful after the medication course has been completed.

However, if dementia is permanent, then a caretaker or family member must be included in the patient's clinical care and education process. Dementia is sometimes associated with medications and illnesses, meaning that eventually the patient returns to normal. But even if the patient doesn't seem to understand, including him or her in the educational process is recommended.

No one knows for certain how much a patient understands; dementia and confusion are difficult to quantify. In a small Swedish pilot study, for example, use of storytelling seemed to help dementia patients remember and make associations with situations they previously had experienced in their lives (Holm, Lepp, & Ringsberg, 2005). Dementia patients may understand more than we think. Even an unconscious patient may hear and understand things we would not think possible, so health care providers should err on the side of including the patient as much as they can.

Learning disorders, such as dyslexia and hyperactivity, affect a person's ability to read. Dyslexic children, for example, cannot recognize words in printed form that may be part of their everyday vocabulary (Schatschneider & Torgesen, 2004). Generally, a dyslexic person is able to read, but does so slowly and inverts many letters. A hyperactive person may not have the patience to sit and read something that takes a long time.

Although studies suggest a high incidence of reading disabilities in children with attention deficit hyperactivity disorder, or ADHD (Palacios & Semrud-Clikeman, 2005), many of these people may not have been diagnosed in school

What's in This Book

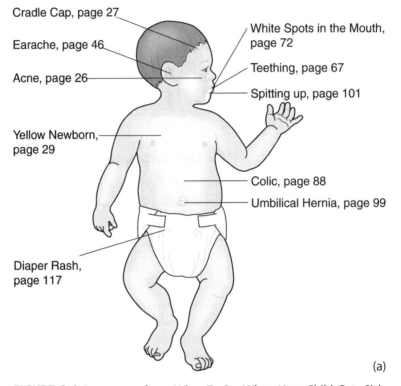

Cradle Cap, page 27

Earache, page 46

Acne, page 26

Yellow Newborn,
page 29

Diaper Rash,
page 117

White Spots in the Mouth,
page 72

Teething, page 67

Spitting up, page 101

Colic, page 88

Umbilical Hernia, page 99

(a)

FIGURE 2.1 Same page from *What To Do When Your Child Gets Sick*, translated into several different languages. This page, shown here in English and translated into Spanish and Chinese (Mandarin), provides those with low literacy skills another option for finding the appropriate page in the book by using the illustration of the child's body. Translations done carefully, using focus groups and other techniques such as back-reads (translating back into the original language and comparing the text to ensure the first translation is appropriate), enhance the usability and credibility of the material. The State of California distributes *What To Do When Your Child Gets Sick* in five languages to all new parents in the state.

Contenido del libro

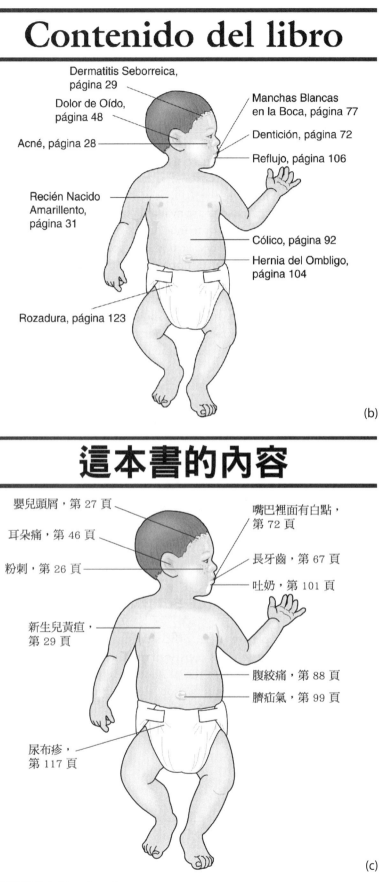

Dermatitis Seborreica, página 29

Dolor de Oído, página 48

Acné, página 28

Recién Nacido Amarillento, página 31

Rozadura, página 123

Manchas Blancas en la Boca, página 77

Dentición, página 72

Reflujo, página 106

Cólico, página 92

Hernia del Ombligo, página 104

(b)

這本書的內容

嬰兒頭屑，第 27 頁

耳朵痛，第 46 頁

粉刺，第 26 頁

新生兒黃疸，第 29 頁

尿布疹，第 117 頁

嘴巴裡面有白點，第 72 頁

長牙齒，第 67 頁

吐奶，第 101 頁

腹絞痛，第 88 頁

臍疝氣，第 99 頁

(c)

FIGURE 2.1 (*Continued*)

and therefore may not have received the additional attention they needed to overcome their disorders. And let's not forget that a patient from another country who speaks another language may still have a learning disorder along with the challenge of acquiring a new language.

The key to helping a person with a learning disorder is to write material in an easy-to-read and easy-to-understand format, accompanied by illustrations in appropriate places. Any symbols that can be used also will be very helpful. If a skill is required of the patient, demonstration and return demonstration are the methods most effective for explaining the skill.

When family members or caretakers are available to assist the patient, they should be included in the care plan. Someone should make sure that the task required of the patient is being performed at home, especially if it is crucial to the patient's health and well-being. For example, a diabetic patient who must measure his or her own blood sugar level and adjust medication based on the results of the test should be reminded and observed completing the task. In fact, those with limited health literacy have been shown to benefit from diabetes education, improving in self-management behavior (Kim, Love, Quistberg, & Shea, 2004). If the patient doesn't live with someone, a reminder phone call is a good idea.

Depression, anxiety, and other affective disorders also can cause reading difficulties. These disorders are usually temporary depending on the symptoms of the disease and the medications taken. Typically, when the disorder is eliminated, so are the reading problems. This is true, however, only if the person could read or write before the symptoms of the disorder appeared.

Similarly, any trauma, stress, or illness can affect a patient's ability to read and understand the written word. If the trauma, stress, or illness is transitory, however, the patient's reading ability should return. Any long-term physical or psychological problem can diminish reading ability, with less than 100% return. Health care professionals must be aware of this fact and take it into consideration when educating patients.

HEALTH LITERACY IN THE OFFICE SETTING

Tools to help the low-literate person in the office setting come in two varieties: human and technological. Human tools consist of family members, caretakers, advocates, interpreters, nurses, staff, and the providers themselves. Nonhuman tools include telephone systems, computers, videos, and written materials of all kinds. Any one of these tools can assist the low-health-literate person in navigating through the health care system and achieving positive health outcomes.

People Who Can Help

Family Members

Family members are critical in the health care process, both for people who read well and for those who cannot read at all. Family members serve as advocates for patients, helping them with each provider they see and often interpreting complicated health care information or directions. A family member who can attend physician appointments and be there at home to help the patient comply with treatment protocols is ideal. If the family member can't be home with the patient, however, telephone calls or periodic visits may achieve the same goal. Family members who understand the reading challenges faced by their loved ones can offer valuable support in a variety of ways.

The most basic support that family members offer is listening to and discussing with their loved one what the provider says in the exam room. Many patients—not just those with low literacy—are confused after an interaction with a health care provider and appreciate another set of ears and eyes to help. If the patient approves, the family member should be included in the office visit. The family member can help read and interpret instructions or written materials that the patient receives.

This help becomes critical if there are follow-up instructions or information regarding radiological or laboratory tests, medications, or referrals to other providers. A family member can facilitate arrangements for making appointments, getting medications, or helping prepare the patient for tests. Such assistance helps patients, providers, and the health system as a whole.

Caretakers

Caretakers can function much as family members do when the patient has no family. Some caretakers care for only one patient at a time and therefore may have more time for assisting a patient with follow-up protocols. Assistance from a caretaker is even more valuable if he or she has some medical knowledge and understands medical terms. Caretakers are valuable to people who have difficulty reading and navigating the health care system.

Advocates

Advocates essentially act as the patient's ambassador, helping the patient when they are needed. Advocates are either paid or work on a volunteer basis. They usually understand the health care system well and can manage the many intricacies associated with obtaining health care. They can interpret language, help with follow-up, clarify directions, question bills, and obtain referral appointments.

Many patients find advocates helpful, though advocates can be especially useful for those who have difficulty reading. Patient advocates in cancer care, for example, have aided in the development of educational dialogues between investigators and patient communities and assisted in streamlining cancer research policies and clinical trials (Collyar, 2005).

Interpreters

Interpreters are used in health care practitioners' offices when the provider speaks a different language from the patient or the patient's family. Health care interpreters are very useful for communicating complex information in a foreign language. Usually they are familiar with medical jargon and terminology and have experience interpreting for a particular health care agency or health care provider (Hwa-Froelich & Westby, 2003). Interpreters can read patient information, interpret patient directions, and help read patient education materials. They are a great support to patients and providers when there is no common language. Normally they stand behind the patient or off to one side and try to interpret the correct meaning of what the provider says. Cultural differences and peculiarities of language can make this practice difficult. (Such issues as the role of interpreters in the health care setting and the special needs of patients with low English proficiency are discussed in chapter 10, Interpreters and Their Role in the Health Care Setting.)

Nurses

Nurses in the provider's office also can be of great help to low-health-literate patients. Nurses have been trained in patient education and adult learning techniques. In addition, they are in a unique position to understand health principles, the target population, and the work environment (Campbell, 1999). Nurses can act as patient advocates or partner with advocates in the community (Morra, 2000). They understand privacy issues and can assist patients with reading and filling out forms. Nurses understand provider referral patterns and can assist patients in arranging appointments.

Furthermore, nurses can explain follow-up instructions, such as preparation for tests or medications, when patients have difficulty understanding them. Many nurses use visual techniques such as pictographs to communicate instructions (Houts et al., 1998). If the nurse in a provider's office knows that a patient has difficulty reading, he or she can offer a variety of resources to assist that patient in getting much-needed health services. Help lines staffed by nurses also provide assistance to low-health-literate patients by telephone (Courson, 2005).

Office Staff

Staff members in the provider's office are key for identifying patients' needs and for assisting low-health-literate patients in getting in to see the provider. They manage the first contact with the patient, which should be handled with care and finesse (Walsh, 2004). Is there a private place in which the patient can tell the receptionist that he or she is having difficulty reading the forms, for example? Is there a location that is private enough so forms can be read out loud to patients with literacy problems? Does the receptionist communicate such information appropriately to nurses and providers, away from the ears of patients in the waiting room?

Dealing with such issues is critical so patients can feel secure during the office visit. The tone set at the beginning of the office visit helps the patient feel comfortable throughout the entire appointment. In this respect, the staff is critical for making office visits a success. Even nonverbal cues sent by the provider and staff can affect patients, either making them feel more tense or putting them at ease (Roter, 2005).

Health Care Providers

If all else fails, the provider usually has the most power to salvage the situation, as we saw at the beginning of this chapter in the story about Mr. Martinez. If the provider knows that the patient has difficulty reading, he or she can communicate in such a way that the patient understands. When dealing with low-literate patients, health care providers must refrain from using medical jargon and must speak slowly, especially when giving instructions. Using the teach-back method is critical. Writing simple directions and using pictographs or videos also can be useful. And it's a good idea to have someone in the office call the patient to see how he or she is doing.

But the most essential part of the equation is having an empathetic health care provider who understands the principles of low-health literacy. It's the provider who sets the tone and philosophy of the office. The provider should offer continuing education to office staff about health literacy and the best way to handle problems with literacy in the office setting. Office personnel cannot judge the patient or label the patient with negative descriptions. The low-health-literate patient is not dumb; he or she just has difficulty reading. Accepting the low-health literate patient in the office and making his or her experience positive are critical components of high-quality care.

Use of Technology

Technology can be an enhancement to patient care, but it also can create additional barriers.

Telephones

Some phone systems place so many obstacles in the way of talking to a live person that the patient becomes angry before he or she has accomplished the purpose of the phone call. Other phone systems are user friendly and assist callers in accessing information in a reasonable time (Baker, 1998). The phone system in the provider's office must be user friendly and adaptable to the various reasons why people call.

For starters, the phone should always be answered by the third ring (Woodson, 2004). If the phone system is automated, the program should answer the call right away. If the patient is put on hold at that time, how long does he or she have to wait to speak to a person on the other end of the phone? Waiting on the phone for a real human being to talk to you can be frustrating. Wait time should be eliminated or reduced if possible. In addition, having multiple choices on a medical office phone system is confusing, especially for older patients and those with literacy problems.

The person on the phone is the patient's first exposure to your office. The voice of that person should be warm and welcoming (Woodson, 2004). In addition, the person who answers the phone should attempt to solve the patient's issue without additional delay. Transferring the caller from one department to another is not an effective means of providing customer service. Someone in the office should take ownership of the patient and his or her issue.

Voicemail, too, can be cold and impersonal (Davidhizar & Shearer, 2000). The best system is to have a person answer the phone and solve the patient's issue without transfers to other individuals. The closer your office can come to this system, the better it will be for patient satisfaction. If you must have voicemail and transfers, someone should make sure that the patient's issue is resolved on the same day (Woodson, 2004).

Internet and World Wide Web

Both the Internet and the World Wide Web can be useful as patient education tools. (The Internet is a massive network of networks that connects millions of computers together globally. The Web, by contrast, is an information-sharing model: the main way information is accessed on the Internet. E-mail is sent over the Internet; the World Wide Web and its Web sites are "surfed" using Web browsers, such as Netscape. The Web features graphics, sounds, text, and video ["The Difference Between," 2006].)

For the low-health-literate patient, use of such technologies presents unusual problems. In observation studies, people with literacy challenges used the Internet differently than did those who read well (Birru et al., 2004). Low-literate patients tend to read every word and do not scan the text on the screen for usable information. Because they plow through every word, they often miss things outside their main view. If a paragraph becomes too complicated, a lower literate reader may simply skip to another area of the text, potentially missing important details.

Some search engines are too complicated for low-literate users. Such patients have a hard time spelling words. They may find the many options presented on a specific topic confusing and check only the first or second link, which may not contain the best material for their needs (Birru et al., 2004).

There are ways to make the Internet and the Web more user-friendly for low-literate adults. (Use of Web-based technologies with low-health-literate patients is discussed in chapter 9, Using Alternative Forms of Patient Communication.) A key point to remember is that health care providers should not discount computer technologies when it comes to helping low-literate patients. In fact, Internet-based consultation may act as a complement to regular health care (Umefjord, Hamberg, Malker, & Petersson, 2006). Clinicians should at least be aware of the various methods for making Web-based sources more useful for those with literacy problems.

Medical Devices

Other technologies can be helpful to patients if developed and used appropriately. If the patient must take a device home, for example, the provider should make sure the patient knows how to use it properly. If the patient has questions or needs help troubleshooting the device, he or she should be given phone numbers to call. Some physiological monitoring devices are now used routinely in disease management programs. Low-literate patients are good candidates for these newer techniques if they are clearly explained and adequate follow-up care is provided.

Use of Written Materials

If written materials are used, clinicians should make sure they are easy to use and easy to understand. Patient education materials are best written at a third-, fourth-, or fifth-grade reading level (Weiss & Coyne, 1997). Brochures from pharmaceutical companies and other commercial medical companies are usually too difficult for the low-literate person to use. A review of patient education materials produced by the American Academy of Family Physicians, for example, found that the materials on average were written at a ninth-grade level, which is too high for the average American reader (Wallace & Lennon, 2004). Numerous studies of patient education materials have reached the same conclusion. These materials should be rewritten so that all patients, regardless of their reading ability, can use them.

Although some people feel that easy-to-read materials are *too* simple for the literate person, very few people—even those with advanced skills—complain that such materials are not useful, as we mentioned in chapter 1. But let's reiterate the point here: all patients seem to like and prefer easy-to-read materials, perhaps because these materials get their point across without too much unnecessary or irrelevant information. If you want to know what to do for a bloody nose, you might not care about the *why* of the bloody nose. You just want to know what action to take to stop the bleeding. Simply put, easy-to-read health materials are more practical. (Various methods for assessing the literacy levels of patient education materials are discussed in chapter 7, Designing Easy-to-Read Patient Education Materials.)

Patient education materials needn't be written in prose; other kinds of materials also can be considered. After all, efforts to simplify written materials may not be enough on their own to increase patient understanding (Wilson, Brown, & Stephens-Ferris, 2006). Pictographs, models, medication calendars, videotapes, and audiotapes are just a few of the many alternatives to the written word that are available (AMC Cancer Research Center, 1994).

Patient–Provider Interaction

The patient first encounters the office at the reception area. Typically, this is where forms and more forms are given to the patient to complete. Why do we need all these forms? The only forms that should be given to the patient at the outset are the ones that *must* be completed. Among such required forms, of course, is the HIPAA Notice of Privacy Practices. Furthermore, the receptionist should ask *all* patients whether they need help in completing the forms. That way, patients will never be preselected as low literate.

The patient should be given help in completing forms in a private location. It might be embarrassing for low-literate patients if other patients overhear their questions and answers. A patient handbook that is easy to read and easy to use may also be helpful. It could address many of the typical questions asked by patients. Patients could take the handbook home and read it there or have someone in their family read it to them.

When the patient and provider are together, the provider should ask, "What questions or concerns do you have?" While taking a social history, the provider also should ask, "Are you satisfied with how well you read?" This question will give the patient an opportunity to discuss any reading problems.

Written instructions for the patient should be easy to follow. The provider might want to discuss the instructions with the patient, the patient's family, or a patient advocate. The patient should give permission for such a discussion to take place, but having the provider ensure understanding with family members or advocates may be the only way to ensure follow-through on directions for low-literate patients. If the patient is required to adhere to complicated medical instructions, a family conference may be needed.

Providers should use the teach-back method, asking patients to describe in detail what they will do with respect to medications or prescribed treatment regimens after returning home. Asking "Do you understand?" is rarely helpful because it is easy for the patient simply to respond *yes*. Providers should instead ask patients to say how they might explain their problem to a friend. Having the patient actually demonstrate a skill (when and how to take a certain medication, for example) is the best way to evaluate his or her ability and understanding.

When patients are ready to leave the office, make sure they have written instructions that are simple to read and easy to understand. The most common problem with written instructions is that too much information is included in them. Ask yourself what is *crucial* for the patient to understand, and then leave out all the "nice-to-know" information. Always include a telephone number for the patient to call in case he or she becomes confused or needs more information. Including the patient's family or an advocate is useful at this point in the teaching process. In fact, as long as the patient agrees to it, giving health-related information to more than one person whom the patient trusts is always a good idea.

Finally, it is important to follow up with patients about their progress. A telephone call from the nurse may be helpful and can answer questions that have arisen since the patient's visit. (Telephone medicine and telephone triage are discussed in chapter 6, Improving Patient–Provider Communication.) Patients usually like some type of follow-up, even if it is not a face-to-face office visit. Telephone calls are convenient, fast, and cost effective. Also, patients and their families appreciate the extra caring and effort that a phone call from health care providers suggests.

Referrals and Ancillary Services

Many patients are referred to other specialists and ancillary services from their primary care provider. For the low-health-literate patient, these referrals can cause feelings of fear and anxiety, evoking questions and concerns. Who are these specialists? Will they recognize that I have difficulty reading? Will there be help for me in the office? What will they want me to do? Will I understand? These and other questions could deter the patient from making the appointment or seeking the care of the ancillary provider.

For this reason, providers, nurses, and staff at the patient's primary care office should take responsibility for alleviating the patient's fears. If the patient approves, for example, the specialist or ancillary provider can be told of the patient's difficulty in reading. Someone who speaks the patient's native language could be made available to interpret at the other office. Language can be kept at a simple level with no medical jargon. If the patient is required to read, a family member or patient advocate may wish to attend the appointment along with the patient. If that's impossible, information should be written in very simple language and given to the patient to take home. At this point, follow-up telephone calls are especially important to ensure that the low-health-literate patient understands what further actions are required.

When patients do not want their primary care providers to mention their difficulty with reading to specialists or ancillary providers, they should be encouraged to tell the other provider about their reading difficulty on their own. We must recognize that there is a great deal of shame associated with not being able to read; many patients with low literacy try desperately to hide the fact. Specialist appointments are often difficult to obtain, however, so patients should be encouraged to share information freely and to use every clinical resource at their disposal.

Armed with important information about a prospective patient's literacy level, specialists and other ancillary providers can seek the best treatments and not be at a disadvantage. And because medical instructions, patient education materials, and prescriptions all require that a patient read to some degree, low-health-literate patients can receive the highest quality care if office staff, providers, and ancillary providers all know about their reading level and any special needs they have.

THE HOSPITAL ENVIRONMENT

Hospital environments are not health-literacy friendly. Outside signage, for example, is difficult to understand even for people who read well. Directional signs use medical jargon with few universal symbols. Such terms as *emergency department, radiology, surgery*, and *admissions* are difficult to read and understand, yet they are used regularly in parking lots and other places to direct people to the appropriate area of the hospital (Rudd, 2004). How many people can read and understand these terms? How many are translated into other languages? When was the last time you saw a directional sign in Spanish? As Rudd notes, "The tools intended to help the public gain entry into, and make their way around, a hospital are of little use to the visitors and non-professional staff for whom they have (at least in part) been designed. In other words, words do get in the way" (Rudd, 2004, p. 23).

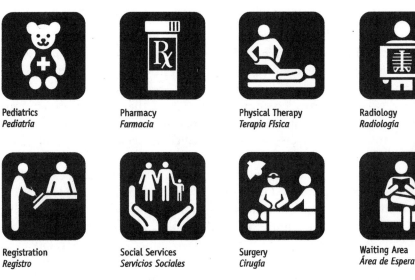

Pediatrics
Pediatría

Pharmacy
Farmacia

Physical Therapy
Terapia Física

Radiology
Radiología

Registration
Registro

Social Services
Servicios Sociales

Surgery
Cirugía

Waiting Area
Área de Espera

FIGURE 2.2 Universal symbols from *Hablamos Juntos*. With support from the Robert Wood Johnson Foundation, *Hablamos Juntos* worked with the Society for Environmental Graphic Design to develop and test 28 symbols like those above. Seventeen were understood by at least 87% of multilingual testers, testers arrived at their destination faster using symbols than when they relied on word signs to direct them, and nearly 9 out of 10 testers said they could understand more than half of the symbols. *Source:* "Universal Health Symbols Provide Direction for Many in Hospitals," Robert Wood Johnson Foundation Press Release, December 14, 2005.

Placing universal symbols for medical areas on signs would make them easier for everyone to understand. Pictures of an x-ray or ambulance or clear, simple line drawings can be used to denote special areas. Instead of using words like *nephrology*, which are common in the hospital environment, "kidney doctor" might be easier to understand. In fact, all medical terminology should be translated into common language. Signage inside and outside the facility should be changed to incorporate symbols, pictographs, or common language. This may take time and effort, but should be done at all hospitals as soon as possible.

Initiatives such as those by the national program *Hablamos Juntos* to create patient-friendly symbols should be encouraged. With support from the Robert Wood Johnson Foundation and help from the Society for Environmental Graphic Design, *Hablamos Juntos* developed and tested 28 symbols for use in hospitals and other health care facilities (Figure 2.2). Hopeful that hospitals nationwide will consider incorporating the symbols into their signage, the group also has developed the *Universal Symbols in Health Care Workbook*, a how-to guide for hospital CEOs, administrators, and other professionals who are interested in improving the readability of signs and symbols they use ("Universal Health Symbols," 2005). For more information, visit the *Hablamos Juntos* Web site at http://www.hablamosjuntos.org.

Having the physician's name on signs also may be helpful (Rudd, 2004). Often patients recognize their own physician's name, but not the medical department in which he or she works. In other words, though I might know that my physician is Dr. Green, I don't necessarily know that Dr. Green is a neurologist.

Forms are another major obstacle for those who have difficulty reading. Most hospital forms are written with the legal profession rather than the lay reader in mind. Forms are sometimes written at a college level and rarely follow any of the principles of writing for low literacy (Schwartzberg, VanGeest, & Wang, 2005). Medical jargon, small fonts, little white space, and legalese all frustrate the poor reader, yet they are common in many medical forms. (Principles of writing for low-literacy patients are described in chapter 8, Principles of Writing for Low Literacy.)

Many people cannot understand informed consent, for example, and have no idea they are signing for surgery that may remove an organ. A well-known example is the experience of Toni Cordell Seiple, who lost her uterus 30 years ago when she was intimidated by an informed consent document and failed to seek further instruction. Her surgical "repair" for a prolapsed uterus turned out to be a hysterectomy, a word she says her gynecologist never used (Rubin, 2003). In the rush of admissions, anxiety about the hospitalization and the unknown adds to a patient's confusion. When the words don't come easily, anxieties only increase. And when patients don't know what to ask, outcomes such as Seiple's hysterectomy are much more likely to occur.

Patients must read many things when they are admitted to the hospital. In the room itself, for example, there are any number of signs and notices. The name of the nurse or aide caring for the patient is usually posted. Instructions for telephone or television use, instructions for how to call the nurse, instructions for how to elevate the bed—all require literacy skills. There may be descriptions of oxygen or other treatments the patient will experience. For the patient who cannot read, such signs and notices create anxiety. And when patients are embarrassed by their inability to read, they may refuse to ask for help, thereby compounding the problem.

Patient instructions and educational materials create additional obstacles for those with low literacy. We give patients a vast number of materials to read, including menus, descriptions of tests, medication instructions, health education materials, and pharmaceutical information. Poor readers may never use many of them. When staff members feel that they have educated patients simply by giving them such materials, a miscommunication has occurred that can cause increased morbidity and more cost to the patient and the system as a whole. (Clinical errors, miscommunication, and how to avoid them are discussed in chapter 4, Understanding and Avoiding Medical Errors, and chapter 6, Improving Patient–Provider Communication.)

Nurses and other professionals working in hospitals have a responsibility to ensure that patients understand the information they need for their health and well-being. It's not enough simply to review written materials with our patients: we must educate them at their level and with their abilities in mind, making sure the materials are accessible and useful. (The pros and cons of using testing to assess patients' literacy levels—as well as several less formal assessments—are discussed in chapter 3, Assessing Patients' Literacy Levels.)

Team meetings with physicians and other health professionals may be required to discuss the difference between information patients *must* know and information it is *nice* for them to know. *As mentioned earlier, we are obligated to limit the information we provide patients to what is absolutely necessary.* We must rewrite health-related information in a format that can be understood by the low-literate patient.

Hospital diversity committees should take on the issue of low health literacy. All forms, patient education materials, videos, audiotapes, and other materials should be made simple and easy to read. This is especially true for legal documents, such as informed consent and advance directives forms. It has become increasingly clear, too, that hospitals face substantial liability with respect to how they treat low-health-literate patients (Liss, 2002). In other words, there is a clear financial interest in devising literacy solutions that work.

A good first step would be for the hospital diversity committee to coordinate efforts to review, rewrite, and monitor all forms that the hospital uses. The hospital attorney may be part of the diversity committee, but at the very least he or she should be involved in any efforts to revise written documents. Most important, the hospital attorney must understand the problem of low health literacy and be willing to seek creative solutions.

*   *   *

What this chapter demonstrates is that all environments in health care must be user friendly. Having health education materials, signs, forms, and other media in a low-literate format is not just the right thing to do—it is good business. Carefully assessing our patients' literacy abilities and seeking to meet their individual needs is time well spent. Even when clinicians are busy with their routine work, they must make time for each patient. Although the primary physician's office is a good starting point, work must be done with specialists, allied health providers, and clinicians in the hospital. All places where patients seek health care must cooperate to bring down the level of educational materials. Only with a concerted effort can we make a difference in our patients' ability to understand.

REFERENCES

AMC Cancer Research Center, Centers for Disease Control and Prevention. (1994). *Beyond the brochure: Alternative approaches to effective health communication.* Denver, CO: Author. Retrieved January 29, 2006, from http://www.cdc.gov/cancer/nbccedp/bccpdfs/amcbeyon.pdf

Baker, D. W., Parker, R. M., Williams, M. V., Pitkin, K., Parikh, N. S., Coates, W., et al. (1996). The health care experience of patients with low literacy. *Archives of Family Medicine, 5*(6), 329–334.

Baker, L. P. (1998). Communicate with patients using common office equipment. *Journal of Medical Practice Management, 14*(2), 78–82.

Birru, M. S., Monaco, V. M., Charles, L., Drew, H., Njie, V., Bierria, T., et al. (2004). Internet usage by low-literacy adults seeking health information: An observational analysis. *Journal of Medical Internet Research, 6*(3), 5. Retrieved November 24, 2005, from http://www.jmir.org/2004/3/e25

Blackburn, G. L. (2005). Teaching, learning, doing: Best practices in education. *American Journal of Clinical Nutrition, 82*(1 suppl), 218S–221S.

Campbell, K. N. (1999). Adult education: Helping adults begin the process of learning. *American Association of Occupational Health Nurses Journal, 47*(1), 31–40.

Chase, T. M. (2001). Learning styles and teaching strategies: Enhancing the patient education experience. *SCI Nursing, 18*(3), 138–141.

Collins, J. (2004). Education techniques for lifelong learning: Principles of adult learning. *Radiographics, 24*(5), 1483–1489.

Collyar, D. (2005). How have patient advocates in the United States benefited cancer research? *Nature Reviews Cancer, 5*(1), 73–78.

Courson, S. (2005). Telephone nurse triage. *PA State Nurses Association.* Retrieved December 13, 2005, from http://www.panurses.org/search1.cfm?filename=membersite/articles/profdevelop/profdev_telephonetriage.htm

Davidhizar, R., & Shearer, R. (2000). The effective voice mail message. *Hospital Materials Management Quarterly, 22*(2), 45–49.

Gamonal, P. (2003). *Adult education: Creating learning programs for adults in your organization.* Retrieved January 5, 2006, from http://www.ravenwerks.com/leadership/adulted.htm

Holm, A. K., Lepp, M., & Ringsberg, K. C. (2005). Dementia: Involving patients in storytelling—a caring intervention: A pilot study. *Journal of Clinical Nursing, 14*(2), 256–263.

Houts, P. S., Bachrach, R., Witmer, J. T., Tringali, C. A., Bucher, J. A., & Localio, R. A. (1998). Using pictographs to enhance recall of spoken medical instructions. *Patient Education and Counseling, 35*, 83–88.

Hwa-Froelich, D. A., & Westby, C. E. (2003). Considerations when working with interpreters. *Communication Disorders Quarterly, 24*(2), 78–85.

Kim, S., Love, F., Quistberg, D. A., & Shea, J. A. (2004). Association of health literacy with self-management behavior in patients with diabetes. *Diabetes Care, 27*, 2980–2982.

Kolb, D. A. (1984). *Experiential learning: Experience as the source of learning and development.* Englewood Cliffs, NJ: Prentice-Hall.

Lieb, S. (1991, Fall). Principles of adult learning. *Vision.* Retrieved January 21, 2006, from http://honolulu.hawaii.edu/intranet/committees/FacDevCom/guidebk/teachtip/adults-2.htm

Liss, S. I. (2002). *Literacy, health, and the law: An update of legal rights for low health literate patients.* Philadelphia: Health Promotion Council of Southeastern Pennsylvania, Inc.

Morra, M. E. (2000). New opportunities for nurses as patient advocates. *Seminars in Oncology Nursing, 16*(1), 57–64.

Padberg, R. M., & Padberg, L. F. (1990). Strengthening the effectiveness of patient education: Applying principles of adult education. *Oncology Nursing Forum, 17*(1), 65–69.

Palacios, E. D., & Semrud-Clikeman, M. (2005). Delinquency, hyperactivity, and phonological awareness: A comparison of adolescents with ODD and ADHD. *Applied Neuropsychology, 12*(2), 94–105.

Parikh, N. S., Parker, R. M., Nurss, J. R., Baker, D. W., & Williams, M. V. (1996). Shame and health literacy: The unspoken connection. *Patient Education and Counseling, 27*, 33–39.

Principles of adult learning & instructional systems design. Arlington, VA: National Highway Institute. Retrieved January 15, 2006, from http://www.nhi.fhwa.dot.gov/download/material/420018/RM/420018.pdf

Roter, D. L. (2005). How effective is your nonverbal communication? *Conversations in Care Web Book* (chapter 2). Retrieved December 2, 2005, from http://www.conversationsincare.com/web_book/chapter02.html

Rubin, R. (2003, April 30). Doctor-patient language gap isn't healthy. *USA Today*. Retrieved January 14, 2006, from http://www.usatoday.com/life/2003–04–30-medical-language_x.htm

Rudd, R. E. (2004). Navigating hospitals. *Literacy Harvest, 11*(1), 19–24. Retrieved January 30, 2006, from http://www.lacnyc.org/resources/publications/harvest/HarvestFall04.pdf#search='rima%20rudd%20navigation%20study%20hospital

Schatschneider, C., & Torgesen, J. K. (2004). Using our current understanding of dyslexia to support early identification and intervention. *Journal of Child Neurology, 19*(10), 759–765.

Schwartzberg, J. G., VanGeest, J. B., & Wang, C. C. (Eds.). (2005). *Understanding health literacy: Implications for medicine and public health.* Chicago: American Medical Association Press.

Sobero, R., & Giraldo, G. P. (2004, May). *Beyond translations: Culturally adapting and developing low-literacy materials.* Paper presented at Clinical and Educational Solutions to Low Health Literacy, Institute for Healthcare Advancement Third Annual Health Literacy Conference, Anaheim, CA.

The difference between the Internet and the World Wide Web. (2006). *Webopedia.* Retrieved March 10, 2006, from http://www.webopedia.com/DidYouKnow/Internet/2002/Web_vs_Internet.asp

Umefjord, G., Hamberg, K., Malker, H., & Petersson, G. (2006). The use of an Internet-based Ask the Doctor Service involving family physicians: Evaluation by a web survey. *Family Practice, 23*(2), 159–166.

Universal health symbols provide direction for many in hospitals [press release]. (2005, December 14). Fresno, CA: The Robert Wood Johnson Foundation. Retrieved January 20, 2006, from http://www.diversityconnection.org/userdocs/uploads/5_PRSign.pdf

U.S. Department of Education, Office of Vocational and Adult Education. (2004). *Adult Education and Family Literacy Act: Program year 2002–2003: Report to Congress on state performance.* Retrieved January 10, 2006, from http://www.ed.gov/about/reports/annual/ovae/2003adulted.pdf

Wallace, L. S., & Lennon, E. S. (2004). American Academy of Family Physicians patient education materials: Can patients read them? *Family Medicine, 36*(8), 571–574.

Walsh, A. L. (2004). Managing your practice's first impression: The process of front-desk reengineering. *Journal of Medical Practice Management, 19*(5), 264–271.

Weiss, B. D., & Coyne, C. (1997). Communicating with patients who cannot read. *New England Journal of Medicine, 337*(4), 272–274.

Wilson, F. L., Brown, D. L., & Stephens-Ferris, M. (2006). Can easy-to-read immunization information increase knowledge in urban low-income mothers? *Journal of Pediatric Nursing, 21*(1), 4–12.

Woodson, C. (2004, May). *Promoting health literacy via the patient-friendly office.* Paper presented at Culture, Language, and Clinical Issues: Operational Solutions to Low Health Literacy, Institute for Healthcare Advancement Third Annual Health Literacy Conference, Anaheim, CA.

Yahya, F. M. (2002–2004). Back translation. *Arabic Freelance: The translation office of Fuad M. Yahya.* Retrieved February 11, 2006, from http://www.arabicfreelance.com/back.html

3

ASSESSING PATIENTS' LITERACY LEVELS

Sometimes you just have to break down the barriers and get right to the root of the problem. This is not always easy to do; professional roles and all manner of barriers exist in the patient–provider relationship that can inhibit the way we communicate, keeping us from achieving the understanding we need to treat patients effectively.

Allan Hixon, MD, assistant professor of family medicine at the University of Connecticut School of Medicine, relates a story about a 38-year-old patient, Mrs. P., who stopped taking her asthma medicine and ended up in the emergency department several times. She also inexplicably had run out of her prescription inhalers and tablets. His line of questioning was not yielding any information, and his frustration was growing. In fact,

> The more specific my questions about her medications became, the more confusing her answers were.
>
> I realized we were not communicating well, so I stepped back and probed for stressors. "How are things at home? How is your husband, how is your job, how are your kids?" All were reportedly fine. Then I asked about her childhood. "Where did you grow up and attend school? How many years of school did you complete?" She told me 2 years. "Did you ever have trouble with reading?" She said she had never learned.
>
> "How do you know how to take your medicines?" She told me she could read numbers, so when she saw the numeral "2," for example, she would take two pills or perhaps take one pill two times a day. In addition, she said that sometimes her kids would read for her. Suddenly, we were beginning to understand each other.
>
> I was able to simplify her medications to one combination inhaler, and I took extra time to explain how to use it properly. She repeated the message to me and to the medical student, and we each got a hug from our patient as she left the examination room (Hixon, 2004, p. 2077).

Information is power, or so the saying goes. Understanding a situation provides one with an advantage. In health care, the advantage in understanding patients' health literacy levels, and tailoring communication and education to that level, can strengthen the patient–provider relationship, as illustrated in the story about Dr. Hixon and Mrs. P.

When it comes to the issue of health literacy assessment, however, there is a very real struggle in health care between practicality and necessity: the practicality of applying some sort of literacy testing method for every patient versus the necessity of having this information. How do providers resolve this very real issue?

There is no easy answer. Patients in general expect any testing to be done by the health care provider. They also expect testing to produce results about the state of their body systems and to be used in their diagnosis. Literacy testing in the provider's office can have an unnatural feel to it, and many patients may be put off if the testing is not introduced properly, explained carefully, and conducted in a respectful manner.

After all, traditional tests, such as x-rays, blood tests, scans, and other diagnostic tests, directly benefit the patient. Results from such tests are used by the provider to rule out certain diagnoses, and they provide valuable information that moves the question "What's wrong with me?" closer to resolution. Medical and clinical tests are tools in an arsenal used by health care providers to help the patient.

Tests of patient literacy levels, however, may not be, at least in the mind of the patient, so directly beneficial to them. The patient may be thinking, "How well I read is not at issue here; your concern should be the pain I'm feeling in my stomach." And, in some ways, this is an unassailable assumption. It is the responsibility of the provider to diagnose, communicate, and treat. Although the patient–provider relationship is just that—a relationship—providers must understand the basic premise brought to the patient–provider encounter: that the locus of expertise resides with the practitioner, not the patient, and the patient needn't prove his or her abilities in an encounter in which the practitioner is expected to "perform." Expecting the patient to submit to a literacy test may fall outside the patient's expectations or comfort zone, raise suspicions unnecessarily, and be disorienting to the patient.

The flip side of the health literacy assessment coin is the provision of appropriately written patient education materials. Once we know that the patient can only read at a sixth-grade level, are we providing him or her with materials that reflect this fact? More information on designing patient materials appears in chapter 7, Designing Easy-to-Read Patient Education Materials, but knowing that patients need special attention in this regard begins with an understanding of their literacy level.

Patient communication and education fall along a continuum. At one end is the first contact with the health care provider—whether it's a regularly scheduled appointment, a call with a complaint, or a walk-in or referral from another provider. After this initial contact, patient–provider communication and education continue until a specific moment is reached (e.g., the complaint has been resolved successfully) or indefinitely, in the case of effective management of chronic conditions, such as diabetes, asthma, or high blood pressure.

WHY TEST FOR LITERACY LEVELS?

Successful management of any illness, injury, or disease depends on the ability of the provider to understand what is happening with the patient, the provider's ability to define an effective treatment regimen, and the patient's ability to understand, consent to, and successfully follow that regimen. A breakdown at any juncture in this delicate process can mean failure for an otherwise successful treatment trajectory.

The health care provider is trained—and paid, of course—to identify and manage the disease process, illness, or injury of the patient. Such factors as the patient's inability to understand the treatment regimen, inability to read instructions, lack of motivation, or fear of pain or discomfort are not issues that determine the ability of the health care provider to carry out his or her role.

However, these issues can affect the patient's ability to effectively carry out his or her role in the patient–provider relationship. The successful treatment regimen is only as strong as the weakest link in the relationship. And if patients' literacy skills prevent them from carrying out any of their responsibilities, the likelihood of a successful treatment regimen is diminished greatly.

We know that there is a direct correlation between poor reading skills and poor health (Berkman et al., 2004; Rudd, 2002). So it falls to the health care community to recognize those patients who are at higher risk for health problems because of their lack of reading skills. If by testing patients' reading levels and providing them with materials that are appropriately matched to their reading skills we can save time, money, and perhaps even lives, why wouldn't we?

Answers to this question will vary. But some of the most common objections to the idea of testing patients to determine their reading level include concerns about time and the accuracy of the tests. Some tests can be time consuming, and in an already busy environment, instituting another step in the health care delivery process might seem unrealistic. In addition, scores on tests of literacy may be affected by the patients' mood, their physical or mental condition at the time of the test, or their nervousness simply because it is a test. Furthermore, most health care workers are not trained to assess patients' reading levels, and most assessment tools do not test comprehension. It is also true that asking adults about reading ability can embarrass and alienate them (Mayer, 2003), as mentioned in chapter 2. Dr. Rima Rudd asks that we

> consider how humiliating [a literacy assessment] test might be for someone with low literacy who comes in to see their doctor, especially if [they're] already not feeling well. Most people with low literacy are very embarrassed about it. They don't admit it even to their husbands and wives. Also, they don't always know that they have limited literacy skills. They arrange their lives so that they read what they can (*Law of averages*, 2001).

Similarly, the editors of the Institute of Medicine's *Health Literacy: A Prescription to End Confusion* (2004) emphasize the following:

> Health-care encounters rely on a dialogue between patient and provider that allow[s] the provider to understand symptoms, follow the course of an illness or disease as experienced by the patient, and provide diagnosis and treatment options. Patients are expected to tell their stories, describe their experiences, provide explanations, and obtain help with needed action. Given the importance of speech and speech

comprehension skills to health literacy, the current measures of health literacy that are modeled on previous functional literacy assessment tools do not tap the full scope of health literacy (IOM, 2004, p. 50).

But despite these and similar concerns, the benefits of knowing what your patients need from written materials—and deriving that information from the various assessment tools that are available—outweigh the objections. If you know what your patients need in terms of language, vocabulary, and explanation, you can give it to them. Without that knowledge, you are taking a shot in the dark when you create or distribute written materials.

It is vital that health care providers understand the facts about low health literacy. Toward this end, Doak, Doak, and Root (1996, p. 6) point out a number of misconceptions that health care practitioners may have about those with low literacy skills:

- *Illiterates are dumb and learn slowly, if at all.* False: Illiteracy is more a function of economic status and access to education. Intelligence levels in this population are about average, and many with low literacy skills show exceptional capacity to compensate for their inability to read.
- *Most illiterates are poor, immigrants, or minorities.* False: Although there are correlations between economic status and literacy levels, and more minorities and immigrants, percentage wise, have reading difficulties, the composite profile of the low-literate individual in the United States is that of a White, native-born American.
- *People will tell you if they can't read.* False: Shame is a strong factor in hiding one's literacy status, particularly in the patient–provider relationship. Parikh, Parker, Nurss, Baker, and Williams (1996) discovered in their study of 202 primarily indigent African American patients that two-thirds never admitted their illiteracy to their spouses, and more than half never told their children.
- *Years of schooling is a good measure of literacy levels.* False: One in five people tested in the 1993 National Adult Literacy Survey had a high-school diploma.

DISCLOSURE: THE PATIENT'S PERSPECTIVE

Those with low health literacy skills face a conflict in the health care setting about whether to disclose their low literacy, as we saw in the example of Mr. Martinez in chapter 2. On the one hand, there is a strong inclination to revert to old, ingrained habits (i.e., continuing to hide their illiteracy). On the other hand, there are compelling reasons (e.g., fear of making an uninformed decision, providing incomplete or incorrect information on a form that could adversely affect their health) to make the disclosure.

Concerns of Low-Health-Literate Patients

When in doubt, talk to patients. In a qualitative study of 200 adults enrolled in a community college literacy program, Brez and Taylor (1997) asked adults with low literacy skills how they felt about attempts to assess their literacy levels in a hospital setting. Results from the study showed some common themes.

Risk of Exposure

In most instances, adults with low literacy skills have worked long and hard to hide their illiteracy, usually under stressful circumstances. The risk of exposure—and the resultant or perceived scorn—leads them to develop sophisticated or at least ingrained responses to situations that require them to exhibit literacy skills. Most adults in this situation live in fear of being discovered, as one patient's confession makes clear: "I don't tell anybody or say anything to anybody [about my illiteracy], they might think I'm a bad person" (Brez & Taylor, 1997).

The researchers also cite such common concerns among illiterate adults as feeling embarrassed or appearing stupid. Such patients fear that others will question their role as a competent parent or family provider if their secret is revealed.

Risks of Nondisclosure During Hospitalization

The perceived risks of not telling health care professionals about their low literacy skills during hospitalization induce a stressful quandary and a state of dynamic tension for these adults. The tendency to engage in old habits of avoiding situations that called on their literacy skills, or even lying about their abilities, was offset by the concern that their subterfuge would cause them harm or injury at some point (Brez & Taylor, 1997).

It is particularly painful and poignant when the victim of a literacy dodge is one's own child. One interviewee discussed her internal pain over having given uninformed consent for a surgery for her child in order to avoid having her secret discovered:

> [Illiteracy is] what put me in trouble for my daughter. . . . I feel guilty about it. I have to look at her face and I say, why did I go through with that operation? If I had known what was going to happen. . . . I didn't know what kind of risk was involved (Brez & Taylor, 1997, p. 1043).

Understanding the Hospital as a "Special Place"

There was general agreement among interviewees that the hospital was a place where they felt safe and most willing to divulge their secret. They perceived health care workers and care providers as "knowledgeable and confident; approachable and friendly; understanding and compassionate; and most importantly, trustworthy and respectful of patient confidentiality" (Brez & Taylor, 1997, p. 1043).

The researchers encourage health care providers to take advantage of this bond of trust—while maintaining and upholding the reasons for that trust—by broaching the subject in a gentle and understanding manner. The trust accorded to health care providers helps moderate the fear of disclosure, providing an atmosphere conducive to disclosure and encouraging subsequent assistance with necessary processes. And patients who consult providers they trust report higher levels of satisfaction (Baker, Mainous, Gray, & Love, 2003).

Support for Screening

There is evidence to suggest that patients with low literacy skills may be willing to confide in their health care providers and share their difficulties with reading and understanding. However, the health care provider, not the patient, needs to initiate the first step in this process. In addition, although the study participants stated that they would be amenable to such an approach, emotional reactions to participating in a REALM (Rapid Estimate of Adult Literacy in Medicine) test correlated with how well they did on the test (Brez & Taylor, 1997). One participant who scored much higher than she thought she would was pleased by the experience, whereas another who did not do well was "frightened" (Brez & Taylor, 1997, p. 1044).

Researchers suggest that health care providers be aware of the potential effects that testing can have on patients and ensure that anyone doing formal testing be thoroughly trained in the test's administration. Testing should be done in a private and supportive environment. Those administering the tests should ensure that patients understand that the results are confidential and will be used only to modify information provided to them. Also, researchers and providers should consider the cost of the exam and whether it is appropriate for the target population's age, primary language, and visual acuity (Davis, Kennen, Gazmararian, & Williams, 2005).

Acknowledging differences in literacy levels and determining the related needs of individual patients needn't be accomplished through formal literacy testing, however. In fact, the potential for embarrassing patients must be weighed carefully against the information such testing provides. In many cases—perhaps even in most cases—carefully observing patient behavior can yield all the information you need to successfully match patients with appropriate materials. But you need to know what to look for. Here are some patient behaviors that can indicate lower reading levels:

- Makes excuses for not reading forms or materials (e.g., "I left my glasses at home.")
- Nods "yes" to health care provider's questions
- Asks to take forms home to read
- Doesn't accept, read, or even glance at written materials that are offered
- Fills out forms incompletely or incorrectly
- Brings along family members and passes written materials to them or defers to them on questions involving literacy tasks or skills
- Asks for assistance with filling out forms or other simple tasks
- Demonstrates unexplained agitation, anger, or indifference when presented with forms
- Focuses attention on something other than the materials when the health care provider refers to the form

Another indicator that many providers may miss as a cue for low literacy in their patients is encountered during a review of the patient's medications, according to Davis and colleagues (2005). If patients identify certain medications by opening the prescription bottle and looking at the medication instead of reading the label on the bottle, that could be an indicator of low literacy skills. Similarly, patients who are confused about the way medications are taken or cannot understand why they are taking a certain medication also may be at risk for low literacy skills (Davis et al., 2005; Weiss, 2003).

There are other, less formal ways of determining whether a patient has literacy challenges. One way is to give the patient a brochure for review and then ask questions or request that he or she demonstrate a technique described in the brochure. It's better to ask open-ended questions about consent forms or other materials patients have filled out. That is, instead of questions like "Did you understand everything on the form?" ask open-ended questions such as "Can you describe to me, in your own words, what will happen during this procedure?"

Another method is the direct approach: ask the patient how much schooling he or she has had. Although it has been noted that years of schooling is not an automatic indicator of one's reading ability (Davis et al., 2005; Kirsch, Jungeblut, Jenkins, & Kolstad, 1993), if the patient indicates that the highest grade level completed was the fifth or sixth grade, this answer provides more direct evidence of a lower literacy level or at least an opening for asking further questions about the patient's reading ability.

Certain groups are more likely to have low literacy skills than others; this information can be used by the health care provider to indicate groups to whom the provider should pay attention when looking for signs of low literacy. Results from the 2003 National Assessment of Adult Literacy (NAAL) showed that 55% of adults who scored in the below basic category of the prose literacy section did not graduate from high school, 44% did not speak English before starting school, 39% were Hispanic, 26% were aged 65 years or older, and 20% were African American (National Center for Educational Statistics, 2005).

Any time that a patient sends a direct or indirect cue or signal that he or she has literacy challenges, providers should strive to keep the atmosphere of the encounter caring, comforting, and understanding. Reassure the patient that confidentiality on the issue will be maintained, if that is the patient's desire. However, it's a good idea to exclude other health care providers and educators in the office from that confidentiality. Explain this need to the patient by providing reasons for the exclusion, including the need for others to know so that they can adequately convey health education materials to the patient in the future. As discussed in chapter 2, referral to literacy programs may be an excellent strategy in these instances. If enrolling the patient in a literacy program is a consideration, ensure that the program has been researched and found acceptable ahead of time.

Because of the issue of shame discussed earlier, the moment when the patient's literacy levels are first discussed is an important one. It represents an opportunity for the health care provider to strengthen the bond of trust with the patient. If the provider demonstrates sensitivity and acceptance and does not appear judgmental, the moment can be a positive experience.

For this reason, it is important for clinicians to be aware of their verbal and nonverbal communication at this point. Negative body language, expressed by crossed arms, looking away, and shaking the head, may add to the patient's shame, fear, and perception that he or she is being looked down on. However, positive body language, such as good eye contact, a comforting touch on the arm or shoulder (if appropriate), a slight turn of the head to indicate attention and listening, and other gestures, can help reinforce the perception of a safe and accepting environment.

INSTRUMENTS FOR ASSESSING LITERACY

Although you cannot assume the reading levels of patients, being aware of behaviors that raise a red flag regarding reading ability can help you be more sensitive to possible patients' needs. Such increased sensitivity toward patients and their needs may be all that is necessary for you to provide patients with appropriate written materials. But for cases in which more specific measurements of a patient's literacy are deemed necessary, a number of tests are available. Some of these tests assess reading levels and others assess comprehension.

Reading Tests

WRAT-R3 (Wide Range Achievement Test-Revised 3)

This test is designed to "measure the codes which are needed to learn the basic skills of reading, spelling, and arithmetic." It takes approximately 15 to 30 minutes to administer for each of the three forms. The test comprises three subtests: reading (recognizing and naming letters and words out of context), spelling (writing letters and words from spoken prompts and writing one's own name), and arithmetic (counting, reading number symbols, and solving oral problems and written computations; Wilkinson, 1993).

General uses for this test include comparing the abilities of one person to another, determining learning ability or disability, comparing codes with comprehension in order to provide remedial programs, and informally assessing error patterns in order to plan instructional programs. The test is available online at www3.parinc.com/products/product.aspx?Productid= WRAT3. The cost is $38 for a package of 25 test forms (blue or tan versions).

REALM (Rapid Estimate of Adult Literacy in Medicine)

Designed to broadly assess adults' literacy in the area of medicine, the REALM tests word recognition and correct pronunciation, not comprehension (Figure 3.1). The REALM is a list of 66 medical terms (revised from its original 125-word set) arranged in order of complexity by number of syllables and difficulty of pronunciation. (A shortened version of the test, the REALM-R, uses only eight terms.) To take the test, patients read all of the terms they can. Correct

RAPID ESTIMATE OF ADULT LITERACY IN MEDICINE (REALM)

Terry Davis, PhD, Michael Crouch, MD, Sandy Long, PhD

Chart #   Examine date:

Name: Birth date:

REALM generated reading level: Grade completed:

List 1		List 2		List 3	
Fat		Fatigue		Allergic	
Flu		Pelvic		Menstrual	
Pill		Jaundice		Testicle	
Dose		Infection		Colitis	
Eye		Exercise		Emergency	
Stress		Behavior		Medication	
Smear		Prescription		Occupation	
Nerves		Notify		Sexually	
Germs		Gallbladder		Alcoholism	
Meals		Calories		Irritation	
Disease		Depression		Constipation	
Cancer		Miscarriage		Gonorrhea	
Caffeine		Pregnancy		Inflammatory	
Attack		Arthritis		Diabetes	
Kidney		Nutrition		Hepatitis	
Hormones		Menopause		Antibiotics	
Herpes		Appendix		Diagnosis	
Seizure		Abnormal		Potassium	
Bowel		Syphilis		Anemia	
Asthma		Hemorrhoids		Obesity	
Rectal		Nausea		Osteoporosis	
Incest		Directed		Impetigo	
# of (+) Responses in List 1:		# of (+) Responses in List 2:		# of (+) Responses in List 3:	

LEGEND: (+)=Correct   (-)=Word not attempted   (/)=Mispronounced word   **Raw Score:**

Red Lake Hospital, Red Lake MN 56671
4/98/JMcD

FIGURE 3.1 Excerpt from the REALM (Rapid Estimate of Adult Literacy in Medicine). *Source:* Davis, T. C., Long, S. W., Jackson, R. H., et al. (1993). Rapid Estimate of Adult Literacy in Medicine: A shortened screening instrument. *Family Medicine, 25,* 391–395.

pronunciation of the terms is noted and tabulated (Davis et al., 1993). This test is quick and easy to administer, taking only 2 to 3 minutes by personnel with minimal training. Samples of the REALM are available online at various sites. Contact the author, Terry C. Davis, PhD, to order the test: tdavis1@lsuhsc.edu. Cost is $65.

LAD (Literacy Assessment for Diabetes)

This is a word recognition test composed of three graded word lists in ascending difficulty. It is specific to diabetes and measures patients' ability to pronounce terms they might encounter during clinical visits and in self-care instructions. Administering this test takes minimal time: about 3 minutes. It is a reliable and valid tool for measuring literacy in adults with diabetes. A patient's raw score is scaled to reading grade level (Nath, Sylvester, Yasek, & Gundel, 2001). The test correlates well with the REALM and the WRAT-R3. No information about purchasing this test was found online. The home page for the journal, *The Diabetes Educator,* published by Sage Publications, is http://tde.sagepub. com.

MART (Medical Terminology Achievement Reading Test)

This test is designed to resemble a prescription label with its use of small print size, glossy cover, and medical terminology. Incorporating these elements into the test allows practitioners and researchers to assess patients' ability, or lack of ability, to read the text. Its basic design uses the WRAT as a model.

Unlike the REALM, the MART provides an exact grade level from the converted score, rather than a grade range. The unique design of MART appears to make it less threatening to patients than other literacy tests (Hanson-Divers, 1997). No information was found online for purchasing this test. However, you can visit the Web site of the *Journal of Health Care for the Poor and Underserved,* publishers of the original article, at http://www.press.jhu.edu/journals/ journal_of_health_care_for_the_poor_and_underserved/.

SORT-R3 (Slosson Oral Reading Test-Revised 3)

This test is designed to provide a "quick estimate to target word recognition levels for children and adults." It is a relatively short test to administer, taking only about 5 to 10 minutes, and requires minimal training to administer. The test presents 200 words in ascending order of difficulty. They are grouped into 20-word sets that approximate grade reading levels. The primary use of SORT-R3 is as a screening instrument, but it also can be used to assess a reader's progress, determine an individual's grade level in reading, or determine whether a person needs further diagnostic assessment (Slosson, 1990). Ordering and other information is available from Slosson Educational Publications, Inc., at http://www.slosson.com. The cost is $68 plus shipping and handling fees.

Comprehension Tests

TOFHLA (Test of Functional Health Literacy in Adults)

This test focuses specifically on health literacy, using actual materials patients might encounter as they navigate the health care system (Figure 3.2). It is composed of a reading comprehension section and a numeracy section. The former uses the modified Cloze procedure (eliminating every nth word; e.g., every fifth word, every eighth word) to measure a patient's ability to read and understand prose passages. The latter is a 17-item test using actual hospital forms and labeled prescription vials to test patients' ability to comprehend directions for taking medications, monitoring blood glucose, keeping clinic appointments, and obtaining financial assistance (Parker, Baker, Williams, & Nurss, 1995).

One of the primary strengths of the TOFHLA over other tests is its availability in a Spanish version. The test is available from Peppercorn Books & Press, Inc., at http://www.peppercornbooks.com/catalog. The cost is $60.

PIAT-R (Peabody Individual Achievement Test–Revised)

This instrument, updated in 1998 and called the PIAT-R/NU (Normative Update), is designed to yield a survey of an individual's scholastic attainment. It is an untimed, individually administered, norm-referenced measure of academic achievement. The multiple-choice test was designed to provide wide-range screening in six content areas (Markwardt, 1989). It can be used with individuals in kindergarten through the 12th grade and is available from AGS Publishing, Inc., at http://www.agsnet.com. Costs vary.

Cloze

This test measures an individual's comprehension. Designed by Richard E. Mayer at the University of California, Santa Barbara, the test presents a short text with blanks where some of the words should be. There are typically 20 to 25 blanks in the passage, with every nth word left blank (Mayer, Schustack, & Blanton, 1999). Among the strengths of a Cloze-type test is ease of administration; the person taking the test is simply asked to fill in the blanks.

NVS (Newest Vital Sign)

A new test for literacy developed by Weiss and colleagues (2005) called the Newest Vital Sign, or NVS, uses the nutrition label from the back of a carton of ice cream as the testing vehicle. One of the strengths of the NVS is that it tests both the ability to read and understand text, as well as numbers (numeracy).

Patients are given a paper copy of the nutrition label and asked six questions, four of which require calculations (Figure 3.3). For instance, one question asks, "If you eat the entire container, how many calories will you eat?" To answer the question correctly, respondents must refer to the label, note that there are four servings in the entire container, that each serving contains 250 calories,

PASSAGE A

Your doctor has sent you to have a _____ X-ray.

    a. stomach
    b. diabetes
    c. stitches
    d. germs

You must have an _____ stomach when you come for _____.

    a. asthma   a. is.
    b. empty   b. am.
    c. incest   c. if.
    d. anemia   d. it.

The X-ray will _____ from 1 to 3 _____ to do.

    a. take   a. beds
    b. view   b. brains
    c. talk   c. hours
    d. look   d. diets

THE DAY BEFORE THE X-RAY.

For supper have only a _____ snack of fruit, _____ and jelly,

    a. little   a. toes
    b. broth   b. throat
    c. attack   c. toast
    d. nausea   d. thigh

with coffee or tea.

TOFHLA   **Standard Print Version, English 12 point font**   9

FIGURE 3.2 Excerpt from the TOFHLA (Test of Functional Health Literacy in Adults). *Source:* Parker, R., Baker, D., Williams, M., & Nurss, J. (1995). The Test of Functional Health Literacy in Adults (TOFHLA): A new instrument for measuring patients' literacy skills. *Journal of General and Internal Medicine, 10*, 537–545.

and then understand that they must multiply 250 x 4 to come up with the only correct response, 1,000 calories. (Two other questions do not deal specifically with numeracy skills.)

This process combines the numeracy skills of multiplication with the contextual skills of finding the appropriate pieces of information on the label.

	ANSWER CORRECT?	
	YES	NO
READ TO SUBJECT: This information is on the back of a container of a pint of ice cream.		
QUESTIONS		
1. If you eat the entire container, how many calories will you eat?		
Answer ❑ 1,000 is the only correct answer	_____	_____
2. If you are allowed to eat 60 g of carbohydrates as a snack, how much ice cream could you have?		
Answer Any of the following is correct:	_____	_____
❑ 1 cup (or any amount up to 1 cup)		
❑ Half the container		
Note: If patient answers "2 servings," ask "How much ice cream would that be if you were to measure it into a bowl?"		
3. Your doctor advises you to reduce the amount of saturated fat in your diet. You usually have 42 g of saturated fat each day, which includes 1 serving of ice cream. If you stop eating ice cream, how many grams of saturated fat would you be consuming each day?		
Answer 33 is the only correct answer	_____	_____
4. If you usually eat 2500 calories in a day, what percentage of your daily value of calories will you be eating if you eat one serving?		
Answer 10% is the only correct answer	_____	_____
Pretend that you are allergic to the following substances: Penicillin, peanuts, latex gloves, and bee stings.		
5. Is it safe for you to eat this ice cream?		
Answer ❑ No	_____	_____
6. (Ask only if the patient responds "no" to question 5): Why not?		
Answer Because it has peanut oil.	_____	_____
Total Correct	_____	

FIGURE 3.3 Questions and answers score sheet from the NVS (Newest Vital Sign). *Source:* Weiss, B. D., Mays, M. Z., Martz, W., et al. (2005). Quick assessment of literacy in primary care: The Newest Vital Sign. *Annals of Family Medicine, 3,* 514–522.

Respondents also must understand the relationship between servings per container and the caloric value per serving and know that the answer involves one specific equation: number of servings times calories per serving.

The NVS has several advantages over other tests for literacy. For example, like the TOFHLA, it is available in a Spanish-language as well as an English-language version. For many health care practices, this availability is invaluable, especially if a majority of patients are Spanish-language speakers. Although such patients may have limited abilities to understand English, they may have competence in their native language and do not need special consideration if patient–provider communication is conducted in Spanish.

The NVS's short list of questions, the fact that it is paired with a visual with which most consumers are familiar (or at least for which they have visual recognition), and its short administration time—about 3 minutes—make it ideal for providing a quick take on the patient's literacy skills. Weiss and colleagues acknowledge that the NVS's specificity is "less than optimal," but they note that, if anything, the test may *overestimate* the percentage of patients with limited

Nutrition Facts	
Serving Size	1/2 cup
Servings per container	4

Amount per serving	
Calories 250	Fat Cal 120

	%DV
Total Fat 13g	20%
Sat Fat 9g	40%
Cholesterol 28mg	12%
Sodium 55mg	2%
Total Carbohydrate 30g	12%
Dietary Fiber 2g	
Sugars 23g	
Protein 4g	8%

* Percent Daily Values (DV) are based on a 2,000 calorie diet. Your daily values may be higher or lower depending on your calorie needs.

Ingredients: Cream, Skim Milk, Liquid Sugar, Water, Egg Yolks, Brown Sugar, Milkfat, Peanut Oil, Sugar, Butter, Salt, Carrageenan, Vanilla Extract.

Note; This single scenario is the final English version of the newest vital sign. The type size should be 14-point (as shown above) or larger. Patients are presented with the above scenario and asked the questions shown in Figure 3.3.

FIGURE 3.4 Nutrition label from the NVS (Newest Vital Sign). *Source:* Weiss, B. D., Mays, M. Z., Martz, W., et al. (2005). Quick assessment of literacy in primary care: The Newest Vital Sign. *Annals of Family Medicine, 3,* 514–522.

literacy skills, thereby erring on the side of *underestimating* their literacy skills (Weiss et al., 2005).

Another advantage of a test like the NVS is less obvious. Because nutrition labels play such an important part in our daily wellness activities, most consumers are expected to be able to read and understand them. The fears of taking a specific literacy test may be allayed by questions on the use of such an innocuous item as an ice cream nutrition label (Figure 3.4). Because the test is quick, focused on the patient's comprehension of an everyday item he or she is likely to encounter, and not framed in a more traditional, formal testing context and environment, the test itself may not trigger the same fears evoked by taking a more formal test.

If a test like the NVS can alleviate patients' anxiety without making them feel shame about their lack of literacy skills—offering the health care provider a vital piece of information at the same time—then several major hurdles standing in the way of literacy screening have been overcome.

ENDNOTE: AN ESSENTIAL BALANCING ACT

In the end, perhaps the goal of literacy testing should not be to precisely quantify the literacy level of every patient, as might be achieved when taking a history or measuring blood pressure, height, or weight. A short test or series of logical, research-based assumptions that alert health care providers to potential problems with basic literacy or numeracy skills among their at-risk patients may be enough to change the way they communicate information. Once alerted to their patients' literacy problems, providers can change the techniques they use in patient education and reconsider whatever follow-up strategies they use to ensure that patients appropriately follow treatment regimens.

Testing is a tool, a means to understand more about the patient. But it is also a potential way to identify an issue that causes patients shame and embarrassment. It is imperative that health care providers understand the stigma of illiteracy, as well as the effects it can have on patients' ability to understand their health care status and to participate fully in their own treatment. When health care providers achieve a balance between these two issues—understanding more about the patient and understanding more about the stigma of low health literacy—patient–provider trust can be strengthened; the provider's ability to communicate health-related information in a clear, understandable manner can be increased; and the chances that a prescribed treatment regimen will succeed can be improved dramatically.

REFERENCES

Baker, R., Mainous, A. G., Gray, D. P., & Love, M. M. (2003). Exploration of the relationship between continuity, trust in regular doctors and patient satisfaction with consultations with family doctors. *Scandinavian Journal of Primary Health Care, 21*(1), 27–32.

Berkman, N. D., DeWalt, D. A., Pignone, M. P., Sheridan, S. L., Lohr, K. N., Lux, L., et al. (2004, January). *Literacy and health outcomes* (Evidence Report/Technology Assessment No. 87. AHRQ Publications No. 04-E007-2). Rockville, MD: Agency for Healthcare Research and Quality.

Brez, S. M., & Taylor, M. (1997). Assessing literacy for patient teaching: Perspectives of adults with low literacy skills. *Journal of Advanced Nursing, 25,* 1040–1047.

Davis, T., Kennen, E. M., Gazmararian, J. A., & Williams, M. V. (2005). Literacy testing in health care research. In J. G. Schwartzberg, J. B. VanGeest, & C. C. Wang (Eds.), *Understanding health literacy: Implications for medicine and public health* (pp. 157–179). Chicago: American Medical Association Press.

Davis, T. C., Long, S. W., Jackson, R. H., Mayeaux, E. J., George, R. B., Murphy, P. W., et al. (1993). Rapid estimate of adult literacy in medicine: A shortened screening instrument. *Family Medicine, 25,* 391–395.

Doak, C. C., Doak, L. G., & Root, J. H. (1996). *Teaching patients with low literacy skills* (2nd ed.). Philadelphia: J.B. Lippincott.

Hanson-Divers, E. C. (1997). Developing a medical achievement reading test to evaluate patient literacy skills: A preliminary study. *Journal of Health Care for the Poor and Underserved, 8,* 56–59.

Hixon, A. L. (2004). Functional health literacy: Improving health outcomes. *American Family Physician, 69*(9), 2077–2078.

Institute of Medicine (IOM) of the National Academies. (2004). *Health literacy: A prescription to end confusion.* Washington, DC: National Academies Press.

Kirsch, I., Jungeblut, A., Jenkins, L., & Kolstad, A. (1993). *Adult literacy in America: A first look at the findings of the National Adult Literacy Survey.* Washington, DC: National Center for Education Statistics, U.S. Department of Education.

Law of averages: Casting a wide net in health literacy efforts with Rima Rudd, ScD. 2001. (2003, March). In *Facts of life: Issue briefings for health reporters.* Retrieved September 12, 2005, from http://www.cfah.org/factsoflife/vol8no3.cfm

Markwardt, F. S. (1989). *Peabody Individual Achievement Test–Revised.* Circle Pines, MN: American Guidance Service.

Mayer, G. G. (2003, May). *Writing easy to read, easy to use health information.* Paper presented at Organizational Solutions to Low Health Literacy, Institute for Healthcare Advancement Second Annual Health Literacy Conference, Anaheim, CA.

Mayer, R. E., Schustack, M., & Blanton, W. (1999). What do children learn from using computers in an informal collaborative environment? *Educational Technology, 39,* 215–227.

Nath, C. R., Sylvester, S. T., Yasek, V., & Gundel, E. (2001). Development and validation of a literacy assessment tool for persons with diabetes. *The Diabetes Educator, 27,* 857–864.

National Center for Education Statistics (NCES). (2005). *A first look at the literacy of America's adults in the 21st century* (NCES 2006-470). Retrieved December 16, 2005, from http://nces.ed.gov/NAAL/PDF/2006470.PDF

Parikh, N. S., Parker, R. M., Nurss, J. R., Baker, D. W., & Williams, M. V. (1996). Shame and health literacy: The unspoken connection. *Patient Education and Counseling, 27,* 33–39.

Parker, R., Baker, D., Williams, M., & Nurss, J. (1995). The test of functional health literacy in adults (TOFHLA): A new instrument for measuring patients' literacy skills. *Journal of General Internal Medicine, 10,* 537–545.

Rudd, R. E. (2002). *Health literacy overview presentation.* Retrieved August 27, 2005, from the Harvard School of Public Health, Health Literacy Studies Web site: http://www.hsph.harvard.edu/healthliteracy

Slosson, R. J. L. (1990). *Slosson Oral Reading Tests—Revised 3.* East Aurora, NY: Slosson Educational Publishers.

Weiss, B. D. (2003). *Health literacy: A manual for clinicians.* Chicago: American Medical Association Foundation and American Medical Association.

Weiss, B. D., Mays, M. Z., Martz, W., Castro, K. M., DeWalt, D. A., Pignone, M. P., et al. (2005). Quick assessment of literacy in primary care: The newest vital sign. *Annals of Family Medicine, 3,* 514–522.

Wilkinson, G. S. (1993). *Wide Range Achievement Test—Revised 3.* Wilmington, DE: Jastak Associates.

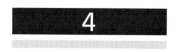

UNDERSTANDING AND AVOIDING
MEDICAL ERRORS

The status quo is not acceptable and cannot be tolerated any longer. Despite the cost pressures, liability constraints, resistance to change and other seemingly insurmountable barriers, it is simply not acceptable for patients to be harmed by the same health care system that is supposed to offer healing and comfort.
—Institute of Medicine
To Err Is Human: Building a Safer Health System (2000, p. 3)

When psychotherapist Carl Rogers, founder of the humanistic psychology movement, first began promoting his innovative ideas about how people could improve the way they communicate interpersonally—a technique he sometimes called "listening with understanding"—the Cold War was in full swing. In 1951, in a speech at Northwestern University, Rogers highlighted the potential benefits of his client-centered therapeutic approach by asking his audience to imagine that a "therapeutically oriented international group" had gone to the leaders of the Soviet Union and told them,

> We want to achieve a genuine understanding of your views and even more important, of your attitudes and feelings, toward the United States. We will summarize and resummarize these views and feelings if necessary, until you agree that our description represents the situation as it seems to you (Rogers, 1961, p. 335).

Indeed, summarizing and resummarizing while actively listening were cornerstones of Rogers's approach. "Then," he continued,

> suppose they did the same thing with the leaders in our own country. If they then gave the widest possible distribution to these views, with feelings clearly described but not expressed in name-calling, might not the effect be very great? It would not guarantee . . . understanding . . . but it would make it much more possible (Rogers, 1961, p. 335).

At the time, this thinking was considered seriously subversive. After all, weren't the Russians the enemy, and weren't we the good guys? What more was there to understand? Many were skeptical, to say the least, that the Soviet Union could be trusted. Others, however, were more hopeful that diplomatic overtures could help reduce tensions between the superpowers. Rogers was an unabashed optimist, and his concept of "listening with understanding," which he believed applied equally well outside the context of psychotherapy, had like-minded people wondering about the possibilities of open, plain communication. What if world leaders sought to understand one another just for the sake of understanding, with nothing to gain but better communication and improved relations? How might the world be different?

Health care providers, charged as we are with safeguarding the well-being of our patients, might ask similarly grandiose questions about the work we do every day. How might true understanding between patients and providers be achieved? What problems could we avoid if we ensured that our patients truly understood their conditions and treatments and were armed with all the information they needed to maximize the healing process? What if we eliminated barriers to effective patient care, such as those that result from errors, miscommunication, and the like?

LISTENING AND UNDERSTANDING

Carl Rogers was a clinical psychologist and a therapist—not a nurse, not a doctor, not a physician's assistant—yet we have much to learn from the penetrating questions he asked. For starters, note that his approach assumes that misunderstanding and miscommunication are basically the norm in human communication: a truism we may be tempted to forget in our high-tech world of e-mail and instant messaging. *The key to avoiding medical errors and for improving patient health outcomes, as we see in this chapter, is better communication, plain and simple.* It is not the only answer, of course, but without good communication, no other clinical safeguards stand much of a chance.

Rogers seemed to grasp that minor breakdowns in communication could lead to crises on a global scale, even to the loss of life. The solution, he firmly believed, was to create a situation "in which each of the different parties comes to understand the other from the *other's* point of view . . . [in order to] gradually [achieve] mutual communication" (1961, p. 336). We know intuitively that communication that isn't mutual really isn't communication at all. The health care provider who does not listen slows the healing process, sometimes stopping it cold, just as the patient who does not understand and does not seek clarification jeopardizes his or her health and wellness.

In this chapter we examine some of the ways plain language and clear health communication can improve patient outcomes, beginning with the problem of medical errors. Along the way we survey some cost pressures and liability constraints, as well as the resistance to change and seemingly insurmountable barriers bemoaned in the epigraph to this chapter. As the Institute of Medicine (IOM) insists, the status quo is no longer acceptable. Avoidable mistakes and obstacles to good patient care—particularly those facing patients with low health literacy—can be minimized. Sometimes the solutions do not come easily, and occasionally they create new problems of their own. Still, to quote the words of the late Strother Martin's character in *Cool Hand Luke* (1967), more often than not "what we have here is a failure to communicate."

Streamlining our systems to make them more computerized may or may not help improve communication. On the other hand, talking to our patients more and knowing more about them, using additional checks and balances, listening carefully to everyone along the entire continuum of care, making sure our patients' questions get answered—these and other approaches almost certainly can improve health care for all Americans, regardless of their literacy level.

Health care is not nuclear disarmament. It is not like international diplomacy or negotiating treaties. But its impact is no less significant, and the implications of its failure are no less profound for untold millions of people. Changing the way patients experience the health system—and changing it for the better—is not an insurmountable task. In fact, changes can come from *within* the system. We can change the way we talk, change the way we teach, even change the way we think. But first we must know what we're up against. That is the intention of this chapter.

Although some negative outcomes are not preventable, we needn't be satisfied with imagining a world in which communication between patients and providers does not break down; it's within our reach to realize such a goal. And reducing errors caused by misunderstandings, miscommunication, and a failure to target those with low health literacy is a good place to start.

MEDICAL ERRORS DEFINED

Various individuals and institutions have attempted to define error in medicine. In its report *To Err Is Human,* for example, the IOM defines error as "the failure of a planned action to be completed as intended or the use of a wrong plan to achieve an aim" (IOM, 2000). Pediatric surgeon and medical researcher Lucian Leape, MD, however, defines error as "an unintended act (either of omission or commission) or one that does not achieve its intended outcomes" (Leape, 1994). Neither definition points fingers or lays blame. The IOM's definition emphasizes failure on the planning end, whereas Leape focuses on the act's being unintended and suggests a failure in terms of outcomes. Both seem on the mark.

Of course, some believe that a satisfactory definition of medical error continues to elude us. In the view of Dovey and Phillips (2004), the terms and definitions we currently use to describe medical errors are "peculiar, unnatural, and un-useful." Be that as it may, for simplicity's sake we refer to the IOM's and Leape's definitions of medical error as touchstones throughout this chapter.

Errors, whether avoidable or unavoidable, cause harm to patients in every kind of health care setting. However, they can be especially devastating to those with low health literacy, who rely even more on the expertise and presumed infallibility of their very human health care providers. Low-health-literate patients are less likely to do their own research or to engage critically with health-related materials they receive. They put their trust in their health care providers, increasing the likelihood that mistakes will go unnoticed until real harm has been done. Those with low health literacy give their doctors and nurses the benefit of the doubt, even if a course of treatment or drug regimen doesn't feel right to them.

THE SCOPE OF THE PROBLEM

How widespread is error in medicine? To properly understand the statistics, it's important to distinguish between *medical error* and *medication error*. Medical errors can take place at any stage in the process of care, from diagnosis to treatment to preventive care (IOM, 2000). Errors that result in injury might be called "preventable adverse events," with an *adverse event* defined as "an injury resulting from a medical intervention . . . [where the event is] not due to the underlying condition of the patient" (IOM, 2000, pp. 3–4). Medical error in general may or may not involve medications, so medication error is a subset of medical error.

According to two large studies, one conducted in Colorado and Utah and one in New York, general medical error accounts for roughly 44,000 to 98,000 deaths per year in the United States (Brennan et al., 1991; Thomas et al., 2000). In fact, Donald M. Berwick, MD, president of the Institute for Healthcare Improvement, notes that these figures, large as they are, may even underestimate the true number of medical errors because they exclude "other areas of care like home care, nursing homes and ambulatory care centers" (O'Connor, 1999).

These data are based on research suggesting that adverse events occur in anywhere from 2.9% (in the Colorado and Utah study) to 3.7% (in the New York study) of hospitalizations. In the Colorado and Utah study, 8.8% of the adverse events led to death; in New York, 13.6% did. In both studies, more than half of adverse events resulted from medical errors that could have been prevented (IOM, 2000).

It's true that these figures represent a relatively small percentage overall. In terms of errors, the average hospital is probably running at an accuracy rate of 99%. That's remarkable. Nevertheless, as Leape notes, even a 99.9% accuracy rate still translates into the equivalent of two unsafe landings at Chicago's O'Hare Airport every day, plus 16,000 pieces of lost mail and 32,000 bank checks deducted from the wrong account every hour (Leape, 1994). We can certainly do better.

MEDICATION ERRORS

Most medical errors, in fact, involve medications; that is, they are mistakes having to do with specific drugs or prescribed treatments, committed either by the health care provider or the patient. These are called *medication* errors. The

National Coordinating Council for Medication Error Reporting and Prevention defines a medication error as

> any preventable event that may cause or lead to inappropriate medication use or patient harm while the medication is in the control of the health care professional, patient, or consumer. Such events may be related to professional practice, health care products, procedures, and systems, including prescribing; order communication; product labeling, packaging, and nomenclature; compounding; dispensing; distribution; administration; education; monitoring; and use (National Coordinating Council, 2002).

By this definition, medication errors are preventable and can occur while the medication is in control of anyone along the health care continuum, from the prescribing physician to the end user. Products, procedures, labels, packaging, gaps in patient education—all conceivably can play a role in bringing about a medication error. With this many variables in play, then, a high risk of error is always present.

One study estimates that 7,000 deaths per year are caused by medication errors, whether the errors occur in or out of the hospital (Phillips, Christenfeld, & Glynn, 1998). That's more than the number of people who die from workplace injuries annually, which a few years ago was estimated to be 6,000 per year (Phillips et al., 1998). In 2002 alone, according to the U.S. Pharmacopeia, 192,477 medication errors were documented in the United States. Of these, roughly 3,200, or 1.7% of the total, resulted in injury (Davis, 2003). About half of all fatal hospital medication errors in 2002 involved senior citizens, those most likely to be disadvantaged by low health literacy.

Quite often, then, medical errors involve drugs and occur when a patient receives the wrong prescription or the wrong dose of a medicine. And although a combination of factors might lead to medication errors, as mentioned earlier, low health literacy on the part of the patient can make matters worse. Imagine a busy pharmacist who fails to verify a physician's handwriting when the name of the medication is difficult to read, and a patient, unable to read well, who does not ensure that the correct medicine is being dispensed.

Something as basic as the name of a drug can lead to errors. According to the Institute for Safe Medication Practices, drug name confusion played a role in 40 documented cases of medication error involving Celebrex, a COX-2 inhibitor for treating arthritis pain, and two other similar-sounding medications used for different purposes that were on the market: Celexa, an antidepressant, and Cerebyx, a seizure medication (Institute for Safe Medicine Practices, 2000). These 40 cases were documented within the first 2 weeks of Celebrex's availability on the market. If everyone in the process is not vigilant, from the doctor to the pharmacist to the patient, whose lack of literacy skills may be a serious impediment, potential problems can and will arise.

General medical errors—including those that involve medications—have a tremendous fiscal impact. In terms of lost income, lost household production, and increased disability and health care costs, preventable adverse events are estimated to cost between $17 billion and $29 billion annually, of which health care expenditures account for more than half (Johnson et al., 1992; Thomas et al., 1999). Two of every 100 patients admitted to a hospital experience a preventable error, increasing hospital costs by $4,700 per admission, or roughly $2.8 million per year for a 700-bed teaching hospital (Bates et al., 1997).

Increased hospital costs alone may be as high as $2 billion for the nation as a whole. However, with more and increasingly complex care taking place in ambulatory settings, outpatient surgical centers, physicians' offices, and community clinics, hospitals treat only a fraction of the population at risk, as Berwick notes (IOM, 2000; O'Connor, 1999). What this means is that medical errors present a problem in any health care setting.

WRONG-SITE SURGERIES AND OTHER DISASTERS

Popular television programs, such as *ER* and *Grey's Anatomy,* sometimes dramatize medical errors specifically as major mistakes made during surgery, such as when a patient has the wrong limb amputated. In fact, that's exactly what happened to Willie King on February 20, 1995, at the University Community Hospital in Tampa. Although he was only joking when he asked surgery personnel if they knew which leg they were going to cut, he awoke from anesthesia to discover that his left leg rather than his right leg had been amputated. Two weeks later the correct leg was removed, leaving King in a considerably more arduous condition than he should have been (Stanley, 1995). Improved communication and additional checks and balances may have helped avoid this disastrous outcome.

Unlike in Mr. King's case, most wrong-site surgery errors actually turn out to be benign or even "warranted by the patient's condition" (Emergency Care Research Institute, 2000). But medical errors are not limited to extreme cases such as having the wrong leg amputated; they can appear in a variety of forms and clinical contexts, as the following examples, each of which constitutes a different kind of error, clearly indicate (*Medical Errors,* 2000):

- Misreading or misunderstanding a prescription label, resulting in the patient taking the wrong medicine or the wrong dose of the medicine, taking drugs at the wrong time, ingesting too many or too few pills, or experiencing harmful interactions, perhaps because contraindications appear in infinitesimal print in a product package insert
- Diagnostic error, such as a misdiagnosis that leads to an incorrect choice of therapy, failure to use an indicated diagnostic test, misinterpretation of test results, and failure to act on abnormal results
- Equipment failure, such as heart monitors that don't work or intravenous pumps whose valves are dislodged or bumped, causing increased doses of medication over too short a period
- Infections originating either in the hospital or after the patient has been discharged

- Blood transfusion-related injuries, such as giving a patient the wrong blood type
- Misinterpretation of medical orders, such as failing to give a patient a salt-free meal ordered by the physician

PLAYING TELEPHONE, TAKING RESPONSIBILITY

Again, the problem with low health literacy is that it drastically increases the likelihood that any of the above errors will take place, thereby increasing the risk that other kinds of mistakes can occur as well. If an interpreter misinterprets a doctor's instructions, for example, non-English-speaking patients are at their mercy, further removed from the original source of the information. It's like a grown-up version of "telephone," the elementary-school game in which children sit in a circle and think of a message they want to communicate. The first child whispers that message into the ear of the child next to him or her, then that child whispers what he or she hears into the next child's ear, and so on. As the message reaches the end of a series of listeners and repeaters and the last child tries to repeat what he or she has been told, often the original message comes out differently, even hopelessly garbled. Needless to say, when health information is conveyed between patients and those who treat them, the stakes are much higher than those in a child's game.

Although placing blame is counterproductive, the chain of responsibility must begin with the health care provider, especially those physicians and nurses on the frontline of patient care. Next in line would be other providers, such as pharmacists and hospice workers, followed perhaps by family members or patient advocates, and then the patient. This by no means absolves the patient from responsibility, of course: armed with good information and the confidence to communicate their needs, patients can circumvent the risk of harmful errors. In fact, patients can learn self-care techniques and take charge of their health care. We can focus on empowering patients with the knowledge they need to achieve the best possible health outcomes, but myriad challenges continue to stand in their way. It is to these challenges that we now turn.

CHALLENGES TO PLAIN LANGUAGE AND EFFECTIVE COMMUNICATION

As mentioned, avoiding medical errors is a difficult task for any patient, but medication error represents a fundamental risk to low-health-literate patients. Though not perfect, use of plain language is a potential solution to this serious problem. In fact, over the years attempts to increase the use of plain language have transformed a fledgling effort by a handful of educators into a full-fledged movement, even a lucrative industry (Balmford, 2002). Scores of books, pamphlets, and articles have appeared to advise their audiences on ways to implement plain language principles in their work and in their writing, whether the topic is medicine, law, marketing, education, real estate, or some other area.

As Carl Rogers would have recognized, however, certain routines, practices, and deeply embedded assumptions stand in the way of plain language communication and improved outcomes for low-literate patients. Carefully considering such obstacles amounts to seeing "the other from the *other's* point of view," much as Rogers recommended for improving interpersonal communication and increasing understanding.

Product Package Inserts

Take, for example, the product package inserts that accompany prescription medications. They include wording required and approved by the U.S. Food and Drug Administration (FDA). Manufacturers write the inserts based on information in the *Physicians' Desk Reference,* or *PDR,* which contains monographs on all FDA-approved drugs. But the *PDR* is written for clinicians, not for lay readers. Where are the package inserts written at the fifth-grade level? They certainly do not accompany the pill capsules, at least at the present time. Only a few words about how to take the medicine generally appear on the bottle itself, and these instructions can be both ambiguous and confusing.

A typical product package insert contains a description of the medication, sections on clinical pharmacology and contraindications, warnings, precautions, and information about adverse reactions, drug overdosing, and dosage and administration. Often the insert includes charts and tables conveying findings from clinical trials of the drug, and these are as difficult to read as the text of the insert itself, which is tiny enough to require a magnifying glass even for relatively young eyes. Of course, this assumes that a lay person with even advanced reading skills would attempt to get beyond sentences such as the following, taken from the "mechanism of action" section of a product package insert for atorvastatin calcium (Lipitor), a drug for lowering cholesterol: "Atorvastatin is a selective, competitive inhibitor of HMG-CoA reductase, the rate-limiting enzyme that converts 3-hydroxy-3-methylglutaryl-coenzyme A to mevalonate, a precursor of sterols, including cholesterol" (Pfizer, 2005).

One might argue that patients can skip over such highly clinical language and focus on what is pertinent, but these documents are shot through with medical jargon, complex sentences, and scientific vocabulary familiar only to those with backgrounds in medicine. Concerned about overdosing? That section of the Lipitor product package insert reads: "In the event of an overdose, the patient should be treated symptomatically, and supportive measures instituted as required. Due to extensive drug binding to plasma proteins, hemodialysis is not expected to significantly enhance atorvastatin clearance" (Pfizer, 2005).

True, this information is intended primarily for physicians prescribing the drug. In fact, in a review of case law concerning whether the package insert and the *PDR* could be used as the "standard of care" in drug liability cases, it was found that doctors who vary from the clinical recommendations in the inserts and the *PDR* basically shift the burden of proof to themselves; that is, they must substantiate their departure from the manufacturer's guidelines (Bradford & Elben, 2001). There is pressure, in other words, for physicians to stand by the language they inherit from the FDA, the *PDR,* and the drug manufacturers themselves, even when it is unclear. Departing too far from it could open the door to a malpractice suit.

In an ideal world, prescribing physicians would read the inserts and the *PDR* and translate the jargon into language the patient could understand. But how many take the time to do so? In chapter 6, Improving Patient–Provider Communication, we discuss some key obstacles to good communication between health care providers and their patients. But let's assume the physician conveys the information accurately, so the patient catches on, and the physician follows the insert's advice when prescribing. Errors still can take place. As gastroenterologist Perry Hookman, MD, notes, the product information section of the *PDR* often includes inadequate dosage information, dosage methods based on clinical studies that are skewed toward higher doses, and no dosing adjustments for elderly patients (Hookman, 1997). In addition, according to Hookman, specific dosages for specific diagnoses are sometimes omitted, and data about side effects in the *PDR* can be "unfocused, inaccurate, and inadequately updated" (Hookman, 1997).

As for Lipitor, information at a lower reading level is available on one of Pfizer Inc.'s many product Web sites (http://www.lipitor.com), as are several questions and answers for consumers that tend to avoid the scientific jargon of the product package inserts. The question is whether the average patient will be enterprising enough to seek out such information on his or her own.

Although it's unclear what percentage of low-health-literate patients use the Internet, the cost of personal computers and Internet access makes them prohibitive for many in the low-literate patient population, and most text-based health information on the Internet is written at a 10th-grade reading level or higher anyway (Birru et al., 2004). This fact may discourage low-literate computer users from relying on the Internet as a source of information, even when access is available for free at schools and libraries.

Without additional written material in an easy-to-read format, patients may simply assume that the product package inserts are authoritative or conclude that the inserts are all that is available to educate them about their medications. How likely are they to read the fine print in these package inserts, let alone to understand them?

HIPAA Notices of Privacy Practices, Informed Consent, and Legalese

Another serious obstacle for low-literate patients has to do with legal requirements in health-related disclosures. In 1996 President Clinton signed into law the Health Insurance Portability and Accountability Act (HIPAA) of 1996, sometimes called the Kassebaum/Kennedy bill, which established new federal regulations for private health plans. Among other things, the law enhanced the portability and continuity of health insurance, strengthened health care fraud and abuse controls, authorized the creation of medical savings accounts, and allowed for the acceleration of death benefits (American Academy of Physical Medicine, 1996).

In April 2003, patients in the United States began receiving HIPAA Notices of Privacy Practices from doctors, hospitals, clinics, pharmacies, and other "covered entities" that use personal health information (Hochhauser, 2003). Although HIPAA rules do not set a goal for the readability level of privacy notice disclosures, some states took the initiative to create documents whose reading levels ranged from the fourth to the sixth grade (Matthews & Sewell, 2002). In a review of 37 privacy notices, however, actual reading levels were found to average much higher: from the second to the fourth year of college. Typically these notices featured too many words per sentence, too many complicated sentences, and too many uncommon words (Hochhauser, 2003).

The Health Resources and Services Administration (HRSA) offers guidelines to aid writers in crafting easy-to-read HIPAA Notices of Privacy Practices. Among its recommendations are to use shorter sentences, to avoid hyphens and compound words, and to give examples to explain "problem" words—plain language practices, one and all. In addition, HRSA offers a thesaurus of common words found in HIPAA, advising those who write the disclosures to substitute words such as *OK* for *authorization, rules* for *regulations, health care records* for *protected medical records,* and so on (*Plain Language Principles and Thesaurus,* 2003). It's certainly a start.

But changing individual words is one thing; adjusting document length is something else. Often federal requirements about the number of topics that must be included in patient forms make writing easy-to-read documents extremely challenging. HIPAA topics must be included in informed consent documents, for example. In addition to the FDA's eight "basic elements" of informed consent and six "when appropriate" elements of consent, as many as 6 to 11 HIPAA privacy topics must be included in informed consent documents, whether they are included in the language of the consent form or they appear as addenda (Hochhauser, 2005a).

Needless to say, such requirements pose a sizeable dilemma to those charged with crafting informed consent forms, especially because they now are under pressure to make the forms readable to the average American. "While they're expected to write consent forms that are compliant with . . . [federal] requirements . . . ," notes reading consultant Mark Hochhauser, PhD, "[consent form writers] must also include up to 25 topics in the consent form, even though a prospective subject's working memory can store only about three to five pieces of information" (Hochhauser, 2005a).

And then there's the communication stumbling block known as legalese, that highly specialized jargon used almost exclusively by lawyers and legislators. Textbooks such as Richard C. Wydick's *Plain English for Lawyers* (1998) and organizations like the Legal Writing Institute have done their best to convert the legal profession to a simpler, easier-to-read prose style, but professionals in a number of disciplines continue to hold out against plain language, as law professor Joseph Kimble notes (1994–1995). Compared with most texts, materials written in legalese are relatively inaccessible—or at least less accessible—to the average American reader. With its convoluted sentences, Latin phrases, and insistence on using such words as *aforementioned, whereas,* and *hereinafter,* legalese poses tremendous difficulties to those at the lowest literacy levels.

Research bears this out. Average readers do better when legalese is rewritten into plain English. In a study of medical consent forms, for example, readers of an unrevised form (that is, a form written in legalese) were able to correctly answer 2.36 comprehension questions out of 5. On the revised form, however, written according to principles of plain language, the participants could answer 4.52 questions out of 5: a 91% improvement. They could do it faster too. The mean response time improved from 2.65 to 1.64 minutes (Kaufer, Steinberg, & Toney, 1983; Kimble, 1994–1995). Unfortunately, more emphasis on plain language has not entirely changed the way things are written. Regulatory guidelines requiring that HIPAA disclosures be written in plain language, for example, are routinely ignored (Hochhauser, 2003). And there are no penalties for noncompliance.

Overdosing and Underdosing: Prescription Bottle Confusion

Even the simplest-sounding instructions on a bottle of prescription medication can be ambiguous to low-literate patients and to those for whom English is not a first language. If a label indicates that a particular medication should be taken three times a day, for example, how are patients supposed to know when exactly to take it? Does the specific hour the drugs are taken make any difference? Would it be reasonable to pace the doses out before lunch, for example, taking one pill every hour on the hour? What about one pill in the morning and two in fairly rapid succession during the evening? And does "four doses daily" mean one should take a dose every 6 hours around the clock or only during waking hours? (*20 Tips,* 2000)

Numbers are not always cut-and-dried; they can be transposed and misinterpreted, especially by older patients. Instructions to "take two pills four times daily," read hastily, might become "four pills two times daily." At any given moment, patients may be under- or overdosing, seriously risking their health.

Similarly, when patients are asked to take a medication "with food," does this mean that they should crush the pills into a powder and roll them into an egg salad sandwich? Some patients, even highly literate ones, have done just that (Mayer, 2002). In fact, making this seemingly harmless mistake could have serious consequences: although most medications can be crushed or opened without affecting their delivery, physically altering the dosage form of other medications can increase side effects or toxicity (*Healthcare Practitioner's Guide,* 1999–2002).

Another issue has to do with foreign words and phrases that are similar to words and phrases in English but mean something different. One example, mentioned in chapter 1, is the word *once,* which in Spanish means "eleven." Spanish speakers who encounter instructions to take a particular medication "once" per day could easily consume 10 pills too many. Corporate marketers have learned this lesson the hard way. When the American Dairy Association wanted to expand its popular "Got Milk?" campaign into Mexico, for example, it was surprised to learn that the best Spanish translation for the slogan was "Are you lactating?" (Gordon, 2003) (For more information about the effects of culture and language on low health literacy, see chapter 5, Factoring Culture Into the Care Process.) Translators must understand the idiosyncrasies of English and take care so that the spirit of certain colloquialisms or idioms survives the translation process.

Many over-the-counter children's medicines come with height and weight dosing charts that guide parents and other caregivers in measuring the right amount of suspension liquid or concentrated drops. Each weight range is assigned a corresponding age range. On the dosing chart for Children's Tylenol (acetaminophen), for example, 24 to 35 pounds corresponds to 2 to 3 years of age, 48 to 59 pounds is paired with 6 to 8 years of age, and so on (McNeill PPC, 2005). (Dosing instructions for children under the age of 2 tend to be omitted because infant doses require a different concentration. Parents are instructed to "consult [their] child's doctor.") However, these dosing charts can cause confusion. When a child does not fit into one of the age-weight categories on the chart, parents sometimes assume that age is the best factor for determining the dosage, whereas researchers have found that weight is the more important criterion (Madlon-Kay & Mosch, 2000).

Liquid measurements pose other challenges as well. In addition to misreading the chart if weight and age don't agree, patients might misinterpret the instructions and confuse teaspoons and tablespoons on the medicine cup. To remedy this, clinicians ought to recommend that patients use more accurate devices, such as an oral dosing syringe (Madlon-Kay & Mosch, 2000; McMahon, Rimsza, & Bay, 1997). In a study of 90 English- and Spanish-speaking families, 100% were able to dose medication correctly when given oral instructions and a syringe with a line marked at the prescribed dose. Eighty-eight percent could do so at follow-up (McMahon et al., 1997).

Unclear Instructions, Illegible Prescriptions

Health care providers must make their instructions clear not only to patients during the clinical encounter but also to pharmacists who fill the prescription. Failing to do so can be both financially costly for the practitioner and dangerous or even deadly for the patient. In one case, a cardiologist was fined $225,000 after he scrawled a prescription that was misunderstood by the pharmacist who filled it (Charatan, 2000). The prescription was for Isordil, a drug for chest pain, but was misread as Plendil, a drug for hypertension. As a result, the patient took twice the recommended daily dose of the antihypertensive medication and died of a heart attack several days later (Charatan, 2000). Misreading a decimal can result in a 10-fold overdose. An order marked as *qd,* doctor's shorthand for "once a day," easily could be read as *qid,* meaning "take four times per day" (Snowbeck, 2001).

Sometimes the provider and the pharmacist must share the blame for medication errors. In 1988, a British court determined that a prescribing physician was 25% liable and the pharmacist who filled the prescription was 75% liable when a patient sued after being prescribed glibenclamide, an oral hypoglycemic agent, instead of the antibiotic amoxicillin for a chest infection (Brahams, 1988). When two or more health care providers fail to communicate, to use the IOM's phrasing, we witness "the failure of a planned action to be completed as intended."

Jokes about physicians' bad handwriting are nothing new, but the truth is that hastily written prescriptions are at the heart of unfortunate outcomes like the ones above. As doctors and nurses see more and more patients, and more similarly named drugs are approved for prescription, an aging population faces increased exposure to medical error.

Illegible writing is a problem in prescriptions, but it can stir up trouble in record keeping as well. A survey of illegible notations on patients' records found an incidence of illegible writings of 1.44% (Gupta et al., 2003)—not a large number, but if extrapolated to the patient population as a whole, the number of affected patients becomes alarming. Older patients and women are most affected by illegible drug notations, but urban practice settings, an increased number of diagnoses and prescriptions written during the office visit, and seeing a family physician or internist are other factors associated with increased chances that at least one illegible drug mention will show up in a patient's record (Gupta et al., 2003).

Health care providers must make sure that their patients understand the reasons why they are being prescribed specific medications. Patients often are asked to continue taking a medication until the bottle is empty and to continue even when their symptoms have dissipated or they've started feeling better. Patients must understand these instructions at the outset. Many are too embarrassed to ask questions once they've left the doctor's office and may let long lines at the pharmacy prevent them from consulting as they should with those dispensing their medications.

Polypharmacy: Managing Multiple Medications

According to the American Public Health Association, the average elderly patient in the United States takes 8.9 medications per day (West-Myers & Hilger, 2004). Many of these elderly patients see more than one doctor; often they are taking medications that could interact with one another, potentially causing serious health complications.

Patients engaged in polypharmacy, or the mixing of more than one drug in a single prescription, should have a reliable method for managing multiple medications. They must track different dosages, come up with a schedule, know whether to take their medications with food, know about drug interactions (especially when using herbs or other forms of complementary and alternative medicine), and so on. Changing medications and transitioning from one medication to another require clarity and good organizational skills. Those with low health literacy may have trouble coordinating their prescriptions among multiple providers and may not take advantage of the services of a pharmacist who can assist them with the task.

SOLUTIONS FOR REDUCING ERROR AND INCREASING CLARITY

Now that we've discussed a number of obstacles in the way of better patient care and clearer understanding for those with low health literacy, let's turn to potential solutions.

First, consider some history. Medical errors were nothing new when the IOM issued *To Err Is Human* (2000). A decade earlier, Lucian Leape and colleagues at Harvard University had begun cataloging medical errors. Reviewing 30,000 inpatient records from 51 New York hospitals, the team found that 4% of patients had been seriously harmed by their providers and that roughly two-thirds of the injuries had been caused by errors (Brennan et al., 1991). Later these figures were extrapolated based on other studies with similar findings, and it was determined that nearly 100,000 deaths occur due to medical errors every year in the United States (Langreth, 2005). Those kinds of numbers began to attract the attention of officials in high places, including the National Academy of Sciences and one of its four component organizations, the Institute of Medicine.

The IOM Quality of Health Care in America Committee was formed in 1998 to develop a strategy for improving health care quality over the coming decade. Addressing issues relating to patient safety, the report the committee produced laid out a national agenda for reducing errors and improving care. "The focus must shift from blaming individuals for past errors to a focus on preventing future errors by designing safety into the system," wrote the committee in the report's executive summary (IOM, 2000, p. 4). This change in focus was one of the first steps toward a systematic solution to the problem of medical error—a problem that Leape and colleagues had helped bring to national attention years earlier.

Several bold recommendations emerged from the IOM report. One was that Congress should create a Center for Patient Safety within the Agency for Health Care Policy and Research; another was that the United States should establish a nationwide reporting system to collect standardized information about adverse events that lead to serious harm or death for patients. Additional recommendations were that the United States should develop voluntary reporting efforts and that Congress should extend peer review protections to data on patient safety and quality improvement (IOM, 2000, pp. 6–9).

That was 1999. Later that same year, in response to the IOM's recommendations, President Clinton directed the Quality Interagency Coordination Task Force (QuIC) to make its own recommendations for improving health care quality and protecting patient safety based on the IOM report (*Medical Errors*, 2000). The QuIC fully endorsed the IOM's call for reducing the number of medical mistakes by 50% over 5 years (*Doing What Counts*, 2000).

The task force took the IOM's recommendations seriously, advising the president to make room in the federal budget for many of them. President Clinton already was amenable to advice about making the public sector run more efficiently. In the previous year, as part of the administration's effort to "reinvent government," the president had sent a memorandum to the heads of all executive departments and agencies in the federal government directing them to use plain language in all new documents after January 1, 1999 (*President Clinton's memorandum*, 1998). It was a victory for the plain language movement. Prospects for reform in health care looked promising.

Yet despite these and other promising developments, administrations come and go and budgets change during wars and other volatile economic times. What can health care providers do on their own to avoid medical errors and to improve communication with their patients?

Communicate Instructions on a Fifth-Grade Level

For starters, whenever possible, patients' instruction sheets should be limited to a single page and should be written at a low grade level, preferably fifth grade or lower (Weiss & Coyne, 1997). Elsewhere we discuss the basic tenets of writing for those with low health literacy, such as using large type, using lots of white space, clustering important information, and using specific and action-oriented instructions (see chapter 7, Designing Easy-to-Read Patient Education Materials, and chapter 8, Principles of Writing for Low Literacy). Although some documents, such as consent forms, have complex requirements that make them harder to translate into easy-to-read English, most documents and sources of information, such as patient education brochures, booklets, questionnaires, and Web sites, can be translated into plain language without much difficulty.

Defining the audience, involving that intended audience in the design of materials, limiting one's objectives, writing the way people actually talk (e.g., by using the active voice, common words, short sentences, and lots of examples), and using a reader-friendly layout and design are among the most effective means for developing easy-to-read patient materials (Doak, Doak, & Root, 1996). Many guidelines are available to help clinicians in their efforts to improve health communications. One is Helen Osborne's *Health Literacy From A to Z: Practical Ways to Communicate Your Health Message* (2005), an up-to-date resource that arranges its advice in alphabetical order, from discussions "about health literacy" to a chapter about adding "zest and pizzazz" to easy-to-read texts.

Trying Something New: Two Product Package Inserts

If product package inserts are too difficult to understand, and inserts written at a fifth-grade level risk excluding information that is legally required or necessary for the patient's understanding, then perhaps two inserts might be included in all medication packaging: one written in legalese and one that can be read and understood by those with lower literacy skills.

It's not a new idea. For some prescription medications, the FDA already requires information sheets designed for lay readers. They are written in plain English and are easier to understand than the typical product package insert. Instead of warning that the antidepressant nefazodone (Serzone) carries a risk of "life-threatening hepatic failure" and "hepatotoxicity," for example, the new FDA-required patient information sheets refer to "serious liver problems" ("Finding Out About the Side Effects," 2005). As of 2004, the government had required plain language handouts for only about 15 drugs (Avorn, 2004), but the private sector is quickly catching on. According to plain language consultant Janet Ohene Frempong, MS, Pfizer Inc. and other pharmaceutical companies and health plans have developed initiatives to produce patients' information that must be written at the sixth-grade level or below (Ohene Frempong, 2005).

When it comes to printed information, it's important to strike a balance between the bare minimum patients *must know* and additional information that is *nice to know* because patients could feel overwhelmed by a proliferation of additional paper warnings. In other words, more paperwork might have the effect of overwhelming the patient rather than simplifying the process of patient education, thereby defeating its original purpose. Those with diminished literacy skills, when faced with what they perceive as an overwhelming amount of material to read, will simply stop reading. As mentioned, a significant problem is that federal law often requires health care providers to cover a minimum number of topics on patient forms, specifically with informed consent documents and privacy disclosures under HIPAA (Hochhauser, 2005b).

Using Visual Aids

Research suggests that patients with low health literacy can benefit from pictorial displays of medications that are accurate in color and size, with graphic illustration of the instructions, including the number of pills to be taken and at what times they should be taken (Kalichman, Ramachandran, & Catz, 1999). No solution is without its share of flaws, however. Research by Parker, Davis, and Wolf suggests that even simple pictographs can be confusing. The investigators interviewed several hundred volunteers of varying reading levels and showed them samples of real warning stickers. A high number of errors occurred across the board, even among those with higher literacy skills (Franklin, 2005).

For example, respondents variously interpreted a yellow label with an icon of the sun with a slash through it, which actually meant "You Should Avoid Prolonged or Excessive Exposure to Direct and/or Artificial Sunlight While Taking This Drug." Some thought it meant the pills should not be taken if *the pills* had been in the sunlight too long; others thought it meant the end user should not leave the medicine out in the sun. A sticker indicating "For External Use Only" misled 90% of those with the lowest literacy levels (Franklin, 2005). If, as Leape notes, a medical error is "an unintended act (either of omission or commission) or one that does not achieve its intended outcomes," we see that even a simple icon can lead to error.

Pictographs are culturally specific, so it's always a good idea to test them first. Using focus groups that include the intended audience can help avoid embarrassing mistakes and ensure that the images are appropriate and properly construed by the patient. In some cultures, for example, diseases are seen as an imbalance of mind and body, whereas in the West they usually are seen strictly in terms of germs and viruses (Cowgill & Bolek, 2003; Osborne, 2005). Such contrasts not only affect the way we must talk about health care with diverse groups but also the associations we should make between diseases and conditions and any visual images we use in relation to them.

Employing the Teach-Back Method

Elements of the teach-back method were evident even in Carl Rogers's emphasis on mutual understanding. In teach-back, the health care provider asks the patient to repeat what he or she has learned during the clinical encounter. Better communication usually takes place in the follow-up exchange, during which any misconceptions can be cleared up. The teach-back method ought to be used in all patient–provider communication to improve patient understanding. Bear in mind, though, that simply repeating information does not guarantee understanding and by no means ensures that the patient remembers it. Notes Hochhauser (2005b), "The success of short-term memory does not guarantee that the same information will be converted to long-term memory; these are two different psychological and biological processes." What's essential is that patients interact with the new information. When people do so, a chemical change takes place in the brain, facilitating long-term memory (Thompson & Greenough, 1989).

With this in mind, a list of strategies follow for building patient interaction into clinical instructions, derived from Doak and colleagues' *Teaching Patients With Low Literacy Skills* (1996, p. 65):

- Ask the patient to tell you about the new information in his or her own words.
- Present a problem: "How/when will you do this when you go home?"
- Ask the patient what problems he or she has or expects to have in terms of compliance.
- Ask questions during a teaching/learning session; dialogue with the patient.
- For written materials, ask questions and leave blanks for patient write-in or check-off, or ask the patient to circle a selected picture.
- For small group instruction, foster interaction between members of the group.

Labels and Calendars

Visual aids such as labels and calendars can be helpful. Pillboxes, for example, should be labeled clearly, perhaps using a color-coded system or divided into the days of the week or the time of day each pill is taken. Illustrations that make sense to patients, whenever they are being used, can help trigger their memories, ensuring that the right medications make it into the right box and are taken at the

Medication Diary

This Medication Diary is a tool to help you keep track of all the medications you take. Having an accurate list of your medications is helpful for your doctors.

When filling out the Medication Diary, be sure to include:
- all of the prescription medications that you take
- all of the over-the-counter medications that you take
- all of the vitamins that you take
- all of the herbal agents that you take

Please be sure to take your Medication Diary with you to your doctor's office or to the hospital.

To complete the Medication Diary:

1. Write in the name of the medication you are taking. Some drugs may have a brand name or generic name. Write in the name of the drug you actually have.

2. Write down the dose you take. Example: 50 mg.

3. Write down how many you take of this medication. Example: 2 tablets, 1 tablet.

4. Write down what times you take the medication. Example: in the morning, at breakfast, at dinner, before bed.

5. Write down why you are taking the medication, for example, high blood pressure. If you are not sure, ask your doctor.

6. If you are no longer taking a medication, simply draw across that entry.

Your Personal Medication Diary

Compliments of:

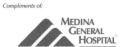

Medication Diary

Medication Name	Dose You Take	How many do you take?	What time(s) do you take this medication?	Why do you take this medication?

Medication Diary for: _____

Allergies: _____

FIGURE 4.1 Medication diary from Medina General Hospital.

right time—especially if patients are using multiple medications. Designating an am/pm pillbox or breaking it down by days of the week also can be effective.

Another way to get organized is to use a medication diary or a medication calendar. Medina General Hospital, in Medina, OH, offers an easy-to-use personal

U.S. PHARMACOPEIA
The Standard of Quality℠

Personal Medication Organizer

Patient Information

Patient's Name: ______ Patient's Birth Date: ______

Address: ______

Telephone Number: ( )

Emergency Contact (Name/Phone Number): ______

Drug and Food Allergies: ______

Health Care Provider's Information

- **PRIMARY PHYSICIAN:** ______ Telephone Number: ( )
  Address: ______
- **SPECIALIST(S):** ______ Telephone Number: ( )
  Address: ______
- **PHARMACY:** ______ Telephone Number: ( )
  Address: ______

	Drug (trade and generic) and over-the-counter product name	Prescribing Physician	Strength (Dosage)	How many times a day and at what time during the day do you take this prescription?	What liquid/food should or shouldn't you take with this medication? Other special instructions?
1					
2					
3					
4					
5					

PSF019G

FIGURE 4.2 Personal medication organizer from U.S. Pharmacopeia (USP).

medication diary on its Web site; the diary is reprinted in Figure 4.1 (Medina General Hospital, 2005). Six easy steps guide the patient through the process of filling out the form. Categories include the medication name, the dosage, how many pills to take, what time to take them, and the reason for taking them. Many medical organizers are available, though not all are written at low literacy levels. Another good organizer is available from the U.S. Pharmacopeia (USP, 2004) (Figure 4.2), though the USP's form is somewhat busier than the version developed by Medina (Figure 4.1). An advantage of the USP form, however, is that it keeps all information, including instructions, down to a single page.

TABLE 4.1 TIPS FOR HELPING PEOPLE REMEMBER TO TAKE MEDICATIONS

1. Place larger, more legible labels on pill bottles or color-code them if the person taking the medication has trouble knowing what they are.
2. Buy an inexpensive pill divider to portion out medications for each day for each medication time. If possible, do this once a week.
3. Set up a specific place to take medications. The kitchen (but not over the stove) is one place people visit every day, and it is generally well lit. Do not store medications in the bathroom, which tends to be warm and moist at bath time and may not have good ventilation.
4. Post reminders and/or place medicines in visible locations.
5. Make sure a readable clock is visible.
6. Draw a large clock and put color codes on it for each medication, matching the colors on the bottles if necessary.
7. Create a chart and check-off system listing the specific times when medications should be taken: morning, mid-morning, noon, dinner, evening before bed, and so on. Customize the list according to the medications taken.
8. Refills: think ahead 3 to 5 days and have refills approved and filled before medications are gone. (West-Myers and Hilger, 2004)

Remembering to take medications is a significant problem for elderly patients, who report using strategies based on external cues, such as bedtime and meals (Spiers & Kutzik, 1995). However, no single strategy seems to work better than any other. Table 4.1, which is derived from West-Myers and Hilger (2004), offers several tips and strategies for helping patients remember when to take their medications.

More Electronic Prescribing, Less Scribbling

Earlier in this chapter we discussed the hazards of illegible prescriptions and hastily scrawled instructions. The Institute for Safe Medication Practices recommends the use of electronic prescribing to reduce medication errors, calling computerized technology a promise but "not a panacea" (Institute for Safe Medication Practices, 2000).

And they're right. In one documented case, a physician using a formulary software system to order electronically from a hospital outpatient pharmacy accidentally chose Occlusal-HP instead of the ophthalmic antibiotic Ocuflox (ofloxacin) from an alphabetical product list and then instructed the pharmacist to "use as directed." Had the pharmacist not counseled the patient on the correct use of the medication, a 17% salicylic acid preparation for wart removal, the patient might have used it for his condition—pinkeye—and perhaps been blinded (Vaida & Peterson, 2002).

Think of the IOM's definition of medical error as "the failure of a planned action to be completed as intended or the use of a wrong plan to achieve an aim." To err is certainly human; at times, though, carrying out a task "as intended" itself can lead to an error. In the case above, the prescription was the "wrong plan" for achieving the end of good care.

Clearly, then, electronic prescribing has limitations. As we saw earlier, however, the potential confusion caused by illegible handwriting poses even greater risks to the patient, necessitating the very same checks and balances. A cautious transition to electronic prescribing emphasizing sufficient checks and balances may be the best approach. For example, pharmacists and patients *both* could double-check each prescription to make sure it is correct and clearly understood by the patient before he or she leaves the pharmacy.

To some extent, of course, double-checking is a standard procedure now, but some busy pharmacists may be less diligent about it than others. Pharmacists filling prescriptions also might ask the patient what he or she intends to use the medication for. Most important, patients should never accept the words "as directed" as their guide on any written prescription or any prescription container until they consult with the pharmacist or verify the accuracy of the medication instructions with their doctor or other health care provider.

Routines and Single, Centralized Sources for Information

All patients, but especially older adults, should be encouraged to establish a routine, taking medications at the same time every day and keeping all medicines in the same place. This applies to everyone who uses prescription or over-the-counter medications, but it is very helpful for people with low health literacy, because it can help them feel more organized and less overwhelmed. Many pharmacies now offer a separate seating area for patient consultations; other health care providers might do well to follow their lead, reserving quiet, private places (preferably away from the examination room) to interact with patients and to ensure clarity and understanding about any medications being prescribed.

One way to establish an effective medication routine in families with older adults is to assign the same person to help with the senior's drug regimen. Doing so avoids the pitfall of having two or more family members duplicate a dose on any given day. After all, overdosing some medicines can be harmful or fatal. In these days of computerized record keeping, older adults should be strongly encouraged to maintain a single pharmacy source, especially if they are using multiple medications. One pharmacy can maintain a single, active database featuring all of the prescribed drugs for an individual patient. Frequenting multiple pharmacies creates unlinked databases and increases the risk that a patient will overdose or use medications that are contraindicated. A pharmacist with a complete picture can check for drug interactions within the system and inform the patient if there are questions about new prescriptions.

ENDNOTE: VIGILANCE AND CLEAR COMMUNICATION

In this chapter we have discussed medical errors and the threat they pose to all patients, regardless of reading ability. As we hope to have shown, patients with low health literacy skills may be especially vulnerable to mistakes and miscommunication. Such obstacles as difficult-to-read product package inserts and confusing prescription bottle instructions continue to stand in the way of good patient care, though effective methods for improving patient outcomes and for reducing various types of error are available, including the wider use of plain language.

Nevertheless, no method for avoiding medical errors is foolproof; human error is a constant threat in the health care system. Take, for example, the potentially disastrous effect of wrong-site surgery discussed earlier. How can it be avoided? In an effort to reduce wrong-site incidents, the American Academy of Orthopedic Surgeons endorses a "sign your site" program, requiring that all surgeons place their initials at the actual operative site on each patient before they ever apply a scalpel (Emergency Care Research Institute, 2000, p. 8). Other strategies to avoid surgical error include continual site specification, a double-check system (including confirmation with the patient of the correct site for surgery), and a verification checklist. But even when each of these strategies is implemented to one degree or another, medical errors have a tendency to creep back in.

At a major hospital in Southern California, for example, a wrong-site surgery took place that was due mostly to breakdowns in communication, not necessarily to a lack of systematic safeguards. A Spanish-speaking patient in her sixties was to have surgery for a medial meniscus tear in her left knee. The outpatient nurse checked her in, marked the correct knee, double-checked that the patient's consent form coincided with that knee, and spoke with the patient through an interpreter, who happened to be the patient's son.

The consent form, which correctly indicated a left-knee arthroscopy, was written in easy-to-understand English. When the surgical nurse, an immigrant from Korea in her mid-fifties who spoke English with a thick accent, arrived to interview the patient, the patient pointed to her right knee when asked which one the surgeon should operate on. At this point the surgical nurse decided that the correct site must be the right one, despite indications on the charts and on the patient's body to the contrary. In the operating room a short time later, the nurse shaved the area around the right knee and applied betadine solution to prepare for surgery, after which she covered the nonoperative leg (including the left knee, which would have been the correct knee) with a blanket. At this point, the surgical scrub tech, whose back had been turned to the patient, proceeded to drape the patient for surgery.

When the surgeon arrived in the operating room, the patient was asleep. Her body was properly draped, with only her right knee exposed. During the operation the surgeon reportedly remarked that there was not as much disease as he thought there would be, but the patient had arthritis in both knees and some evidence of a meniscus tear in the incorrect knee as well. Not until after the operation, when the postoperative nurse told the doctor that the recovering patient was wondering why her right knee was bandaged, did the surgeon realize his mistake. In fact, for a brief time after hearing about the patient's query, he still was quite certain that he'd operated on the left knee.

Following this incident, the surgery staff changed its protocol, deciding to stop and confer with one another and to examine charts before each surgery to ensure that no wrong-site mistakes could be made again (S. Knight, personal communication, November 2005). Of course, at the time the surgeon could have checked the chart himself and examined the patient's other knee. By the same token, the surgery nurse could have verified the information with the interpreter or the outpatient nurse, deferring to the authoritative information in the patient's records. But the point is not to blame anyone; it is simply to underscore the indispensable role played by clear, effective communication.

There is always a need for better and more efficient checks and balances, even if they seem redundant or time consuming. Of course, even the most effective checks and balances do not eliminate the need for unfettered communication between nurses and other clinical staff members, between prescribing physicians and pharmacists, between patients and their health care providers, between patients and their close friends and family members, and even between the friends and family members of patients and the physicians and other providers treating those patients. Our duty as health care providers is to follow the lead of the late Carl Rogers, who advocated "listening with understanding" or "client-centered therapy" in myriad contexts, from international diplomacy to one-on-one communication. If we do so, the result might well be a new patient-centered medicine for the 21st century.

REFERENCES

20 tips to help prevent medical errors: Patient fact sheet. (2000, February). Rockville, MD: Agency for Healthcare Research and Quality. Retrieved October 2, 2005, from http://www.ahrq.gov/consumer/20tips.htm

American Academy of Physical Medicine. (1996). *Health Insurance Portability and Accountability Act of 1996.* Retrieved October 2, 2005, from http://www.aapmr.org/hpl/regulation/hipaa.htm

Avorn, J. (2004). *Powerful medicines: The benefits, risks, and costs of prescription drugs.* New York: Knopf.

Balmford, C. (2002). *Plain language: Beyond a "movement": Repositioning clear communication in the minds of decision-makers.* Retrieved November 25, 2005, from http://www.plainlanguage.gov/whatisPL/definitions/balmford.cfm

Bates, D. W., Spell, N., Cullen, D. J., Burdick, E., Laird, N., Petersen, L. A., et al. (1997). The costs of adverse events in hospitalized patients. *Journal of the American Medical Association, 277,* 307–311.

Birru, M. S., Monaco, V. M., Charles, L., Drew, H., Njie, V., Bierria, T., et al. (2004). Internet usage by low-literacy adults seeking health information: An observational analysis. *Journal of Medical Internet Research, 6*(3), e25. Retrieved November 24, 2005, from http://www.jmir.org/2004/3/e25

Bradford, G. E., & Elben, C. C. (2001). The drug package insert and the PDR as establishing the standard of care in prescription drug liability cases. *Journal of the Missouri Bar, 57,* 5. Retrieved October 15, 2005, from http://www.mobar.org/journal/2001/sepoct/bradford.htm

Brahams, D. (1988). Illegible prescriptions. *Lancet, 1*(8593), 1061.

Brennan, T. A., Leape, L. L., Laird, N. M., Herbert, L., Localio, A. R., Lawthers, A. G., et al. (1991). Incidence of adverse events and negligence in hospitalized patients: Results of the Harvard Medical Practice Study I. *New England Journal of Medicine, 324,* 370–376.

Charatan, F. (2000). Compensation awarded for death after illegible prescription. *Western Journal of Medicine, 172*(2), 80.

Cowgill, J., & Bolek, J. (2003). *Symbol usage in health care settings for people with limited English proficiency* (Hablamos Juntos Report. JRC Design, Hablamos Juntos). Retrieved November 20, 2005, from http://www.hablamosjuntos.org/signage/PDF/pt1evaluation.pdf

Davis, J. L. (2003). Seniors: At risk for medication errors: Patients don't get medications, get wrong dosage. *WebMD Medical News.* Retrieved October 12, 2005, from http://www.webmd.com/content/article/77/90414.htm?lastselectedguid={5FE84E90-BC77-4056-A91C-9531713CA348

Doak, L. G., Doak, C. C., & Root, J. H. (1996). *Teaching patients with low literacy skills* (2nd ed.). Philadelphia: J.B. Lippincott.

Doing what counts for patient safety: Report of the Quality Interagency Coordination Task Force (QuIC). (2000, February). Retrieved November 5, 2005, from http://www.fda.gov/cdrh/humfac/sandiego3.pdf

Dovey, S. M., & Phillips, R. L. (2004). What should we report to medical error reporting systems? *Quality and Safety in Health Care, 13*, 322–323.

Emergency Care Research Institute. (2000). Wrong-site surgery. Risk analysis. *Surgery and Anesthesia, 26.* Retrieved November 2, 2005, from http://www.ecri.org/Patient_Information/Patient_Safety/Surgan26.pdf#search='willie%20king%20wrong%20leg%20amputated

Finding out about the side effects of your prescription drugs. (2005, April). *Harvard Health Letter.* April 2005. Retrieved November 25, 2005, from http://www.health.harvard.edu/newsweek/Finding_out_about_the_side_effects_of_your_prescription_drugs.htm

Franklin, D. (2005, October 25). And now, a warning about labels. *New York Times.* Retrieved October 31, 2005, from http://www.boston.com/yourlife/health/other/articles/2005/10/25/and_now_a_warning_about_labels?mode=PF

Gordon, K. T. (2003). ¿Se habla Español? If you don't already, it's time to start. Tapping the Latino market could translate to increased sales. *Entrepreneur Magazine.* Retrieved November 11, 2005, from http://www.entrepreneur.com/magazine/entrepreneur/2003/june/61944.html

Gupta, A. K., Cooper, E. A., Feldman, S. R., Fleischer, A. B., Jr., & Balkrishnan, R. (2003). Analysis of factors associated with increased prescription illegibility: Results from the National Ambulatory Medical Care Survey, 1990–1998. *American Journal of Managed Care, 9*, 548–552.

Healthcare practitioner's guide to alternative oral dosage forms for the geriatric patient. (1999–2002). Novartis Pharmaceutical Corporation. Retrieved November 18, 2005, from http://www.novartisvin.com/seniorcare/hps/od/HCP_AOD.pdf

Hochhauser, M. (2002, October). Why you can't write a consent form at a sixth-grade reading level. *DIA Forum.*

Hochhauser, M. (2003). Compliance vs. communication: Readability of HIPAA notices. *Clarity 50.* Retrieved November 10, 2005, from http://www.privacyrights.org/ar/HIPAA-Reading.htm

Hochhauser, M. (2005a). Informed consent: Writing? readability? understanding? deciding? *Society of Research Administrators 2005 Symposium Proceedings Book*, 105–114.

Hochhauser, M. (2005b). Memory overload: The impossibility of informed consent. *Applied Clinical Trials, 14*(11), 70.

Hookman, P. (1997). *The Physicians' Desk Reference: Problems and possible improvements.* Retrieved October 27, 2005, from http://www.hookman.com/hc9703.htm

Institute for Safe Medication Practices. (2000). *A call to action: Eliminate handwritten prescriptions within 3 years!* Retrieved October 24, 2005, from http://www.ismp.org/MSAarticles/Whitepaper.html

Institute of Medicine (IOM). (2000). *To err is human: Building a safer health system.* Washington, DC: National Academy Press.

Johnson, W. G., Brennan, T. A., Newhouse, J. P., Leape, L. L., Lawthers, A. G., Hiatt, H. H., et al. (1992). The economic consequences of medical injuries. *Journal of the American Medical Association, 267,* 2487–2492.

Kalichman, S. C., Ramachandran, B., & Catz, S. (1999). Adherence to combination antiretroviral therapies in HIV patients of low health literacy. *Journal of General Internal Medicine, 14,* 267–273.

Kaufer, D. S., Steinberg, E. R., & Toney, S. D. (1983). Revising medical consent forms: An empirical model and test. *Law, Medicine, and Health Care, 11*(4), 155–162,184.

Kimble, J. (1994–1995). Answering the critics of plain language. *The Scribes Journal of Legal Writing, 5.* Retrieved November 10, 2005, from http://www.blm.gov/nhp/main/regtest/kimble.html

Langreth, R. (2005). *Fixing hospitals.* Retrieved November 5, 2005, from http://www.forbes.com/global/2005/0620/054_print.html

Leape, L. (1994). Error in medicine. *Journal of the American Medical Association, 272*(23), 1851–1857.

Madlon-Kay, D. J., & Mosch, F. S. (2000). Liquid medication dosing errors. *Journal of Family Practice, 49*(8), 741–744.

Matthews, T. L., & Sewell, J. C. (2002). *State official's guide to health literacy.* Lexington, KY: The Council of State Governments.

Mayer, G. G. (2002, May). Welcome/introductions. Presented at State of the Art 2002, Institute for Healthcare Advancement First Annual Health Literacy Conference, Anaheim, CA.

McMahon, S. R., Rimsza, M. E., & Bay, C. (1997). Parents can dose liquid medication accurately. *Pediatrics, 100,* 330–333.

McNeill PPC, Inc. (2005). *Children's Tylenol dosage guide.* Retrieved November 17, 2005, from http://www.tylenol.com/page.jhtml?id=tylenol/painex/subchild.inc

Medical errors: The scope of the problem. (2000). Rockville, MD: Agency for Healthcare Research and Quality. Retrieved October 14, 2005, from http://www.ahrq.gov/qual/errback.htm

Medina General Hospital. (2005). *Medication diary.* Retrieved November 20, 2005, from http://www.medinahospital.org/services/Medication_Diary.pdf

National Coordinating Council for Medication Error Reporting and Prevention. (2002). *About medication errors.* Retrieved October 23, 2005, from http://www.nccmerp.org/aboutMedErrors.html

O'Connor, E. (1999, November 30). *Medical errors kill tens of thousands annually, panel says.* Retrieved October 10, 2005, from http://www.cnn.com/HEALTH/9911/29/medical.errors

Ohene Frempong, J. (2005, May). *Panel discussion: Questions and answers in health literacy.* Presented at Culture, Language, and Clinical Issues: Operational Solutions to Low Health Literacy, Institute for Healthcare Advancement Fourth Annual Health Literacy Conference, Irvine, CA.

Osborne, H. (2005). *Health literacy from A to Z: Practical ways to communicate your health message.* Sudbury, MA: Jones and Bartlett Publishers.

Pfizer Inc. (2005). *Lipitor (atorvastatin calcium).* Retrieved November 14, 2005, from http://www.lipitor.com/cwp/appmanager/lipitor/lipitorDesktop?_nfpb=true&_pageLabel=prescribingInformation

Phillips, D. P., Christenfeld, N., & Glynn, L. M. (1998). Increase in US medication-error deaths between 1983 and 1993. *Lancet, 351,* 643–644.

Plain language principles and thesaurus for making HIPAA privacy notices more readable. (2003). Retrieved October 3, 2005, from ftp://ftp.hrsa.gov/hrsa/hipaaplainlang.pdf

President Clinton's memorandum on plain language in government writing. (1998). Retrieved October 7, 2005, from http://www.plainlanguage.gov/whatisPL/govmandates/memo.cfm

Rogers, C. R. (1961). Dealing with breakdowns in communication—interpersonal and intergroup. In C. Rogers, *On becoming a person: A therapist's view of psychotherapy* (pp. 329–337). Boston: Houghton Mifflin.

Rosenberg, S. (1967). *Cool hand Luke* [Motion picture]. United States: Warner Bros.

Snowbeck, C. (2001, June 26). Getting it write: Changing the low-tech way prescriptions and records are written could reduce outpatient medication errors. *Pittsburgh Post-Gazette.* Retrieved November 6, 2005, from http://www.post-gazette.com/healthscience/20010626herror1.asp

Spiers, M. V., & Kutzik, D. M. (1995). Self-reported memory of medication use by the elderly. *American Journal of Health-System Pharmacy, 52*(9), 985–990.

Stanley, D. (1995, February 28). Amputee recovering after wrong leg taken. *Tampa Tribune.*

Thomas, E. J., Studdert, D. M., Burstin, H. R., Orav, E. J., Zeena, T., Willians, E. J., et al. (2000). Incidence and types of adverse events and negligent care in Utah and Colorado. *Medical Care, 38*(3), 261–271.

Thomas, E. J., Studdert, D. M., Newhouse, J. P., Zbar, B. I., Howard, K. M., Williams, E. J., et al. (1999). Costs of medical injuries in Utah and Colorado. *Inquiry, 36*, 255–264.

Thompson, R. F., & Greenough, W. (1988, November 1). Researchers gain insight into how brain remembers. *Philadelphia Inquirer*, p. 8.

U.S. Pharmacopeia (USP). (2004). *Personal medication organizer.* Retrieved October 10, 2005, from http://www.usp.org/pdf/EN/patientSafety/personalMedOrg.pdf

Vaida, A. J., & Peterson, J. (2002). Incomplete directions can lead to dispensing errors. *Pharmacy Times.* Retrieved October 15, 2005, from http://www.pharmacytimes.com/article.cfm?ID=289

Weiss, B. D., & Coyne, C. (1997). Communicating with patients who cannot read. *New England Journal of Medicine, 337*(4), 272–274.

West-Myers, R. J., & Hilger, Z. (2004). *Safely managing medications.* Retrieved October 3, 2005, from http://www.familycaregiversonline.com/newsletter-v-3-04.html

Wydick, R. C. (1998). *Plain english for lawyers* (4th ed.). Durham, NC: Carolina Academic Press.

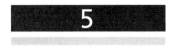

FACTORING CULTURE INTO THE CARE PROCESS

A Hmong child, just 3 months old, is carried through the doors of the Merced Community Medical Center (MCMC) in Merced, CA, by her parents, who speak no English. On this day, October 24, 1982, the only hospital employee who can translate for Hmong patients—and then only falteringly—is a Laotian janitor who is fluent in his native Lao, but not in Hmong. Misdiagnosed with tracheobronchitis rather than epilepsy—her true condition—the infant, Lia Lee, is prescribed an antibiotic and sent home.

Her parents attribute her condition to the slamming of their front door by the baby's older sister. What they call *quag dab peg* in Hmong means "the sprit catches you and you fall down" (Fadiman, 1997, p. 3). In other words, Lia's parents believe that the severe fright caused by the noise made their baby's soul flee her body and become lost to a malignant spirit. For them, Lia's condition is not epilepsy at all, but soul loss. In some respects, however, they believe their daughter has been blessed, that she is a "very special person . . . because she had these spirits in her and she might grow up to be a shaman" (Fadiman, 1997, p. 22).

The doctor who examines Lia on her third visit to the emergency department (ED) recognizes that she has had a severe seizure. His understanding of the condition's origins, however, contrasts sharply with that of the baby's parents, Laotian refugees who have had their many other children delivered at home, usually on a dirt floor.

The story is told by Anne Fadiman in her book, *The Spirit Catches You and You Fall Down: A Hmong Child, Her American Doctors, and the Collision of Two Cultures* (1997). Throughout the book, Fadiman describes a series of miscommunications and frustrating encounters between Lia's parents and the caregivers at MCMC, raising profound questions about the demands of health literacy, the importance of cross-cultural communication, the standards of care in the U.S. health system, and the nature of informed consent.

Lia's devoted and loving parents attempt to cure her through shamanistic interventions and the sacrifice of pigs and chickens, but to no avail. Similarly, nurses visiting the Lees at home do everything *they* can to get Lia's parents to comply with her drug regimen, attempting many of the low-health-literacy approaches discussed in chapter 4 of this book:

> [They] tried putting stickers on the bottles, blue for the morning medications, red for the noon medications, yellow for the night medications. When Lia was taking elixirs, they tried drawing lines on the plastic syringes or medicine droppers to mark the correct doses. When she was taking pills, they tried posting charts on which they had drawn the appropriate pie-shaped fractions. They tried taping samples of each pill on calendars on which they had drawn suns and sunsets and moons. They tried putting the pills in plastic boxes with compartments for each day (Fadiman, 1997, p. 48).

But the missing element in these strenuous efforts to save Lia is cultural understanding. One in five residents in Merced is Hmong, making it virtually impossible for health care workers in the region to treat their patient population adequately when they lack at least some passing familiarity with Hmong practices and beliefs.

According to Fadiman, nurses and other health care providers at MCMC often failed to understand their Hmong patients because of linguistic and cultural barriers, just as the members of Merced's Hmong community were frustrated and perplexed by the health care instructions they regularly received. The result was a nearly unbridgeable communication gap. One physician tells the author,

> Until I met Lia, I thought if you had a problem you could always settle it if you just sat and talked long enough. But we could have talked to the Lees until we were blue in the face—we could have sent the Lees to medical school with the world's greatest translator—and they would still think their way was right and ours was wrong (Fadiman, 1997, p. 259).

Unfortunately, Lia's story ends tragically. After trying everything he can think of to get the Hmong parents to comply with their daughter's anticonvulsant regimen, one of the clinic's supervising pediatricians—a man only "hazily aware" of the religious and cultural reasons for the Lees' noncompliance—notifies Child Protective Services and has Lia placed in foster care. Although the young girl eventually is returned to her parents, she winds up suffering brain death instead of recovering.

One physician with whom the author speaks insists that it is septic shock that destroys Lia's brain, rather than her parents' noncompliance with doctors' orders, but there is little consensus. That's the point. Fadiman takes great pains to be fair to both sides, asking questions without placing blame. Toward the end of the book, the exasperated author laments, "I have come to believe that [Lia's] life was ruined not by septic shock or noncompliant parents but by cross-cultural misunderstanding" (Fadiman, 1997, p. 262).

CHANGING DEMOGRAPHICS

The rapidly shifting ethnic landscape of Merced made it ripe for such misunderstandings. Before 1975, very few Hmong could be found outside Southeast

Asia, whether in California or elsewhere. After the Vietnam War ended, however, more than a half-million Hmong refugees scattered across the globe, settling mostly in the United States. By 2001, roughly 300,000 Hmong people lived in the United States, with 12,000 in Merced alone (Pobzeb, 2001; Thao, 1999).

The story of Lia Lee, though tragic, almost certainly is not unique. From Merced to San Antonio to Boston, such a tragedy has probably happened many times and could easily happen again.

Not all immigrants are refugees, of course, but there is no doubt that the demographics of the United States are changing—and quickly. People from all over the world—Asia, Africa, Central and South America—continue to transform the face of American culture, just as Merced was transformed during the mid-1970s. In the coming years, groups that today constitute a relatively small percentage of the population will represent a much larger share of the country.

If some population projections turn out to be correct, in fact, the definition of a minority may need to change before the end of the century. By 2080, White Americans are expected to make up only 48.9% of the total U.S. population (Catalano, 2003). The need for health care approaches that respond to the challenges of a diverse population soon will reach an all-time high. Our changing landscape underscores the need for culturally aware approaches to health care. Clearly, if dealing with diverse cultures in health care has not yet reached priority status, it certainly will soon.

Even today, understanding the nuances of patients' cultures is more than an exercise in polite interest for health care providers. It is central to overcoming communication barriers related to low health literacy and integral to considering patients' behaviors that could affect their overall health. In addition, it is essential to understanding patients' reactions to prescribed treatments. In other words, understanding patients' cultures is absolutely necessary to providing adequate care.

In the United States, with its multitude of ethnic groups and its diversity of experiences, health care professionals need to increase their awareness of and sensitivity to the cultural identity of their patient population. They need to take steps to understand the impact of culture on their patients' behaviors and experiences as these behaviors and experiences relate to health. Providers need to educate themselves and work to discover their own cultures and their underlying beliefs, values, and attitudes if they hope to provide high-quality care to their patients.

WHAT IS CULTURE?

Defining culture is not an easy task. A review of the literature yields hundreds of possibilities. Krober and Kluckhohn (1978) alone cite more than 160 definitions. One useful definition comes from Leninger (1978), who calls culture the "learned, shared and transmitted values, beliefs, norms and life practices of a particular group that guides thinking, decisions and actions in patterned ways." Culture is important to a discussion of health literacy because it is the lens through which people view and attach meaning to health communication (Institute of Medicine, 2004).

In the broadest sense, then, culture is the context in which we operate. That is, it is our environment and all the things in it. It is where we live: the area of the world, the country, the city, the neighborhood. Culture is the people with whom we interact: our family, our coworkers, our neighbors, our friends. It is the shared ideas to which we are exposed through the television shows and movies we watch, through the music we listen to, through the books we read. It is our background: our ethnicity, our religious beliefs, our personal history and experience. It is our language, our level of education, our political affiliations. Culture is all of these things—and more.

Even the most casual study of culture reveals that the concept is complicated. Two people from the same country will share a great deal culturally. Yet the impact of culture will not be exactly the same for each of them. As doctoral student Amandah Lea so aptly puts it, "Cultural diversity is . . . a reality that exists between and within ethnic groups" (Lea, 1994, p. 308).

Consider two people who live in the same country but in different cities. In some areas of the world, this could very well mean that they speak different languages. It might mean that they eat different foods. It could mean that they follow different religions. Think about how all of these differences might affect how these two people view the world.

Even in the United States, the area in which you live shapes your culture to some degree, despite the notion of America as a melting pot. Some ingredients never dissolve completely.

Los Angeles fashion, for example, is different from the style of dress popular in New York, which is different still from the trends in Miami. The colloquialisms popular in Fargo, ND, are not the same as those of Savannah, GA. A traditional Sunday dinner in New Orleans may be significantly different from what the people in Portland, OR, or Portland, ME, are eating.

And where a person lives is only one of many variables that shape culture. Imagine how different the world might appear to two people with different levels of education or income. Think about how the values and priorities of people change as they enter different phases of their lives, as they gain or lose family and friends, as they witness world events, as they face personal challenges, and as they work toward personal goals. Two people from the same country—or the same city, the same neighborhood, the same street, even the same family—will experience culture just a bit differently.

CULTURE AND PATIENT–PROVIDER INTERACTIONS

Despite how challenging it may be to define culture or to list all of the things that come together to shape the culture of a particular group or individual, the importance of understanding culture cannot be overestimated. Culture shapes our beliefs, our attitudes, and our values. It should come as no surprise, then, that culture exerts considerable and significant influence on health literacy. As we have seen in earlier chapters, health literacy can have a profound effect on the quality of health care. Providers who are aware of the effects of health literacy on patient care and compliance and who endeavor to optimize care for their patients must therefore take into account the effects of culture on their patients.

This is especially important—and, perhaps, especially challenging—in the United States, with its wide range of ethnic backgrounds and its diversity of spoken languages. The 2000 U.S. Census reported more than 211 million Americans of European descent living in America, along with close to 70 million people from other ethnic and cultural groups (U.S. Census Bureau, 2000). These different groups of people have differing ideas about health and wellness, about health care providers and institutions, and about illness and the appropriateness of particular interventions. Add to that the variety of languages and communications styles used by all of these different groups, and the challenge of responding to the cultural component of health literacy begins to appear overwhelming.

Still, to best serve patients, the health care industry as a whole must recognize both that culture plays a role in health literacy and how it does so. After all, it is only by identifying and understanding the components of culture and the way they function in shaping each patient's perspective that health care providers can truly care for their patient population.

CHALLENGES OF THE MULTICULTURAL ENVIRONMENT

The diversity of cultures in the United States poses particular challenges for health care providers committed to providing culturally sensitive and competent care for their patients. Our rapidly shifting demographics underscore the importance of the recognition by health care providers of cultural differences and, perhaps more important, their adopting an approach to patient care that will allow them to "practice with compassion and respect for the inherent dignity, worth, and uniqueness of every individual" (American Nurses Association, 2001).

Flowers (2004) points out that sometimes achieving culturally competent patient care puts providers in the position of supporting patients even when decisions they make are at odds with standard health care practices. She cites as an example the following experience:

> As an emergency room nurse in a small rural hospital, I was present when an elderly Native American man was brought to the emergency room by his wife, sons, and daughters. He had a history of 2 previous myocardial infarctions, and his current clinical findings suggested he was having another. During the patient's assessment, he calmly informed the emergency room staff and physician that, other than coming to the hospital, he was following the "old ways" of dying. He had "made peace with God and was ready to die" and "wanted his family with him" (Flowers, 2004, p. 49).

Despite the patient's expressed wishes, the ED physician ordered intravenous fluids, a dopamine infusion, a Foley catheter, and transfer to the intensive care unit of a regional hospital 3 hours away. The patient died 2 weeks and two code blues later and was intubated and receiving mechanical ventilation for most of that time. No family members were present when he died except his wife. The rest of his family members were unable to afford the cost of traveling to a health care facility that far from home.

This patient's values and beliefs were subordinated to those of the health care providers who made the decisions regarding his treatment. Flowers implies that the patient made clear to the ED staff that he did not want modern, invasive medical practices undertaken on his behalf and that he knew such a decision would ultimately be fatal. If nothing else, it seems obvious that the patient was very clear about the fact that having his family with him when he died was important to him.

Yet at the end of his life this patient was being kept alive by machines, and his family was hours away. No doubt the ED physician who cared for him had the best of intentions. No doubt he or she followed standard practices in treating this patient. Nevertheless, the physician's decisions were at odds with the patient's wishes. And it was the physician's values and beliefs—not those of the patient—that were given the most weight.

Cultural Competence

Stories like these underscore the importance of developing an approach to patient care that factors culture into the decision-making process. Admittedly, the influence of culture on the health care process is neither easily identified nor easily managed. However, the importance of identifying and managing that influence increases even as the task becomes more difficult. As providers deal with increasingly diverse patient populations, it becomes more and more important that they recognize the effects of culture on their patients' thought processes and behaviors and that they prepare themselves to address this influence.

To begin, providers need to recognize that their role is, as it has always been, to provide effective patient care. Recognizing the effect of culture in health care scenarios does not alter that objective; in fact, it serves as an opportunity to fulfill it more completely. Instead of looking at culture as a stumbling block to patient understanding or compliance, perhaps health care providers should view it as a means of connection. Understanding a patient's culture and its potential impact on his or her understanding, beliefs, and comfort level allows a provider to connect to that patient on a level that is more likely to result in competent care and compliance with instructions.

Cross and colleagues (1989) define cultural competence as "a set of congruent behaviors, attitudes, and policies that come together in a system, agency, or amongst professionals and enables that system, agency or those professionals to work effectively in cross-cultural situations." The National Medical Association (n.d.) explains in its *Cultural Competence Primer* that culture is "the application of cultural knowledge, behaviors, clinical and interpersonal skills that enhances a provider's effectiveness in patient care." Similarly, the U.S. Department of Health and Human Service's (DHHS's) Culturally and Linguistically Appropriate Services (CLAS) standards define cultural competence as "the capacity to function effectively as an individual and an organization within the context of cultural beliefs, behaviors, and needs presented by consumers and their communities" (IOM, 2004).

Based on these and similar views of cultural competence and an appreciation of the role of culture in provider–patient interactions, the Institute of Medicine (IOM), in *Speaking of Health: Assessing Health Communication Strategies for Diverse Populations* (2002), identifies the following components of cultural competence:

Cultural Awareness

The IOM notes that a deliberate, cognitive process of recognizing cultural beliefs, values, and practices is a necessary part of the approach of all health care providers who wish to work with and to be sensitive to the culture of their patients (IOM, 2002). This process includes providers' recognition of their own culture, which is necessary to ensure that they do not unknowingly impose their beliefs, values, or patterns of behavior on patients (Leninger, 1978).

Cultural Knowledge

Health care providers have a responsibility, in developing a culturally sensitive approach to patient interactions, to take measures to educate themselves about the worldviews of various cultures (IOM, 2002). Campinha-Bacote (2002) and Purnell (1998) have identified four stages in this process of education: unconscious incompetence, conscious incompetence, conscious competence, and unconscious competence.

Unconscious incompetence refers to the state of being unaware of a personal lack of cultural knowledge. At this point, health care providers do not realize that there are cultural differences between themselves and their patients.

Conscious incompetence refers to the state of being aware of a lack of knowledge about other cultures. Such awareness may be the result of formal training on cultural diversity, reading articles on the topic, or personal experience with patients from other cultures. At this stage, says Campinha-Bacote (2002), providers have "the 'know that' knowledge, but not the 'know how' knowledge." They know that culture is an important aspect of health care, but they do not yet know how to use this knowledge.

Conscious competence refers to the state of intentionally learning about different cultures and providing culturally responsive care.

Unconscious competence refers to a health care provider's ability to spontaneously provide culturally responsive care to patients from various cultural backgrounds (Campinha-Bacote, 2002).

Cultural Skill

To be culturally competent, a health care provider's approach to patient interactions must enable him or her to collect data and perform physical histories that are both thorough and culturally sensitive (IOM, 2002).

Cultural Encounter

This component of cultural competence refers to direct interactions between providers and patients despite the fact that they may have different cultural backgrounds. The more health care providers interact with patients from culturally diverse backgrounds, the more opportunities they have to refine their approaches to these groups (IOM, 2002).

Not all concerns affecting health care are cross-cultural, of course. As we learned in chapter 1, most of those with low-health-literacy skills are White, native-born Americans. In other words, low health literacy is not exclusively a product of differences in language or ethnic background. It is not a problem that affects only immigrants or non-native English speakers. Health literacy concerns and efforts certainly need to take into account these groups of people, but they are not exclusive to them. Similarly, the idea of cultural competence has implications outside the arena of health literacy. Educators and employers, for example, might benefit from an examination of the components of cultural competence described above.

Still, health literacy efforts are undeniably aided by an understanding of cultural competence. Davis and Voegtle (1994) illustrate how health care providers' failure to pay attention to cultural differences in their patients can lead to misdiagnosis, lack of patient cooperation, poor use of health resources by patients, and patient alienation. Given the seriousness of the cultural component, the IOM's explanation of cultural competence is significant because it gives practitioners a framework for developing and evaluating approaches to patient care.

Taking Care Not to Oversimplify

There are some potential pitfalls when it comes to striving for culturally competent patient care. One is the tendency to oversimplify. Making assumptions about a patient's beliefs, values, or attitudes based on his or her appearance, religious preference, or last name leads to stereotyping. And stereotyping, however unintentional, is at odds with the concept of culturally competent patient care.

For example, not all Latino patients share similar beliefs about health and illness. To assume that you know about the attitudes of a particular patient because of his or her ethnic background is to ignore important differences between and within ethnic groups. Latinos could be first-generation immigrants from Colombia or fifth-generation Mexican Americans in California. Different Latino patients will have different levels of acculturation, which will affect their beliefs and behaviors. Their citizenship or refugee status will affect their beliefs, too, as will the length of time they have lived in the United States.

Within any cultural group there are numerous variations. Geographic region, religious affiliation, socioeconomic level, gender, and level of education—among other factors—all affect patients and may result in differences among people who might otherwise appear similar. Among immigrant groups, the degree of acculturation of an individual patient also affects his or her culture. For example, Mexican Americans with higher levels of acculturation to U.S. society may be more likely to agree that patients should be directly informed of their conditions, as opposed to those with lower acculturation levels, who see decision making in health care as the province of their families (Beauchamp & Childress, 1994). Because these differences result in variations in health literacy level and affect the quality and success of patient care, providers must be aware of them.

COMMON CULTURAL ELEMENTS THAT AFFECT HEALTH CARE

With so many different elements informing culture, there is no single list of ways in which culture might affect health care. Just as the exact nature of culture varies with each individual, so too does its impact on health care. How can health care providers begin to understand culture? How can they use an understanding of culture to optimize health care for patients?

It seems logical to begin at the point where culture and health care intersect. Therefore, we focus on those elements of culture that are most likely to influence the patient–provider relationship. Of course, it is not possible to completely separate one cultural component from others: they are intertwined, and a discussion of one naturally leads to a discussion of others.

Language

Language is perhaps the most obvious component of culture. It serves as a connection to others and as a means of transmitting cultural beliefs and values from one person or one generation to the next. In some cases, it can be argued that language actually shapes cultural beliefs and values. Thus, although health literacy and its impact on health care are not related solely to language issues, health care providers must give particular attention to the challenges that language poses. If health care providers are committed to achieving a culturally competent model for patient care, they must consider the impact of language.

Just as native English speakers have different levels of health literacy, patients whose native language is not English will have varying levels of health literacy in their native language. In cases in which the patient has adequate health literacy in his or her native language, the solution seems relatively simple: provide care in the patient's native language or through interpreters and translated materials. (For more about the use of interpreters, see chapter 10, Interpreters and Their Role in the Health Care Setting.)

However, when a patient's health literacy level is low even in his or her native language, the obstacles presented by differences in language are compounded. Merely translating the words of the health care provider into the patient's language does not ensure that the patient will understand the meaning of those words.

For the health care industry, the problem of language differences extends beyond the exam room and permeates the entire health care experience. For example, as we discussed in chapters 1 and 2, a basic understanding of written language is necessary simply to find one's way to the appropriate department in a hospital. Imagine the challenges patients face when the signs pointing the way to "lab" or "maternity" or "surgery" are printed in a language different from their own. How much harder must it be if, even in their native language, patients do not know what those words mean? How do they figure out where to go?

Family Relationships and Experiences

Family is a major influence that shapes an individual's culture. Shared experiences, roles within the family structure, and the current state of relationships among family members all influence the patient and, by extension, the patient–provider interaction. Although an individual patient may walk into his or her doctor's office unaccompanied by other family members, the attitudes and beliefs shaped by family background, relationships, and values remain present. A culturally aware approach to patient care necessarily respects the power of familial ties while maintaining a focus on providing the best possible patient care.

Aspects of family life such as ethnic background and socioeconomic standing are important and relevant for finding the best course of treatment for a particular patient, but they are not the only factors associated with the family that affect a patient's health care experience.

In addition to these rather broad family attributes, health care providers are called on to be sensitive to the patient's individual family experience. Part of a culturally competent approach to patient care is an understanding of the family's past experiences with the health care community, which can reveal important information about a patient's knowledge or attitude toward particular medical interventions.

Consider the case of a female patient whose mother, sister, grandmother, and aunt all died of breast cancer. Such a tragic family history could understandably cause such a patient to experience fears about her own health. These fears might make her seek out genetic testing or even prophylactic mastectomy. On the other hand, her fear could create an attitude of denial or hopelessness that leads her to avoid taking such necessary preventive steps as getting regular mammograms.

Providers also should strive to understand and work with their patients' beliefs concerning the role of institutionalized health care and the health care provider. Obviously, such beliefs are shaped, to a large degree, by the beliefs of the patient's family. Knowing, for example, that a particular family turns to the medical community only after employing traditional remedies should provide important information to the provider when a member of that family shows up in the examination room. And understanding the family's expectations regarding the role of health care professionals versus the role of the family provides some direction when it comes to communication.

In some cultures, for example, patients will have a whole network of people on whom to rely in times of illness, and they may feel more comfortable and recover more quickly when they are allowed to use that support system (Shubin, 1980). In such situations, health care professionals actively work to optimize patient care when they seek ways to understand and honor the role of family in health care. However, to make use of this network of care for a particular patient, providers first need to recognize that it is part of his or her culture.

Allowing family members to participate in a patient's health care can have more immediate advantages as well. For example, when dietary changes are part of the suggested treatment plan, a patient may best be served if health care providers explain the importance of those changes to the person who prepares the patient's meals. In many cases, that person will be a family member and not the patient. In addition, there are times when information from family members gives health care providers insight into a patient's recovery or overall well-being. An undiagnosed case of depression, for example, might hinder a patient's recovery from surgery or illness. The patient may not be forthcoming in admitting his or her struggle with depression, but other members of the family might.

And consider the case of a woman who, after undergoing surgery to remove a brain tumor, assumed that the nausea and vomiting she was experiencing was "normal" and so did not mention those symptoms at her follow-up visit with her physician. It was only after her daughter brought them to the physician's attention that the patient learned that these discomforts were not normal and were, in fact, the result of excessive fluid on her brain.

These scenarios highlight the potential for improved patient care that exists when health care providers adopt an approach that allows them to take advantage of their patients' family ties and that opens a line of communication with family members.

Sex and Gender

The very fact of being male or female will influence a person's experience with the health care environment. Gender is one of the major determinants of health because certain illnesses or diseases are more likely to affect one sex than the other. In addition, certain behaviors that have been shown to affect health, like using tobacco or drinking alcohol, are associated with gender-based patterns.

Yet medical research has been criticized for devoting more resources to studying men than women. Doyal (1995, p. 17) observes,

> Both the priorities and the techniques of biomedical research reflect the white male domination of the profession. Bias has been identified in the choice and the defini-tion of problems to be studied, the methods employed to carry out the research, and the interpretation and application of results. . . . There has been relatively little ba-sic research into non-reproductive conditions that mainly affect women. . . . Where health problems affect both men and women, few studies have explored possible differences between the sexes in their development, symptoms and treatment.

For a long time, the male body was treated as the norm, and information gathered from studies based on men was applied to women without much consideration for biological differences. Until relatively recently, for example, clinical drug trials were conducted on men only. Once the research was completed, the medical community applied the results to women as though they were just smaller men—and without having asked the necessary questions about how a woman's different chemical or cellular makeup might lead to different results.

In the 1980s, activist groups in the United States began to push for the right of women to participate in clinical trials in the same numbers as men, arguing that female patients should have the same opportunities to reap the potential benefits of the drugs being tested. They also called for changes in research methods to ensure that the knowledge gained would be of equal value to men and women (Mastroianni, Faden, & Federman, 1994). In addition to achieving gender equity, these activist groups claimed that such changes would be more efficient because drugs tested only on men might turn out to be more or less potent in women. Including women in appropriate numbers during the initial testing of drug treatments would bring these differences to the forefront early on, they argued, and preclude the squandering of resources and the delivery of inappropriate care.

Legislation such as the Women's Health Equity Act (1990) required all federally funded projects to include women and men (and members of different ethnic groups) in numbers appropriate to the problem being studied. Some other countries, including Canada, Australia, and South Africa, have implemented similar guidelines, but ridding medical research of gender bias is by no means a worldwide priority. Doyal (2003) points out that a survey of British medical schools uncovered the lack of a systematic approach to gender issues and health. It found that, although individual schools might offer a course here or there having to do with gender and health, those courses are not consistent from school to school. And there is little effort to connect the ideas taught in the courses to broader public programs.

Far from being a problem just for those in research and education, the issue of gender differences in health care affects all aspects of patient care. Interestingly, certain inequalities in care seem to be self-imposed by patients themselves. For instance, gender may influence how long a patient will wait before seeking treatment. Studies report that men may find it more difficult to accept or admit to illness; therefore, they may delay seeking medical advice (Cameron & Bernardes, 1998; Sabo & Gordon, 1995; Watson, 2000).

Equally significant is the difference in care that men and women receive once they do seek medical treatment. Numerous studies from different countries have shown that health workers may diagnose male and female patients differently, even when the symptoms and clinical findings are similar. Shaw, Hachamovitch, and Redberg (2000) suggest that providers may choose different treatment for men than they do for women in what appear to be identical clinical situations.

For example, according to McKinley (1996), health care professionals are more likely to miss myocardial infarctions in women under age 65 than in men of the same age. In addition, women are less likely to receive certain procedures (e.g., coronary angioplasty, acute catheterization) even though these interventions are equally effective for both sexes (Mark, 2000; Wenger, 1997). Other studies show that women on kidney dialysis are less likely than men to be offered transplants (Held et al., 1988).

In addition to gender disparities, we must consider gender relationships within different ethnic communities. These relationships can differ dramatically, affecting the expectations that members of various communities have about health care. More traditional cultures, such as those in the Middle East and some Latin countries, for example, tend to place men at the center of decision making about reproduction.

Recent surveys in Honduras found that roughly one-quarter of women and men reported male-centered decision-making attitudes and behaviors related to family planning use or family size (Speizer, Whittle, & Carter, 2005). Honduran women who lived in less urbanized areas, had less than a secondary education, or had medium or low socioeconomic status were more likely to live in a household where men made reproductive decisions and to believe that men alone should make such decisions. Education was an important factor in the study: the least educated Honduran men were more likely to support and practice male-centered decision making.

Similar patterns emerge in studies of patients in Middle Eastern countries. In a survey of Egyptian men and women, for example, only 41% of married women responded that their views about family planning carried any weight in the household, whereas a majority of those polled (60.4%) said they thought family planning decisions should be made by both partners (Govindasamy & Malhotra, 1996).

Still, ideals and practices are not always the same. Health care providers caring for patients from other cultures should understand traditional views about reproduction and differences in power between the sexes, especially when advising patients about personal health decisions, such as which birth control methods to use. Some cultures are considerably more conservative about sexual functioning than are others. In fact, according to some studies, migration to and residence in the United States do not necessarily alter traditional beliefs. In contrast with their nonmigrant peers, for example, Mexican women in the United States were found to average higher emotional consonance with their partners, but lower relationship control and sexual negotiation power (Parrado, Flippen, & McQuiston, 2005).

Should health care providers and community workers play a role in encouraging more equitable relations between the men and women for whom they care? Opinions are mixed. "Telling women to talk with their husbands about reproductive decision making would probably be unhelpful in places where prevailing gender norms do not encourage this type of communication," note Speizer and colleagues (2005, p. 137). Nevertheless, making gender-based power an integral feature of sexual and reproductive health programs could offer advantages for women and men (Blanc, 2001). In any event, both men and women should be aware that some traditional beliefs and practices could have a detrimental effect on the quality of their health care and their lives.

For example, more equitable decision making may encourage safer sex through the wider use of condoms. Among mostly Latina women at an urban community health center in Massachusetts, those with high levels of power as measured by the Sexual Relationship Power Scale (SRPS) were five times more likely than women with low levels to report consistent condom use (Pulerwitz, Amaro, De Jong, Gortmaker, & Rudd, 2002). In a sample of women at risk for HIV and other sexually transmitted diseases recruited from clinics and community locations in Atlanta, Los Angeles, Oklahoma City, and Portland, OR, more than half reported that they share power with their partner (Harvey, Bird, Galavotti, Duncan, & Greenberg, 2002). Although relationship power was not associated with condom use in the study, women who reported that they made decisions about using condoms alone or with their partner were more likely to use condoms than those who reported that their partner made those decisions.

Health beliefs also may differ between men and women of different ethnicities and different cultural backgrounds. A study comparing the beliefs of African American women and White women about breast cancer offers one case in point. In the study, African American women were more likely to believe in chance or to depend on powerful others (i.e., other people in their lives to whom they attributed power and wisdom) for their health. Perceived susceptibility to cancer, doubts about the value of early diagnosis, and beliefs about the seriousness of breast cancer all were significantly associated with powerful other scores among African American women. Although no relationship was found between health beliefs and years of education in African American women, White women with the least education were more likely to believe that death was inevitable with a cancer diagnosis (Barroso et al., 2000).

By approaching patient interactions with an informed and expanded view, health care providers can adapt explanations of illnesses and treatments so they are more meaningful for patients. For example, the need to immediately report adverse reactions to drug therapies, rather than "toughing it out," should be emphasized because contrasting notions about pain behavior could have clinical relevance. In a study comparing beliefs about pain behavior held by Japanese and by Euro-Americans, female participants were found to consider pain behaviors (such as the verbal expression of pain) more acceptable than were male participants (Hobara, 2005). Differences were found across cultures too: compared with both male and female Japanese, Euro-Americans rated pain behaviors in both sexes as more acceptable.

Awareness of cultural norms is key to successful patient management. Gender differences affect the health care system, and patients with low health literacy—especially women operating under the demands and assumptions of traditional cultures—may be less confident about communicating their needs or beliefs with their providers. Seals (2005, p. 2) notes that "traditionally, in the formal healthcare system, 'women's health' has focused almost exclusively on childbearing and reproductive organ-related problems or disease." Discrepancies such as these, he says, point to the impact of culture and the traditional role of women.

Today, the health care field is challenged to redefine women's health. In doing so, health care providers must take into account the impact of sex and gender on the health care experience of all patients, both male and female. Similarly, they must recognize the inherent risks patients face by virtue of their biology, as well as the pressures they face while operating in a world that values, say, stoicism in men or assumes that heart disease is a man's disease. A first step for health care providers is to understand that beliefs about sex and gender are not the same from culture to culture—or even within the same or similar cultures—and that awareness about such differences goes a long way toward dealing appropriately and adequately with them.

Race and Ethnicity

Over the past several decades, the United States has made numerous advances in the area of racial and ethnic equality. For many, it may be tempting to point to these gains as evidence that the problem of inequality is adequately "on the radar" of the nation's political and institutional powers. But despite improvements, raised awareness, and other positive developments, disparities still exist. And health care is one area in which ethnic inequality remains particularly apparent and important.

A disproportionate number of minorities are afflicted with diabetes and cardiovascular disease, for example. They have higher infant mortality rates and lower rates of childhood immunization than Whites. Overall, statistics indicate that, at least as far as health is concerned, minorities have not yet achieved equality. Consider the following research findings:

- African Americans, American Indians, Hawaiians, Indians, Pakistanis, Mexicans, South and Central Americans, and Puerto Ricans are 1.4 to 3.6 times more likely to present with advanced (stage IV) breast cancer than are non-Hispanic Whites (Li, Malone, & Daling, 2003).
- African American females experience higher death rates from breast cancer than any other racial or ethnic group, even though Whites experience higher incidence rates (National Cancer Institute, 2003).
- For early-stage lung cancer, the rates of surgery and of 5-year survival are lower for African Americans than for Whites. However, for those who undergo surgery, survival rates are similar despite racial differences. This suggests that the lower survival rates among African Americans could be due to the lower rate of surgical treatment (Bach, Cramer, & Warren, 1999).
- Data collected from January to September 2002 via a National Health Interview Survey reveal that, of people aged 65 years and older who were surveyed, 60% of White non-Hispanics had received a pneumococcal vaccination at some point. Yet in the same age group only 35% of African American respondents and 25% of Hispanic respondents had ever received a pneumococcal vaccination (National Center for Health Statistics, 2003).

Even in light of these findings, which point so clearly to the fact that full equality in the realm of health care has not yet been achieved, misperceptions abound. A 1999 Kaiser Family Foundation survey on public perceptions of the quality of care received by other ethnic groups compared to Whites makes this clear. More than two-thirds (67%) of Whites surveyed indicated that they believed African Americans received the same quality of care that they did. More than half of Whites surveyed (59%) reported that they believed Latinos also received the same quality of care (Kaiser Family Foundation, 1999).

Health care providers are not above having misperceptions about ethnicity and health care quality. In a survey conducted in 2001, only 29% of the physicians who participated thought that people were treated unfairly by the health care system "very or somewhat often" based on their racial/ethnic background. Those who acknowledged disparities usually attributed them to patient characteristics, such as insurance (or lack thereof), education, or personal preferences (Kaiser Family Foundation, 2002).

On the other hand, a Commonwealth Fund 2001 Health Care Quality Survey focusing on patient perceptions revealed that Blacks, Hispanics, and Asians were more likely than Whites to believe that they would receive better medical care if they belonged to a different race. Members of these groups also felt that medical staff judged them unfairly or treated them disrespectfully because of their race or fluency in English (Johnson, Saha, & Arbelaez, 2004).

Health care providers must educate themselves about such disparities and examine their own beliefs and behaviors to identify ways that their own culture might be contributing to the overall environment of inequality. It is the least that those who are truly committed to providing care that is not only culturally competent care but also the best care for all patients can do. By recognizing how your culture affects your treatment of patients, you can adapt your approach if necessary.

In addition to these rather high-level effects of race and ethnicity on health and health care, culture also can have an impact on individual patients and the interactions health care providers have with them. For example, research suggests that Latino patients have a tendency to be forthcoming with their symptoms and are generally comfortable with conventional treatments. Japanese patients, on the other hand, may be more closed-lipped about their symptoms (Shiba & Oka, 1996). They may be reluctant to divulge information if they feel nervous or uncomfortable with the provider (e.g., because of the provider's age, gender, tone of voice, gestures, or other factors), and they often prefer homeopathic remedies to more conventional treatments.

Recognizing these culturally based differences in the way patients behave may not change a diagnosis or a treatment plan, but it can offer health care providers a perspective with which to examine inconsistencies between the information obtained from an interview with the patient and the results of clinical tests.

Ethnicity also may affect patients' attitudes toward the role their health care providers ought to play. Although White, native-born Americans of European descent tend to believe that they should be involved in decisions regarding their own health and treatment, patients of other backgrounds sometimes prefer that their providers act as experts who make the best possible decisions on behalf of their patients (Salimbene, 2000).

In Russian medicine, for example, it is not unusual for a physician to decide a patient's level of life support without consulting the patient or the patient's family (Karakuzon, 2002). For Russian immigrants or even U.S.-born patients of Russian descent, this desire for health care professionals to make the decisions related to patient care could come into play. Health care providers working with such patients should be aware of cultural differences among them and act accordingly.

Legal requirements and an emphasis on informed consent have led to a "full disclosure" health care environment in the United States. This attitude of giving patients complete information regarding their conditions, treatments, and prognoses may be at odds with the values of many patients. The families of terminally ill Hispanic, Chinese, and Pakistani patients, for example, may prefer to keep knowledge of their loved one's condition from them, even refusing to translate diagnosis and treatment options at times (Kaufert & Putsch, 1997). Directly informing a patient of a cancer diagnosis is seen as cruel in some Asian cultures (Holland, Geary, Marchini, & Tross, 1987; Matsumura et al., 2002).

Some patients believe that it's the job of the health care provider to help them hold on to hope. Often they expect providers to withhold terminal diagnoses or to avoid discussions regarding end-of-life care. Filipino patients, for example, may feel that talking about end-of-life care denigrates the belief that God determines each person's fate (Yeo & Hikuyeda, 2000). The Navajo even believe that talking about illness or death is dangerous because words may become reality. Chinese patients, too, may be reluctant to discuss such topics because of their belief that doing so may become a self-fulfilling prophecy.

Ethnicity influences the role that family plays in a given patient's health care experience. In some cultures, the family is given considerable input in this area. According to Beauchamp and Childress (1994), for example, Koreans and Mexican Americans are more likely to agree that family members, and not just the patient, should make decisions about life support. In Asian cultures, illness is viewed as a family—rather than an individual—event. In Asian families, concern for the patient is mirrored by an equal concern for the family (Candib, 2002).

Home Remedies and Complementary and Alternative Health Care

In 1993, Eisenberg and colleagues published a landmark study on alternative therapy use in the United States. In it, they defined alternative therapies as "medical interventions not widely taught at United States medical schools or generally available at United States hospitals" (Eisenberg et al., 1993, p. 246). The National Library of Medicine (NLM) Medical Subject Heading (MeSH) considers complementary and alternative medicine (CAM) therapies to be "therapeutic practices which are not currently considered an integral part of conventional allopathic medical practice" (National Library of Medicine, 2005).

The definition goes on to explain that CAM therapies "may lack biomedical explanations but as they become better researched some (physical therapy, diet, acupuncture) become widely accepted whereas others (humors, radium therapy) quietly fade away, yet are important historical footnotes." Therapies are considered *complementary* when used in addition to conventional treatments and *alternative* when used instead of conventional treatment. The National Center for Complementary and Alternative Medicine, or NCCAM, the federal government's lead agency for scientific research on CAM therapies, defines them as "a group of diverse medical and health care systems, practices, and products that are not presently considered to be part of conventional medicine" (NCCAM, 2002).

Regardless of the definition used, most people would not be surprised to learn that research indicates an increase in the use of CAM therapies in the United States in recent years. In the 1993 study, Eisenberg and colleagues found that 34% of those surveyed had used some form of CAM therapy in the previous year. In fact, visits to providers of CAM therapies outnumbered those to primary care physicians that year (Eisenberg et al., 1993).

In a follow-up study, Eisenberg and colleagues (1998) reported that the use of CAM therapies had increased to 42.1% of patients and that patients' total out-of-pocket expenditures for CAM therapies had more than doubled. In May 2003, a study in the journal *Pediatrics* reported the results of a study of 142 families and their use of non-FDA-regulated herbal products and home remedies with pediatric patients. Forty-five percent of the caregivers who participated in the study admitted to giving their children an herbal product (Lanski, Greenwald, Perkins, & Simon, 2003).

Today, mainstream television programming is peppered with advertisements for herbal remedies claiming to address the symptoms of the common cold and influenza. The local grocery store sells supplements that are supposed to help with ailments ranging from jet lag to eczema. An Internet search for "natural health care" will turn up tens of millions of Web sites discussing, promoting, or selling remedies for ear infections, hypertension, menopause symptoms, high cholesterol, and other health problems.

It is true that some therapies originally considered unconventional by mainstream medicine are becoming more widely accepted. However, patients still face potential dangers when they engage in the use of certain alternative treatments. Some herbal therapies, for example, may have potentially harmful side effects and adverse interactions with other medication (Lanski et al., 2003). The herbal and "all natural" product ephedra has been linked to cardiovascular problems, and some researchers have suggested a relationship between kava kava use and hepatotoxicity (U.S. Food and Drug Administration, 2002). Some patients report that, although they do not avoid mainstream medicine, they tend to use herbal remedies in conjunction with conventional treatments, often without consulting their providers regarding possible interactions between the therapies (Ngo-Metzger et al., 2003).

Other CAM remedies may prove benign but ineffective. The problem is that manufacturers are not required to prove that their herbal products are safe or effective before they put them on the market (Lanski et al., 2003). Therefore, in some cases, patients are just wasting their money on products that do not address their physical complaints. In other cases, by using herbal therapies, unsuspecting patients may be engaging in behavior that is actually detrimental to their health.

Alternative therapies such as cupping and coining may not be dangerous, but they could affect a patient's health care. Ngo-Metzger and colleagues (2003) point out that bruises left by such procedures can be mistaken by health care providers as indicators of hematological diseases or signs of abuse. Such misunderstandings could lead to misdiagnosis or unnecessary testing for the patient.

In the study by Lanski and colleagues, the therapies used included aloe plant juice, echinacea, sweet oil, and even such unusual products as pine needles, turpentine, and cow chips. Most significant to a discussion of health literacy is the fact that, of all the people interviewed in this study, 77% did not believe or were uncertain whether herbal products produced side effects. Sixty-six percent were unsure or thought that herbal products did not interact with other medicines. What's more, only 45% of participants who reported giving herbal products to their children said they had discussed the use of those products with their children's primary health care provider. Instead, according to 80% of those participants who admitted to using alternative remedies, family and friends were their sources of information (Lanski et al., 2003).

Despite this and similar studies that indicate a high rate of herbal medicine use in the United States, health care providers underestimate the prevalence of the use of such remedies among their patient base. This is partly because patients report having encountered negative reactions from Western clinicians when broaching the subject of alternative therapies, as in the following example:

> I [a Chinese woman] told the doctor, "I am taking some angelica and ginseng. Do you think it is OK?" The doctor said, "I don't know Chinese medicine.... You should be responsible for the results if you take them!" After that I did not dare mention Chinese medicine again (Ngo-Metzger et al., 2003, p. 48).

Experiences such as these can cause patients to be more reluctant to disclose CAM use with their health care providers. But the resulting discrepancy between actual patient behavior and health care providers' perceptions is problematic.

For optimal patient care, then, health care providers should approach patients' health beliefs and practices with respect, screen patients for the use of herbal products and alternative treatments, and discuss with them the possible implications of using CAM therapies with conventional treatments.

Spiritual Beliefs and Values

The intersection of medicine and spirituality is of increasing concern and interest among those in the medical community. In the past, patients' beliefs about the spiritual or supernatural dimension of illness were considered irrelevant at best; at worst they were looked down on as ridiculous. Today, however, U.S. medical schools offer classes on medical ethics in various faiths and the beliefs of non-Western religions.

Such education does not make health care professionals experts in religion, however, and this poses a problem for them. On the one hand, most patients want physicians to ask about their spiritual beliefs in at least some instances (McCord et al., 2004). Patients in one study believed that information concerning their spiritual beliefs would assist their health care providers in encouraging hope (67%), giving medical advice (66%), and changing medical treatment (62%; McCord et al., 2004). In addition, King and Bushwick (1994) found that 70% of patients would welcome physician inquiry into their religious beliefs, 55% would appreciate silent prayer, and 50% believe their physician should pray with them.

It would be easy to assert that health care professionals have no business dealing with their patient's spirituality. After all, they are not experts in religion or spirituality. Many see the study of medicine as logical and factual, not spiritual. What such a position fails to take into account, however, is that, regardless of the religious or spiritual attitudes of health care providers, religion and spirituality permeate all aspects of life for patients who are devout. Quite often in the United States, the religious and spiritual beliefs held by patients affect their health care decisions and practices.

Perhaps the most obvious example of religion informing health care decisions is that of Christian Scientists, who may choose prayer rather than medical treatment for healing. But that is not the only example. Other faiths also affect a patient's health care choices. Jehovah's Witnesses do not accept blood transfusions; they request nonblood alternatives instead. The religious beliefs of Roman Catholics might make certain fertility treatments (e.g., in vitro fertilization) undesirable because they conflict with church doctrine. For some Jewish families, the decision of whether to circumcise their infant boys is as much a question of faith and tradition as it is a medical decision.

If religion and belief affect the medical decisions of the followers of these faiths, imagine the conflict that religious beliefs pose for followers of those faiths who are further removed from the history of Western medicine. The Mien and Hmong Vietnamese groups, for instance, see health care providers who do not intrude on the body as the ultimate healers. Consequently, they often resist invasive medical techniques (LaBorde, 1996). In fact, we saw just such beliefs playing out in the passages from Anne Fadiman's *The Spirit Catches You and You Fall Down* (1997).

All patients, even those who do not belong to or believe in a particular religion or spiritual practice, make decisions about what is medically or morally good according to a specific worldview or thought tradition. When religion and spirituality are part of the patient's tradition, the effect on his or her health care is compounded. Providers have much to gain from an understanding of their patients' beliefs. "The individual's search for his or her good is generally and characteristically conducted within a context defined by those traditions of which the individual's life is a part," explains ethicist Alisdair MacIntyre (1984).

What, then, is the appropriate role for the health care provider when it comes to the patient's spirituality? Should providers listen to patients' concerns without comment? Should they respond with affirmation and counsel? What if patients ask them to pray, as 50% of patients believe they should (King & Bushwick, 1994)? And what if patients ask them to participate in or assist in healing rituals? What if these rituals contradict standard medical care? What if they conflict with the beliefs of the health care providers themselves?

Patient Views of the Health Care System and Providers

Interestingly, though it seems logical that culture would influence patients' views of the health care system and health care providers, interviews with patients reveal that any dissonance they perceive in patient–provider interactions is more generic in nature (Shapiro, Hollingshead, & Morrison, 2002). Complaints about excessive waiting time are common among patients, for example, as is the notion that doctors don't really listen.

Other patients' dislikes, according to Shapiro and colleagues (2002), include providers acting like they know it all, treating patients as ignorant, minimizing patients' complaints or not taking them seriously, using technical language, being dismissive of patients' efforts to research their own conditions, and telling patients not to use homeopathic remedies.

BODY LANGUAGE/NONVERBAL CUES

It has been estimated that in a typical conversation between two people, fully two-thirds of all meaning exchanged is transmitted on a nonverbal level (Brill, 1973). That means that the spoken word is not the primary method of communication for people engaged in conversation, as we might be tempted to think.

This fact has interesting implications for health care providers, both in their role as transmitters of information and in their role as collectors of information. Clinical efficacy hinges heavily on good communication. To successfully treat their patients, providers must understand and must be understood. It therefore behooves providers to become students of body language.

After all, if our own body language is communicating information to the patient, we should be sure the information is correct and that it supports the message we want to get across. Conversely, if a patient's body language represents a means to increased understanding of his or her condition, we would not want to miss a chance to understand our patients that much better.

Certain gestures have been shown to reflect particular attitudes or beliefs. Some of those gestures and their corresponding "meanings" are shown in Table 5.1. However, no gesture can be assumed to have the same meaning in every situation. A given body movement may be culturally defined. Nodding the head up and down generally signals agreement or "yes" in most parts of the world, but in regions of India it means the opposite. The reverse is true, too: shaking the head from side to side generally indicates disagreement or "no," but in India it can mean "yes." In fact, in India a head wiggle can serve many purposes, from acknowledging a friend to giving thanks.

Nonverbal communication is affected by culture both when it is transmitted and when it is received. This is illustrated in the example of the Indian head wiggle just mentioned. Our response to a nod or shaking of the head is culture specific. In Iran, Nigeria, Australia, Bangladesh, and elsewhere, the "thumbs up" gesture is considered rude and obscene; in the United States it signals thanks or approval. Koreans point with their middle finger, which at first might seem disconcerting to a Westerner. In Japan, tipping your head backward and sucking

TABLE 5.1 WHAT SOME OF YOUR PATIENTS' GESTURES MIGHT SUGGEST

A complete lexicon of nonverbal communication would contain far too many entries to detail here. However, because health care professionals can benefit from an understanding of the gestures they are most likely to encounter when interacting with patients, some of those gestures and their possible meanings are identified below.

Crossed arms can be an indication of a desire to isolate or protect oneself. It can also show a person's defiance or rejection of what is being said. In some cases, this gesture is indicative of a person's desire to be heard (Nierenberg and Calero, 1971).

Touching the nose can indicate confusion if it occurs in response to being asked a question. This gesture is often accompanied by the person squirming or physically withdrawing (Scheflen, 1972).

Nail biting, thumb sucking, wringing hands. All of these gestures can be seen as signs of nervousness and a need for reassurance.

Silence may be an expression of hostility.

Covering the mouth may indicate that the speaker has said something he or she considers to be embarrassing or taboo (Scheflen, 1973).

Outstretched hands. When a person extends his or her arms with palms facing up, the gesture may be an expression of feelings of helplessness or resignation (Scheflen, 1973).

Biting the lips, fidgeting. These and similar gestures may be indications that the person is nervous.

Shrugging the shoulders may indicate indifference.

Lifting the eyebrows can be an indication of doubt.

---

air through your teeth means "no" or that something is difficult. Those wishing to learn more about nonverbal communication in various cultures should consult Roger E. Axtell's *Gestures: The Do's and Taboos of Body Language Around the World* (1991), a breezily written introduction to gestures and body language across the globe.

What, then, are the implications of nonverbal communication for health care providers? There are many. In terms of health literacy, we now realize that both the patients' and the health care providers' cultures come into play in ways that might be unconscious, but still are significant.

PROVIDERS AS RECEIVERS OF NONVERBAL COMMUNICATION

Compassionate and careful health care providers need to take the available information regarding nonverbal information into account when dealing with patients. In their role as receivers of patients' information, as contained in medical histories, explanations of symptoms, and reports of compliance with prescribed remedies, health care professionals can use information about nonverbal communication to understand their patients more fully. In addition to helping providers understand possible discrepancies in meaning between the nodding and shaking of their patient's head, knowledge of nonverbal communication can offer another means to ensure that they receive their patients' messages accurately.

This is not to say that all health care professionals are duty bound to become experts in the field of nonverbal communication. However, those professionals who interact with patients should become more sensitive to nonverbal communication, especially when it appears to conflict with what is being said. For instance, when working with a patient whose culture places a premium on quietly enduring suffering or working through pain, a provider should be more sensitive to possible nonverbal signals of discomfort even if the patient reports feeling fine.

PROVIDERS AS TRANSMITTERS OF NONVERBAL COMMUNICATION

As a health care provider, you invariably send nonverbal messages that become infused with extra importance. Your patients look to you for information, and it is important to realize that the information you impart is not transmitted wholly by your words. In an ideal situation, your nonverbal behavior will complement your spoken message, but if you ignore the impact of nonverbal communication, such an oversight can end up undermining or even contradicting your words.

Why should you bother to worry about body language and facial expressions? Why not just expect patients to listen to your words and take their meaning at face value? Because you do not want to run the risk of being misunderstood. You want to put your patients at ease and optimize their understanding of your words. A study by DiMatteo, Taranta, Friedman, and Prince (1980) suggests that health care providers who can accurately interpret their patients' nonverbal messages and who can themselves express emotions nonverbally have patients who are more satisfied. A number of studies also suggest a direct correlation between effective provider–patient communication and patient compliance with care instructions and drug regimens (Betancourt, Carrillo, & Green, 1999; DiMatteo, 1995; DiMatteo, Hays, & Prince, 1986; Winnick, Lucas, Hartman, & Toll, 2005).

Health care providers who understand their own nonverbal behavior, then, may be able to use it to improve communication with their patients, thereby improving patients' outcomes. After all, improved patient–provider communication contributes to patients' understanding of instructions, illness, and treatments. And when patients understand what their health care providers are asking them to do—whether it is taking an antibiotic three times a day or scheduling a follow-up appointment in 2 weeks—they are in a better position to comply. (For more about communicating with low-literate patients during the clinical encounter, see chapter 6, Improving Patient–Provider Communication.)

TOWARD A CULTURALLY COMPETENT PRACTICE

Of course, it would be impossible to imagine every possible scenario that might present itself in the course of a patient–provider interaction. Even more impossible would be any attempt to consider all the cultural variations on those scenarios. Yet health care professionals are challenged to establish individual and group approaches that work for patients of diverse cultures.

Directions: Use your Web browser to print this page to a printer. (Note: You may need to use Page Setup in your browser to set the left and right margins to .25 inches or less if the printout is missing text from the right side edge.) Then, with paper in hand, select A, B, or C for each numbered item listed.

A = Things I do frequently
B = Things I do occasionally
C = Things I do rarely or never

PHYSICAL ENVIRONMENT, MATERIALS, AND RESOURCES

____ 1. I display pictures, posters, and other materials that reflect the cultures and ethnic backgrounds of children and families served by my program or agency.

____ 2. I insure that magazines, brochures, and other printed materials in reception areas are of interest to and reflect the different cultures of children and families served by my program or agency.

____ 3. When using videos, films, or other media resources for health education, treatment, or other interventions, I insure that they reflect the cultures of children and families served by my program or agency.

____ 4. When using food during an assessment, I insure that meals provided include foods that are unique to the cultural and ethnic backgrounds of children and families served by my program or agency.

____ 5. I insure that toys and other play accessories in reception areas, and those which are used during assessment, are representative of the various cultural and ethnic groups within the local community and the society in general.

COMMUNICATION STYLES

____ 6. For children who speak languages or dialects other than English, I attempt to learn and use key words in their language so that I am better able to communicate with them during assessment, treatment, or other interventions.

____ 7. I attempt to determine any familial colloquialisms used by children and families that may impact on assessment, treatment, or other interventions.

____ 8. I use visual aids, gestures, and physical prompts in my interactions with children who have limited English proficiency.

____ 9. I use bilingual staff or trained/certified interpreters for assessment, treatment, and other interventions with children who have limited English proficiency.

____ 10. I use bilingual staff or trained/certified interpreters during assessments, treatment sessions, meetings, and other events for families who would require this level of assistance.

____ 11. When interacting with parents who have limited English proficiency I always keep in mind that:

____ * limitations in English proficiency are in no way a reflection of their level of intellectual functioning.

____ * their limited ability to speak the language of the dominant culture has no bearing on their ability to communicate effectively in their language of origin.

____ * they may or may not be literate in their language of origin or English.

____ 12. When possible, I insure that all notices and communiqués to parents are written in their language of origin.

____ 13. I understand that it may be necessary to use alternatives to written communications for some families, as word-of-mouth may be a preferred method of receiving information.

VALUES AND ATTITUDES

____ 14. I avoid imposing values that may conflict or be inconsistent with those of cultures or ethnic groups other than my own.

____ 15. In group therapy or treatment situations, I discourage children from using racial and ethnic slurs by helping them understand that certain words can hurt others.

____ 16. I screen books, movies, and other media resources for negative cultural, ethnic, or racial stereotypes before sharing them with children and their parents served by my program or agency.

____ 17. I intervene in an appropriate manner when I observe other staff or parents within my program or agency engaging in behaviors that show cultural insensitivity, bias, or prejudice.

____ 18. I understand and accept that family is defined differently by different cultures (e.g., extended family members, fictive kin, godparents).

____ 19. I recognize and accept that individuals from culturally diverse backgrounds may desire varying degrees of acculturation into the dominant culture.

____ 20. I accept and respect that male-female roles in families may vary significantly among different cultures (e.g., who makes major decisions for the family, play and social interactions expected of male and female children).

Figure 5.1 Cultural Competence Self-Assessment. Although the focus of this self-assessment is on encouraging culturally diverse and culturally competent services for children with disabilities or special health care needs, it applies in most any human service setting.

___ 21. I understand that age and life cycle factors must be considered in interactions with individuals and families (e.g., high value placed on the decisions of elders or the role of the eldest male in families).

___ 22. Even though my professional or moral viewpoints may differ, I accept the family/parents as the ultimate decision makers for services and supports for their children.

___ 23. I recognize that the meaning or value of medical treatment and health education may vary greatly among cultures.

___ 24. I recognize and understand that beliefs and concepts of emotional well-being vary significantly from culture to culture.

___ 25. I understand that beliefs about mental illness and emotional disability are culturally based. I accept that responses to these conditions and related treatment/interventions are heavily influenced by culture.

___ 26. I accept that religion and other beliefs may influence how families respond to illnesses, disease, disability, and death.

___ 27. I recognize and accept that folk and religious beliefs may influence a family's reaction and approach to a child born with a disability or later diagnosed with a physical/emotional disability or special health care needs.

___ 28. I understand that traditional approaches to disciplining children are influenced by culture.

___ 29. I understand that families from different cultures will have different expectations of their children for acquiring toileting, dressing, feeding, and other self-help skills.

___ 30. I accept and respect that customs and beliefs about food, its value, preparation, and use are different from culture to culture.

___ 31. Before visiting or providing services in the home setting, I seek information on acceptable behaviors, courtesies, customs, and expectations that are unique to families of specific cultures and ethnic groups served by my program or agency.

___ 32. I seek information from family members or other key community informants that will assist in service adaptation to respond to the needs and preferences of culturally and ethnically diverse children and families served by my program or agency.

___ 33. I advocate for the review of my program's or agency's mission statement, goals, policies, and procedures to insure that they incorporate principles and practices that promote cultural diversity and cultural competence.

There is no answer key with correct responses. However, if you frequently responded "C," you may not necessarily demonstrate values and engage in practices that promote a culturally diverse and culturally competent service delivery system.

(*Source:* Adapted from *Promoting Cultural Competence and Cultural Diversity in Early Intervention and Early Childhood Settings.* June 1989. Revised 1993, 1996, 1999, 2000, and 2002. Tawara D. Goode, Georgetown University Center for Child and Human Development, University Center for Excellence in Developmental Disabilities Education, Research, and Service. Washington, D.C.: National Center for Cultural Competence. Reprinted with permission. Available at: http://gucchd.georgetown.edu/nccc/nccc7.html.)

Figure 5.1 *(Continued)*

Guidelines for More Culturally Competent Care

Although there are no easy, one-size-fits-all answers, there are some guidelines that health care professionals can follow as a first step toward developing culturally competent behaviors in patient–provider interactions. Adopting these behaviors will go a long way toward optimizing those interactions and contributing to more successful outcomes.

Conduct a Cultural Self-Assessment

Every health care professional brings to the patient–provider relationship his or her personal culture, as well as the culture of the medical environment. It's a lot to manage, but understanding which areas of your practice, knowledge, or behavior could be improved is a logical first step. Such tools as the *Cultural Competence Self Assessment,* developed by Tawara D. Goode of the Georgetown University Child Development Center and presented in Figure 5.1, can help (Goode, 2002).

Do Some Homework

Look back over your records for the last few months to determine which cultural groups your patients came from. Without much effort, you should be able to learn a little about each of those cultures. It should not be hard to do, and your efforts are sure to be rewarded with greater understanding among your patients and an increased ability to ask meaningful questions and to gather significant information.

Make Your Office Culturally Comfortable

Try to find magazines and newspapers of cultural interest to your patients or in their native language. In addition, assess whether the signs and posters on your waiting room walls are meaningful to them. If you serve patients from Asia or the Middle East, consider having tea available (Salimbene, 2000). Such small touches can go a long way toward making patients feel welcomed and understood.

Respect Cultural Differences

This means more than simply paying lip service to tolerance and acceptance. It means acknowledging and adapting to the fact that different cultural groups may have very different ideas about certain issues. For example, different cultural groups have varying ideas about what is appropriate in nonverbal communication, such as eye contact and proximity. Westerners may view eye contact as a sign of interest and respect, but some cultural groups believe that it is disrespectful to make eye contact with those who are older or in a position of authority.

Although it may not be possible to predict accurately how each patient will feel about these topics, it is possible to research and become more aware of the differences in body language among the different cultural groups in your community. In all situations, it is a good rule of thumb to take cues regarding nonverbal communication from patients.

Keep Language Simple

Avoid using unnecessary jargon or offering extraneous information. Keep in mind that some cultures view "small talk" as inappropriate. It's best to use *who, what, when, where, why, how,* and *which* questions to gather information. If your patient's response seems irrelevant or vague, rephrase your question in simpler terms (Salimbene, 2000).

Ask Questions That Will Help Determine Your Patient's Beliefs and Behaviors

Often, newly admitted hospital patients are simply asked whether they are affiliated with a specific religious denomination. But Joan E. Kub, PhD, RN, a professor of nursing who also has studied theology, believes that it may be more helpful for nurses to formulate specific questions about patients' religious practices and the importance of religion in their lives (Blum, 2004). Such information, she says, can aid nurses in helping patients stay connected to their religious affiliation. According to previous studies, religious affiliation has been associated with better health outcomes and increased longevity, coping skills, and quality of life (Blum, 2004; Levin, 1996).

Never Dismiss or Ridicule Patients' Beliefs

Even if you think they are misguided, a patient's beliefs can affect his or her health and compliance with treatment. For example, a patient's belief that he or she has been hexed or is being punished by a supernatural power may result in poor compliance with your treatment plan because that patient may believe there is nothing you can do to cure the illness (Salimbene, 2000).

Do What You Can to Accommodate the Patient's Family

Do not become annoyed if a patient brings friends or family along to the appointment. In many cultures, decisions regarding health are routinely made only after consulting with family members. By accepting and respecting this cultural behavior, you can improve your relationship with your patient and increase his or her confidence in you as a health care provider (Salimbene, 2000).

Respect Cultural Beliefs That Affect How Bad News Should be Delivered

Patients' preferences regarding the delivery of bad news can vary with ethnic background (Lee, Batal, Maselli, & Kutner, 2002; Searight & Gafford, 2005). In some cultures it is not considered appropriate to give a poor prognosis directly to the patient. In others, certain words (e.g., cancer) are never used. In cases such as these, it's best to follow the advice of the patient's family about how much to disclose and how to present the information (Salimbene, 2000). Some cultures even believe that the act of articulating bad news is connected with poor outcomes (Lee, Batal, Maselli, & Kutner, 2002; Searight & Gafford, 2005).

Carrese and Rhodes (1995) point out, for example, that the Navajo concept of *hozho* (harmony) influences communication and dictates that providers and patients alike speak and think in a positive way because doing otherwise would be a violation of Navajo values. Lee, Back, Block, and Stewart (2002) believe that such attitudes may be more widespread than many providers realize. If these researchers are correct, it is a good argument in favor of increased attention on the part of health care providers to the differences between their own cultural beliefs and those of their patients.

Be Aware of the First Impression You Make

You should strive to appear polite, professional, and unhurried when interacting with patients. Something as simple as shaking hands on first meeting a patient can help create a foundation of trust. Handshakes signal respect and consideration, and studies confirm that a firm handshake contributes to the formation of a favorable impression (Chaplin, Phillips, Brown, Clanton, & Stein, 2000).

When taking a physical history or talking to patients, try to sit down. This simple gesture goes a long way toward communicating to patients that you are interested in what they have to say. It says that you have the time to listen to what patients have to say, to answer any questions they may have, and to fully explain whatever information or instructions you need to communicate. Such behavior by providers also allows patients to relax. It signals to them that their provider will not rush them (Baile et al., 2000).

During All Interactions With Patients, Look Like You Are Listening

First of all, turn toward your patient and lean slightly forward. Do this even if you are using an interpreter to communicate with the patient. This posture strongly suggests interest and engagement. Unless you know that eye contact makes your patient uncomfortable, look at your patient when you speak to him or her. Although it is true that cultural attitudes toward eye contact vary, most patients will feel more comfortable and connected with you if you look at them during the encounter. Eye contact is an important and effective means of establishing rapport with patients from most cultures (Baile et al., 2000).

Another way to make a connection with patients is to touch them on the arm. If the patient is comfortable with it, you may even choose to hold his or her hand (Baile et al., 2000). Avoid looking distracted: thumbing through files or gazing off into the distance may be interpreted as a lack of interest or as a lack of attention or ability. An exception to this rule is if the patient begins to cry. In that case, offer a tissue and look away until the patient has regained his or her composure (Roter, 2005).

Avoid doing anything that might be distracting. If you have a habit of blinking or rolling your eyes, for example, try to keep it in check during interactions with patients. Habits like these can make patients feel that you're not giving them your full and undivided attention. If for some reason you might need to engage in a potentially distracting behavior—say you suffer from allergies that cause you to clear your throat frequently—explain this to your patient at the beginning of your meeting.

Maintain a Neutral Stance

Avoid crossing your arms, which can be interpreted as annoyance or defensiveness. Doing so creates a barrier between you and your patient when you should be establishing rapport. Also, try to avoid crossing your legs. This may be the most comfortable way for you to sit, but to some patients it seems too comfortable or laid back. Instead, try to sit with your knees and feet as close together as feels natural and comfortable. If you are standing, avoid shifting your weight from one foot to the other. This movement comes across as anxious, signaling a desire to finish the conversation. Either of these impressions could make your patient feel dissatisfied with your care.

Smile

Be aware of your own facial expressions throughout your interactions with a patient. Do not be offended if the patient does not return your smile, however. It could be that he or she is trying to be polite. In some cultures (e.g., Korean), smiling at strangers and authority figures is considered rude (Theiderman, 2003).

Understand That Some Patients May not Want to Make Decisions About Their Own Health Care

Lee, Back, et al. (2002) state that older patients and those with certain ethnic backgrounds prefer *less* control over decision making rather than *more*. Wanting to participate in health care decisions is a uniquely White American cultural trait. The researchers also suggest that it is all right and even preferable to share personal recommendations with patients (Lee, Back, et al., 2002). Asking the opinions of patients whose culture places physicians in the role of expert may shake their trust (Salimbene, 2000). However, when you do articulate your own opinions, be careful to reveal any personal biases that influence your thinking (Lee, Back, et al., 2002).

Discovering a patient's preference for information may be as simple as asking him or her about it (Baile et al., 2000). For example, health care providers can ask patients, "How would you like me to give the information about the test results? Would you like me to give you all the information or sketch out the results and spend more time discussing the treatment plan?" If patients do not want to know the details, providers can offer to answer future questions or talk to a relative or a friend (Baile et al., 2000).

Patients who expect their health care providers to be authoritative may ask, "What do you want me to do?" A culturally sensitive and appropriate response might be something like, "Well, if it were me, I would choose X, but I'm required by law to have you make the final decision" (Salimbene, 2000).

Communicating Instructions

Given that roughly 7,000 deaths per year result from medication errors (Phillips, Christenfeld, & Glynn, 1998), it is reasonable to devote some attention to ensuring that patients understand their medication instructions. As we saw earlier, cultural differences between patients and their providers can contribute to misunderstandings and to patients' low health literacy.

The most obvious example occurs when the language of the patient is different from that of the health care provider. In such cases the services of a trained interpreter are invaluable. Often, members of the patient's family accompany the patient and can act as interpreters, but patients may prefer that trained professionals—not just someone who happens to be bilingual—interpret for them (Baker, Parker, Williams, Coates, & Pitkin, 1996).

In cultures in which respect for elders is important, having children interpret can alter family dynamics and cause discomfort in patients (Ngo-Metzger et al., 2003). As we see in chapter 10, Interpreters and Their Role in the Health Care Setting, family members simply are not trained to interpret medical terminology. Relying on them to accurately relay medical information can result in just the opposite, creating the potential for error. In addition, counting on family members to bridge the language gap between patient and provider can put an unnecessary burden on them. They may not always be available to accompany the patient to health care appointments.

A study comparing different methods of interpretation and patients' satisfaction with the health care interaction revealed that patients who use professional interpreters report levels of satisfaction equal to that of patients who are treated by bilingual providers (Lee, Batal, et al., 2002). On the other hand, patients who use family members or nonprofessional interpreters (e.g., bilingual nurses, technicians, receptionists) to communicate with providers report lower levels of satisfaction (Lee, Batal, et al., 2002).

Instructions in Print

Low health literacy affects patient understanding of provider instructions, beginning with the means used to communicate. When language is a barrier, verbal communication is fraught with challenges. Without a skilled translator, written instructions are not any better. In fact, written instructions often fall short, even when they are crafted in the patient's native language. The problem, as outlined in chapter 1 and elsewhere in this book, is a mismatch between the reading level of the material and the reading level of the patient.

Studies on print materials developed for patients' education have established that the reading levels of these materials usually fall in the high school, college, or graduate school range (Rudd, Moeykens, & Colton, 2000). Yet patients for whom these materials are intended read at much lower levels.

When print material is not written in the patient's native language, there are other obstacles to understanding. Securing a translation of the material may do no good: there is always the risk that translators might not accurately relay the information.

Nontext Resources

One way to get around this problem is to use print materials that rely on illustrations rather than text. Studies show that nontext-based media can effectively convey health care information to patients with low health literacy (Schloman, 2004). Pictographs, videos and DVDs, computer-based CDs, audiotapes, and *fotonovelas* are examples of nontext-based materials that have been used to communicate successfully with patients of varying cultures and languages. Such media rely on the ability of photographs and illustrations to improve comprehension among patients with low literacy—an ability that has been observed by researchers (Michielutte et al., 1992).

The main reason these media work in the context of health care is that they reduce the burden of presenting numerous details and explanations in text. Effectively prepared illustrations emphasize important points and motivate patients to read what little text is present. When words are not sufficient to accurately capture the message, illustrations bring an additional dimension to the material (Doak, Doak, & Root, 1996). Yet illustrations, like language, have the drawback of being affected by culture. For pictographs, videos, and other materials focused on illustration to work, the images must conform to the patient's way of perceiving, identifying, and interpreting them (Fuglesang, 1973).

CULTURE AND PATIENT CARE: FROM BELIEFS TO BROCHURES

From beliefs to brochures, the impact of culture on health care is evident. With so many components and so many variables, culture can be hard to define and even harder to analyze. But its effects on health care are significant; no study of health care practices can ignore them. More importantly, no approach that seeks to optimize patient care and outcomes can ignore them. Culture permeates the health care experience. Providers therefore are challenged to recognize the effects of culture and to adopt systematic approaches that respect patients' individual culture while delivering the best possible care.

REFERENCES

American Nurses Association. (2001). *Code of ethics for nurses.* Washington, DC: ANA Publishing.

Axtell, R. E. (1991). *Gestures: The do's and taboos of body language around the world.* New York: John Wiley & Sons.

Bach, P. B., Cramer, L. D., & Warren, J. L. (1999). Racial differences in the treatment of early-stage lung cancer. *New England Journal of Medicine, 341*(16), 1198–1205.

Baile, W. F., Buckman, R., Lenzi, R., Glober, G., Beale, E. A., & Kudelka, A. P. (2000). SPIKES—a six-step protocol for delivering bad news: Application to the patient with cancer. *Oncologist, 5*(4), 302–311.

Baker, D. W., Parker, R. M., Williams, M. V., Coates, W. C., & Pitkin, K. (1996). Use and effectiveness of interpreters in an emergency department. *Journal of the American Medical Association, 275*, 783–788.

Barroso, J., McMillan, S., Casey, L., Gibson, W., Kaminski, G., & Meyer, J. (2000). Comparison between African American and White women in their beliefs about breast cancer and their health locus of control. *Cancer Nursing, 23*(4), 268–276.

Beauchamp, T. L., & Childress, J. F. (1994). *Principles of biomedical ethics* (4th ed.). New York: Oxford University Press.

Betancourt, J. R., Carrillo, J. E., & Green, A. R. (1999). Hypertension in multicultural and minority populations: Linking communication to compliance. *Current Hypertension Report, 1*(6), 482–488.

Blanc, A. K. (2001). The effect of power in sexual relationships on sexual and reproductive health: An examination of the evidence. *Studies in Family Planning, 32*(3), 189–213.

Blum, K. I. (2004). Toward meeting the spiritual needs of the terminally ill. *Johns Hopkins Nursing, 2*, 2. Retrieved March 7, 2006, from http://www.son.jhmi.edu/JHNmagazine/archive/fall2004/pages/bench2bedside.html

Brill, N. T. (1973). *Working with people.* New York: J.B. Lippincott.

Cameron, E., & Bernardes, J. (1998). Gender and disadvantage in health: Men's health for a change. In M. Bartley, D. Blane, & G. Davey Smith (Eds.), *The sociology of health inequalities* (pp. 115–134). Oxford, England: Blackwell Publishers.

Campinha-Bacote, J. (2002). *The process of cultural competence in the delivery of healthcare services: A culturally competent model of care* (4th ed.). Cincinnati, OH: Transcultural C.A.R.E. Associates. Retrieved November 7, 2005, from http://www.transculturalcare.net

Candib, L. M. (2002). Truth telling and advance planning at the end of life: Problems with autonomy in a multicultural world. *Families, Sytems, and Health, 20*, 213–228.

Carrese, J. A., & Rhodes, L. A. (1995). Western bioethics on the Navajo reservation: Benefit or harm? *Journal of the American Medical Association, 274*(10), 826–829.

Catalano, J. (2003). *Nursing now: Today's issues, tomorrow's trends* (3rd ed.). Philadelphia: F.A. Davis.

Chaplin, W. F., Phillips, J. B., Brown, J. D., Clanton, N. R., & Stein, J. L. (2000). Handshaking, gender personality, and first impressions. *Journal of Personality and Social Psychology, 9*(4), 110–117.

Cross, T., Bazron, B., Dennis, K., & Isaacs, M. R. (1989). *Towards a culturally competent system of care: A monograph on effective services for minority children who are severely emotionally disturbed* (Vol. 1). Washington, DC: CASSP Technical Assistance Center.

Davis, B. H., & Voegtle, K. H. (1994). *Culturally competent health care for adolescents: A guide for primary care providers.* Chicago: AMA Department of Adolescent Health.

DiMatteo, M. R. (1995). Patient adherence to pharmacotherapy: The importance of effective communication. *Formulary, 30*(10), 596–598, 601–602, 605.

DiMatteo, M. R., Hays, R. D., & Prince, L. M. (1986). Relationship of physicians' nonverbal communication skills to patient satisfaction, appointment noncompliance, and physician workload. *Health Psychology, 5*, 581–594.

DiMatteo, M. R., Taranta, A., Friedman, H. S., & Prince, L. M. (1980). Predicting patient satisfaction from physicians' nonverbal communications skills. *Medical Care, 18*(4), 376–387.

Doak, L. G., Doak, C. C., & Root, J. H. (1996). *Teaching patients with low literacy skills* (2nd ed.). Philadelphia: J.B. Lippincott.

Doyal, L. (1995). *What makes women sick: Gender and the political economy of health.* London: Macmillan Press.

Doyal, L. (2003). *Gender innovation and medical education in Europe.* Unpublished review of medical schools in Europe funded by the European Commission's 5th Framework Programme on Women and Science. Available from l.doyal@bristol.ac.uk

Eisenberg, D. M., Davis, R. B., Ettner, S. L., Appel, S., Wilkey, S., Van Rompay, M., et al. (1998). Trends in alternative medicine use in the United States, 1990–1997: Results of a follow-up national survey. *Journal of the American Medical Association, 208*(18), 1569–1575.

Eisenberg, D. M., Kessler, R. C., Foster, C., Norlock, F. E., Calkins, D. R., & Delbanco, T. L. (1993). Unconventional medicine in the United States: Prevalence, costs, and patterns of use. *New England Journal of Medicine, 328*(4), 246–252.

Fadiman, A. (1997). *The spirit catches you and you fall down: A Hmong child, her American doctors, and the collision of two cultures.* New York: Noonday Press.

Flowers, D. L. (2004). Culturally competent nursing care: A challenge for the 21st century. *Critical Care Nurse, 24*(4), 48–52.

Fuglesang, A. (1973). *Applied communication in developing countries: Ideas and observations.* Stockholm, Sweden: Dag Hammarskjold Foundation.

Goode, T. D. (2002). *Promoting cultural competence and cultural diversity in early intervention and early childhood settings.* Georgetown University Center for Child and Human Development-University Center for Excellence in Developmental Disabilities Education, Research & Service. Retrieved October 24, 2005, from http://gucchd.georgetown.edu/nccc/nccc7.html

Govindasamy, P., & Malhotra, A. (1996). Women's position and family planning in Egypt. *Studies in Family Planning, 27*(6), 328–340.

Harvey, S. M., Bird, S. T., Galavotti, C., Duncan, E. A., & Greenberg, D. (2002). Relationship power, sexual decision making and condom use among women at risk for HIV/STDs. *Women's Health, 36*(4), 69–84.

Held, P., Pauly, M., Bovberg, R., Newman, J., & Salvatierra, O., Jr. (1988). Access to kidney transplantation: Has the United States eliminated income and racial differences? *Archives of Internal Medicine, 148*, 2594–2600.

Hobara, M. (2005). Beliefs about appropriate pain behavior: Cross-cultural and sex differences between Japanese and Euro-Americans. *European Journal of Pain, 9*(4), 389–393.

Holland, J. L., Geary, N., Marchini, A., & Tross, S. (1987). An international survey of physician attitudes and practice in regard to revealing the diagnosis of cancer. *Cancer Investigations, 5*, 151–154.

Institute of Medicine (IOM) of the National Academies. (2002). *Speaking of health: Assessing health communication strategies for diverse populations.* Washington, DC: National Academies Press.

Institute of Medicine (IOM) of the National Academies. (2004). *Health literacy: A prescription to end confusion.* Washington, DC: National Academies Press.

Johnson, R. L., Saha, S., & Arbelaez, J. J. (2004). Racial and ethnic differences in patient perceptions of bias and cultural competence in health care. *Journal of General Internal Medicine, 19*(2), 111.

Kaiser Family Foundation. (1999, October). *Survey of race, ethnicity and medical care: Public perceptions and experiences.* Washington, DC: Author.

Kaiser Family Foundation. (2002, March). *National survey of physicians.* Washington, DC: Author.

Karakuzon, M. (2002). Russia. In D. Crippen, J. K. Kilcullen, & D. F. Kelly. (Eds.), *Three patients: International perspectives on intensive care at the end-of-life* (pp. 67–72). Boston: Kluwer.

Kaufert, J. M., & Putsch, R. W. (1997). Communication through interpreters in healthcare: Ethical dilemmas arising from differences in class, culture, language, and power. *Journal of Clinical Ethics, 8*, 71–87.

King, D. E., & Bushwick, B. (1994). Beliefs and attitudes of hospital inpatients about faith healing and prayer. *Journal of Family Practice, 39*, 349–352.

Krober, A., & Kluckhohn, C. (1978). *Culture: A critical review of concepts and definitions.* New York: Krauss Reprint Co. [Originally published 1952]

LaBorde, P. (1996). *Vietnamese cultural profile* [online]. *EthnoMed.* Retrieved November 10, 2005, from http://www.ethnomed.org/ethnomed/cultures/vietnamese/vietnamese_cp.html

Lanski, S. L., Greenwald, M., Perkins, A., & Simon, H. K. (2003). Herbal therapy use in a pediatric emergency department population: Expect the unexpected. *Pediatrics, 11,* 5.

Lea, A. (1994). Nursing in today's multicultural society: A transcultural perspective. *Journal of Advanced Nursing, 20,* 307–313.

Lee, S. J., Back, A. L., Block, S. D., & Stewart, S. K. (2002). Enhancing physician-patient communication. *Hematology, 2002,* 464–483.

Lee, L. J., Batal, H. A., Maselli, J. H., & Kutner, J. S. (2002). Effect of Spanish interpretation method on patient satisfaction in an urban walk-in clinic. *Journal of General Internal Medicine, 17,* 641–646.

Leninger, M. (1978). Transcultural nursing theories and research approaches. In M. Leninger (Ed.), *Transcultural nursing* (pp. 31–51). New York: Wiley.

Levin, J. S. (1996). How religion influences morbidity and health: Reflections on natural history, salutogenesis, and host resistance. *Social Science & Medicine, 43*(5), 849–864.

Li, C. I., Malone, K. E., & Daling, J. R. (2003). Differences in breast cancer stage, treatment, and survival by race and ethnicity. *Archives of Internal Medicine, 163*(1), 49–56.

MacIntyre, A. (1984). *After virtue: A study in moral theory* (2nd ed.). Notre Dame, IN: University of Notre Dame Press.

Mark, D. B. (2000). Sex bias in cardiovascular care: Should women be treated more like men? *Journal of the American Medical Association, 283*(5), 659–661.

Mastroianni, A., Faden, R., & Federman, D. (Eds.). (1994). *Women and health research: Ethical and legal issues of including women in clinical studies* (Vols. 1 and 2). Washington, DC: National Academy Press.

Matsumura, S., Bito, S., Liu, H., Kahn, K., Fukuhara, S., Kagawa-Singer, M., et al. (2002). Acculturation of attitudes toward end-of-life care: A cross-cultural survey of Japanese Americans and Japanese. *Journal of General Internal Medicine, 17,* 531–539.

McCord, G., Gilchrist, V. J., Grossman, S. D., King, B. D., McCormick, K. E., Oprandi, A. M., et al. (2004). Discussing spirituality with patients: A rational and ethical approach. *Annals of Family Medicine, 2*(4), 356–361.

McKinley, J. (1996). Some contributions from the social system to gender inequalities in heart disease. *Journal of Health and Social Behavior, 37,* 1–26.

Michielutte, R., Bahnson, J., Dignan, M. B., & Schroeder, E. M. (1992). The use of illustrations and narrative text style to improve readability of a health education brochure. *Journal of Cancer Education, 7,* 251–260.

National Cancer Institute (NCI). (2003). *Cancer health disparities: Fact sheet.* Retrieved November 3, 2005, from http://www.nci.nih.gov/cancertopics/factsheet/cancerhealthdisparities

National Center for Complementary and Alternative Medicine (NCCAM). (2002, May). *What is complementary and alternative medicine?* (NCCAM Publication No. D156). Retrieved November 20, 2005, from http://nccam.nih.gov/health/whatiscam

National Center for Health Statistics. (2003, March 19). Early release of selected estimates based on data from the January-September 2002 National Health Interview Survey. Retrieved November 19, 2005, from http://www.cdc.gov/nchs/about/major/nhis/released200303.htm

National Library of Medicine (NLM). (2005, October 13). *Medical subject headings.* Retrieved November 20, 2005, from http://www.nlm.nih.gov/mesh

National Medical Association. (n.d.). *Cultural competence primer.* Retrieved November 10, 2005, from http://www.ohiokepro.com/providers/physician/changepacket/Cultural/

NMAPrimer.pdf#search='the%20application%20of%20cultural%20knowledge,
%20behaviors,%20clinical%20and%20interpersonal%20skills%20that%20enhances
%20a%20provider's%20effectiveness%20in%20patient%20care'

Ngo-Metzger, Q., Massagli, M. P., Clarridge, B. R., Manocchia, M., Davis, R. B., Iezzoni,
L. I., et al. (2003). Linguistic and cultural barriers to care: Perspectives of Chinese and
Vietnamese immigrants. *Journal of General Internal Medicine, 18,* 44–52.

Nierenberg, G. I., & Calero, H. H. (1971). *How to read a person like a book.* New York:
Hawthorn.

Parrado, E. A., Flippen, C. A., & McQuiston, C. (2005). Migration and relationship power
among Mexican women. *Demography, 42*(2), 347–372.

Phillips, D. P., Christenfeld, N., & Glynn, L. M. (1998). Increase in U.S. medication-error
deaths between 1983 and 1993. *Lancet, 351,* 643–644.

Pobzeb, V. (2001, August 24). *Hmong population and education in the United States
and the world.* Retrieved December 6, 2006, from http://www.uwec.edu/minkushk/
2001_Hmong_Population_and_Education_in.htm

Pulerwitz, J., Amaro, H., De Jong, W., Gortmaker, S. L., & Rudd, R. (2002). Relationship
power, condom use and HIV risk among women in the USA. *AIDS Care, 14*(6),
789–800.

Purnell, L. (1998). Transcultural diversity and health care. In L. Purnell & B. Paulanka (Eds.),
Transcultural health care: A culturally competent approach (pp. 1–6). Philadelphia: F.A.
Davis.

Roter, D. L. (2005). How effective is your nonverbal communication? *Conversations
in Care Web Book* (Chapter 2). Retrieved December 2, 2005, from http://www.
conversationsincare.com/web_book/chapter02.html

Rudd, R., Moeykens, B. A., & Colton, T. C. (2000). Health and literacy: A review of
medical and public health literature. In J. Comings, B. Garners, & C. Smith. (Eds.),
Annual review of adult learning and literacy (pp. 158–199). New York: Jossey-Bass.

Sabo, D., & Gordon, D. (1995). *Men's health and illness: Gender, power and the body.*
Thousand Oaks, CA: Sage.

Salimbene, S. (2000). *What language does your patient hurt in? A practical guide to culturally
competent care.* Amherst, MA: Diversity Resources, Inc.

Scheflen, A. E. (1972). *Body language and social order.* Englewood Cliffs, NJ: Prentice-Hall.

Scheflen, A. E. (1973). *How behavior means.* New York: Gordon Breach.

Schloman, B. (2004). Information resources column: Health literacy: A key ingredient for
managing personal health. *Online Journal of Issues in Nursing.* Retrieved November 14,
2005, from http://nursingworld.org/ojin/infocol/info_13.htm

Seals, A. A. (2005). Gender differences in health care: The need for women's cardiovascular
health initiatives. *Northeast Florida Medicine.* Retrieved December 6, 2006, from
http://www.dcmsonline.org/jax-medicine/2005journals/Diabetes/diab05b-
genderheart.pdf

Searight, H. R., & Gafford, J. (2005). Cultural diversity at the end of life: Issues and
guidelines for family physicians. *American Family Physician, 71*(3), 515–522.

Shapiro, J., Hollingshead, J., & Morrison, E. H. (2002). Primary care resident, faculty, and
patient views of barriers to cultural competence, and the skills needed to overcome
them. *Medical Education, 36,* 749–759.

Shaw, L. J., Hachamovitch, R., & Redberg, R. F. (2000). Current evidence on diagnostic
testing in women with suspected coronary artery disease. *Cardiology Review, 8*(1), 65–
74.

Shiba, G., & Oka, R. (1996). *Japanese Americans. Culture and nursing care: A pocket guide.*
San Francisco: University of California.

Shubin, S. (1980). Nursing patients from different cultures. *Nursing, 10*(6), 79–81.

Speizer, I. S., Whittle, L., & Carter, M. (2005). Gender relations and reproductive decision making in Honduras. *International Family Planning Perspectives, 31*(3), 131–139.

Thao, P. (1999). *Mong education at the crossroads.* New York: University of America Press.

Theiderman, S. (2003). *Seeing applicants accurately: Bridging cultural gaps.* Retrieved October 8, 2005, from http://www.thiederman.com/articles_detail.php?id=67

U.S. Census Bureau. (2000). *United States Census 2000. Profile of general demographic characteristics.* Washington, DC: Author.

U.S. Food and Drug Administration. (2002). Kava-containing dietary supplements may be associated with severe liver injury. *FDA CFSCAN Consumer Advisory.* Retrieved November 27, 2005, from http://vm.cfsan.fda.gov/~dms/addskava.html

Watson, J. (2000). *Male bodies: Health, culture and identity.* Buckingham, England: Open University Press.

Wenger, N. (1997). Coronary heart disease: An older woman's health risk. *British Medical Journal, 315,* 1085–1090.

Winnick, S., Lucas, D. O., Hartman, A. L., & Toll, D. (2005). How do you improve compliance? *Pediatrics, 115*(6), e718–e724.

Yeo, G., & Hikuyeda, N. (2000). Cultural issues in end-of-life decision making among Asians and Pacific Islanders in the United States. In K. Braun, J. H. Pietsch, & P. L. Blanchette (Eds.), *Cultural issues in end-of-life decision making* (pp. 101–125). Thousand Oaks, CA: Sage.

6

IMPROVING PATIENT–PROVIDER COMMUNICATION

In Jeff Kane's book, *How to Heal: A Guide for Caregivers* (2003), he tells the story of Ellen, a woman generally quite nervous about her health who had had a biopsy after finding a lump in her breast. When the results were available, a nurse called Ellen at home to inform her that the "biopsy was negative." Hearing only the word *negative* and not understanding the true purport of the nurse's words, the woman went into something like shock, "having taken the message as confirmation of her most morbid fears" (24). When her husband, Dave, came home and tried to talk to her, Ellen was unresponsive, staring into space as though she'd lost her mind. Worried that his wife may have had a stroke, Dave rushed her to the emergency department (ED) to have her examined.

Naturally, the physician on duty could find nothing wrong with Ellen, but he did ask Dave if his wife had been having any health problems. Dave responded that Ellen had recently had a biopsy, so the doctor thought perhaps that she did have cancer and that a tumor had metastasized, affecting her brain. Among other tests, then, he ordered a spinal tap to get a sample of Ellen's spinal fluid.

Things just got worse from there. Spinal taps can be painful (and in this case the procedure was unnecessary), but Ellen developed a common side effect: a massive headache. She then had an anaphylactic reaction to the painkiller that was prescribed to her and she lost consciousness. Kane writes:

> She awoke the next morning in the intensive care unit. A neurologist examined her there and afterward offered a startling diagnosis: transient global amnesia. "All that means," the doctor explained, "is that you were probably stressed something fierce, and it pretty literally blew your mind. In other words, no brain tumor, no disease. You can expect your memory to return within a few days" (Kane, 2003, p. 24).

When Ellen finally learned that a negative biopsy was one in which no cancer had been found, naturally she was shocked, but relieved. "I still can't believe all that happened to me," she summarizes. "I wasn't sick with *anything*, but I felt like I'd been yanked out of my life and locked in a trunk. I'd hate to think what people go through who get diagnosed for real" (Kane, 2003, p. 24).

Had the nurse explained Ellen's news more completely and clearly, perhaps adding "so this means you're in the clear, no cancer," or had she eliminated the phrase "biopsy was negative," what happened to Ellen might have been avoided. Says Kane:

> When you give a patient any kind of news, all terms should be explained. We use so many emotionally loaded words in medicine. Often the patients hear one word and utterly blank out; they don't hear anything at all after that. For this woman, that one word—*negative*—knocked over the whole line of dominoes. But what happened was easily avoidable (Jeff Kane, MD, personal communication, December 2005).

Yet hindsight is 20–20, as we often hear. Surely the nurse didn't realize that her message could be misunderstood so completely. She probably had no idea that Ellen had stayed up the night before either, seriously agonizing over the "miserable gantlet she was surely about to run" if her biopsy revealed that she had breast cancer (Kane, 2003, p. 23). But in this case, effective communication was hindered by at least two factors: use of the telephone, which provides no opportunity for face-to-face exchange in the context of conveying sensitive health information, and the use of jargon. Did Ellen even understand what a biopsy was? If the information had been delivered to Ellen in person, would the nurse's facial expression or body language have clearly indicated that her news was positive? Was Ellen simply afraid to ask for clarification for fear of appearing stupid, or did she react the way she did because she was shocked?

Perhaps it's wrong to speculate. Nevertheless, Ellen's story is especially poignant for those patients with low health literacy—patients who might similarly be baffled by terms they cannot understand. As we saw in chapter 4, the effects of medical miscommunication can be devastating. Add to the mix some measure of low health literacy, and the powder keg can blow entirely. In this case, luckily, Ellen turned out to be alright. She probably had no amnesia and certainly had no breast cancer. But gaps in her communication with a nurse, her husband, and two physicians nevertheless led to a painful, traumatic experience. As we've learned thus far in this book, steps can and should be taken to ensure that patient–provider communication is clear, culturally appropriate, and tailored to the patient's abilities.

WHAT IS EFFECTIVE COMMUNICATION?

At its most basic, interpersonal communication involves the sending and receiving of messages between two or more people. It is not linear, but circular, with each person sending and receiving messages and encoding and decoding them in a unique way. These messages might be auditory, visual, tactile, olfactory, or any combination of these. The way we dress, walk, smile, and touch all contribute consciously and unconsciously to the messages we send.

We communicate through various channels or media (e.g., face-to-face and through electronic means, such as the computer or telephone), and we must contend with "noise" that distorts and interferes with our messages: anything from the hum of an air conditioner to a speech impediment to the recipient's closed-mindedness. Our intended messages are sent and received in a variety of times and contexts, from bad jokes told immediately after learning of the illness of a friend to stories shared in baseball stadiums and rock concerts. Messages have effects on the listener and have an ethical dimension, with some being more "right" or more "wrong" than others (DeVito, 1986, pp. 4–12).

Our primary concern in this chapter is with the interfering noises of patients' low health literacy and health care providers' poor communication skills in the context of the patient–provider relationship. What are the effects when messages are sifted through a patient's particular cultural, linguistic, and life experiences? In what ways is communication diminished or distorted when a nurse, physician, or physician's assistant does not realize that his or her message has been misconstrued? How might we maximize the beneficial effects of our messages and minimize the potential damage of misunderstanding? What does it mean to communicate health information clearly to patients?

Consider the following comparison between two explanations offered by a doctor to a patient who has found a lump in her breast—precisely the situation in which Ellen found herself in the story conveyed at the outset of this chapter:

> VERSION 1: You have a lesion in your mediastinum that is two centimeters. We need to perform a fine-needle aspiration in order to rule out metastatic adenocarcinoma to a lymph node.

> VERSION 2: You have a small lump inside your chest. The way to figure out what it is, is to stick a small needle in it. It is important to do this so we can know how to give you the best treatment (Davis et al., 2002).

The first explanation, dense and clinical, is targeted toward a patient with at least an 11th-grade reading level; the second, clearer and in much plainer language, might be understood by someone with a third-grade reading level (National Women's Health Resource Center, 2004). Although a patient could certainly be confused by the second version and have follow-up questions, the chances that he or she will misunderstand the doctor's message have been reduced. Perhaps, as we have already mentioned, this is the first step toward improving communication: simplifying language by eliminating jargon.

TALKING TO PATIENTS, LISTENING TO PATIENTS

But there is much more to good communication, and health care providers have a powerful incentive to convey their messages clearly, ensuring that all clinical encounters are mutually understandable. The reason is simple. *Better communication leads to improved health outcomes.* When communication is clear and well functioning, patients and their health care providers are more satisfied, resulting in fewer complaints and fewer patient-initiated lawsuits (Haas, Leiser, Magill, & Sanyer, 2005). Health care providers should refrain from interrupting their patients, instead concentrating on the practice of active listening.

Engaging in active listening is easier said than done. Too often, for example, doctors redirect patients' initial descriptions of their concerns, choosing a single problem on which to focus before fully exploring the patient's spectrum of concerns (Marvel, Epstein, Flowers, & Beckman, 1999). Having a good understanding of the patient's agenda and expectations and engaging in participatory decision making can improve compliance and follow-through and help reduce fears of serious illness and complaints at follow-up (Heisler, Bouknight, Hayward, Smith, & Kerr, 2002; Jackson & Kroenke, 1999).

Low-literate patients often feel overwhelmed by information about their illness and tend to ask fewer questions than do those with higher literacy skills (Mayeaux et al., 1996). In the typical clinical encounter, patients with low health literacy have trouble determining what information their health care providers need and what information might be irrelevant. They often lack the health care vocabulary to report symptoms accurately and may convey information illogically or in a jumbled order (Williams, Davis, Parker, & Weiss, 2002). Caregivers who are aware of these difficulties can be more patient and effective communicators, listening and asking the right questions.

Effective communication is not a one-way street, with health care providers lecturing and offering information on one end and patients passively receiving wisdom on the other. To illustrate, let's turn again to Jeff Kane, MD, director of psychosocial education at the Sierra Nevada Cancer Center and author of the book *How to Heal* (2003), from which we shared the story of Ellen, who misunderstood the word *negative*. Kane notes that some physicians still hold to an outmoded concept of patient–physician communication. Some years back, while preparing to speak before a large group of doctors about his clinical practice, which involves facilitating cancer patient support groups, Dr. Kane was chatting with the internist who was going to introduce him. Their exchange went something like this:

"Exactly what is your practice?"
"Basically," said Dr. Kane, "I listen to patients."
"Hey, that's what I do. I spend almost all my time talking to my patients."

Notes Dr. Kane: "I didn't comment on his choice of words." Still, despite the fact that Dr. Kane's autobiographical notes were in front of the internist—notes that made it clear that Dr. Kane saw his job as *listening* to patients—the internist introduced his colleague using these words: "Dr. Kane's practice is mainly talking to patients. . . ."

Kane calls the inability to distinguish between talking and listening "the Dreaded L-Block, a virtually neurological aversion to listening." An acupuncturist friend of Kane's had a similar aversion. When asked to assess his communication skills, he informed Dr. Kane, "I consider myself good at it. I tell my clients everything. I tell them exactly what I'm going to do and not do, what to expect, and how to get hold of me if they have any concerns" (Kane, 1996, p. 112).

Of course, it's a good thing when health care providers are attuned to the needs of their patients, communicating information in ways the patients can understand and making themselves available for further questions. But communicating with patients—especially those with low health literacy—requires knowledge, skills, and practices that transcend the prescription of Dr. Kane's acupuncturist friend. Among such practices are the use of open-ended questions, the effort to remain silent as the patient attempts to explain symptoms or voice concerns, and the use of teach-back exchanges in which the patient explains back to the physician what he or she has learned or what he or she will do next.

CHALLENGES TO EFFECTIVE ORAL COMMUNICATION

In *Overcoming Communication Barriers in Patient Education* (2001), Helen Osborne, MEd, discusses strategies for communicating with members of groups who have special communication needs, including those who have difficulty reading, older adults, the visually and hearing impaired, those who speak little English, and people from other cultures. According to the National Assessment of Adult Literacy (NAAL) of 2003, 46% of those adults who scored in the below basic level on prose literacy had one or more disabilities, compared with 30% of adults in the overall survey population (National Center for Education Statistics, 2005).

Other factors standing in the way of effective patient–provider communication, according to Weiner, Barnet, Cheng, and Daaleman (2005), include insufficient time during scheduled office visits, competing incentives such as the pressure to generate more revenue, and limited opportunities for interaction and the exchange of information outside the context of the standard office-based visit.

Part of the problem is simply the way physicians talk to patients. Using audiotape analysis to describe communication patterns in primary care, Roter and colleagues (1997) studied 127 physicians and 537 patients coping with ongoing problems related to various diseases. Five distinct communication patterns emerged: (1) narrowly biomedical, in which the physician asked closed-ended questions and engaged in exclusively biomedical talk during the visit (32%); (2) expanded biomedical, which was similar to the first pattern but with moderate levels of psychosocial discussion added in (33%); (3) biopsychosocial, in which psychosocial and biomedical topics were discussed in roughly equal proportions (20%); (4) psychosocial, which consisted mostly of psychosocial exchange (8%); and (5) consumerist, which was characterized by patient-initiated questions and plenty of physician information-giving (8%; Roter et al., 1997).

Let's take a moment to discuss the biomedical model, which has been the accepted clinical model for the last 300 years or longer. The biomedical model holds that all illnesses can be explained by physical processes; that is, that they are separate from the mind. Those who embrace this model hold that psychological and social processes are largely independent of disease, and vice versa.

Many criticize the biomedical model as reductionist, charging that it emphasizes illness over health. Patients can have wide-ranging responses to the same treatment, a phenomenon that the biomedical model has trouble explaining.

In the biopsychosocial model, by contrast, diagnosis requires attention to biological, psychological, and social factors, and does not assume that the mind and body are separate (Collier, n.d.). Some clinicians, such as Hinz (2000), recommend keeping to a biopsychosocial approach during patient interviews to help build a partnership with the patient.

Ironically, in the above study by Roter and colleagues (1997), biomedically focused visits—those in which language was the most formal and exchanges tended to feature clinical jargon—took place most often with sicker, older, and lower income patients (the very patients who probably desire a consumerist approach) by younger, usually male physicians. Physician satisfaction was lowest in the narrowly biomedical pattern, perhaps because caregivers could sense that patients were confused or dissatisfied, even if they failed to ask questions or seek clarification. By contrast, physician satisfaction was highest in the consumerist pattern.

Patients in the study, however, were more satisfied with the psychosocial pattern (Roter et al., 1997). Why didn't patients agree with physicians and prefer the consumerist pattern? It is not entirely clear. It could be that when physicians rely too heavily on a consumerist pattern, patients feel that the physician is not in control of the discussion, but believe he or she ought to be.

Whatever the reason, there is a clear mismatch between what health providers assume patients know and what patients really know. Although 63% of patients in one study were aware that the term *metastasis* meant that cancer was spreading, only half (52%) understood that the phrase "the tumor is progressing" was not good news (Chapman, Abraham, Jenkins, & Fallowfield, 2003). In the same study, 94% of those sampled knew where their lungs were, but only 46% were able to locate their liver. High confidence ratings in the study suggest that asking if patients understand is likely to overestimate comprehension because respondents generally were confident that they understood the terms they were asked about.

Similarly, it was assumed that Ellen, the woman who had the biopsy, knew what a biopsy was and understood the meaning of the word *negative* in the context of her reported test results. This is why teach-back and other methods that open up two-way communication and create a patient–provider dialogue are usually better for determining patient comprehension than asking yes–no questions, such as "Do you understand?"

How can patients be encouraged to get more involved in their medical care? According to Street, Gordon, Ward, Krupat, and Kravitz (2005), patient participation in medical encounters depends on a complex interplay of personal, physician, and contextual factors. The researchers measured the degree to which patients asked questions, were assertive, and expressed their concerns, as well as the degree to which physicians used partnership-building and supportive talk (such as praise, reassurance, and empathy) in patient interactions. In their analysis of 279 physician–patient interactions, educated and White patients tended to be more active participants than did other patients. The vast majority of active participation behaviors (84%) were patient-initiated rather than prompted by partnership-building or supportive talk from the physician, but more active participants received better communication from the physicians. Clinical setting and the physician's communicative style were the strongest predictors of patients' participation. The researchers concluded that health care providers could encourage patients' involvement by using partnership-building and supportive communication more frequently (Street at al., 2005).

OTHER FACTORS TO CONSIDER

Not all efforts geared toward improving patient–physician communication will work, of course. A randomized, controlled trial designed to determine whether a 10-hour communication skills program titled "Thriving in a Busy Practice: Physician-Patient Communication" could improve general patient satisfaction found that the program was unsuccessful (Brown, Boles, Mullooly, & Levinson, 1999). Occasionally such failure is due to physicians not wanting to hold themselves accountable for communication problems, instead attributing them to the patient and blaming such factors as lack of adherence or patients' unreasonable demands (Levinson, Stiles, Inui, & Engle, 1993).

Patients vary with respect to their communication needs, especially during the initial contact with their health care provider. In a study by Greene, Adelman, Friedmann, and Charon (1994), for example, older patients were found to prefer encounters in which there was physician supportiveness and shared laughter, they were questioned about and given an opportunity to provide information on their own agenda items, and physicians provided some structure for the first meeting through use of questions worded in the negative. Extra care should be taken with older patients because they process information more slowly and are more likely to suffer from hearing loss or other chronic conditions that diminish their ability to absorb complex health-related information (Safeer & Keenan, 2005).

Communication issues transcend language. Just because a patient speaks Spanish and his or her nurse speaks Spanish, for instance, does not necessarily mean the two are communicating. All the same communication obstacles apply: the patient may not understand jargon the nurse uses, the two may have radically different education levels or socioeconomic status, and the patient may have literacy problems in his or her own native language. Sometimes patients and providers speak the same language but a different dialect, or have trouble understanding one another because of a marked age difference. Some patients also may attach different meanings and emotional charge to terms the provider uses.

As we saw in chapter 5, we should not underestimate the potential for cross-cultural miscommunication in all its forms. Even how we talk about disease in relation to our body can vary from culture to culture, as Jeff Kane explains.

> When Americans have conflicts with their children, they might say something like, "I'm having trouble with my kids." A Mexican explaining similar circumstances is more likely to clutch his or her chest when uttering the words, perhaps pointing to his or her *corazón* [heart] to suggest the depth of emotion he or she is feeling. In clinical practice, then, it's not always clear whether pain a Mexican patient is talking about is literal or figurative. . . . Dealing with patients anywhere, it's important to understand how conscious they are of metaphors and how seriously they take them.

In my line of work, I want to get to the metaphorical level—where meaning is made and suffering treated—as soon as possible. If the person already recognizes that process within herself, we have a head-start advantage. But some folks, regardless of tongue and culture, aren't even aware of their imaginary life. . . .

Not long ago I asked a cardiologist friend, "Do some patients strike you as suffering the heartache of life as much as medical angina?" He looked at me as though I'd just asked him something in Urdu. It wasn't his disagreement with my notion as much as his certainty that *heartache* and *angina* inhabit different, totally incongruent worlds (J. Kane, MD, personal communication, December 2005).

Factors other than language, then, can be equally powerful in facilitating or interfering with cross-cultural communication. Age, gender, and communication style, just to name a few examples, may all have played a role in the decision of one 43-year-old Spanish-speaking woman not to undergo careful monitoring following her diagnosis of transitional cell carcinoma, or cancer of the bladder. Three years after her initial diagnosis (when she underwent a transurethral resection), the patient made an appointment with a second urologist, Dr. Gabal, who was younger and, unlike the woman's previous physician, female. The patient told Dr. Gabal that she did not continue seeing the other urologist because he could not answer her fundamental question: *Why does this keep happening to me?*

Through a Spanish-speaking interpreter, Dr. Gabal explained that she, too, could not fully answer such a question and that sometimes the origins of disease are not clear even to the finest, most competent physicians. More important, Dr. Gabal sat and listened without judgment to the woman's story, spending more time with her than she might have with other patients.

When the woman originally came to see Dr. Gabal, after 3 years without treatment, she said she had been bleeding for roughly a month. Soon she had a second transurethral resection to remove the cancer from her bladder. (Stage 0 and stage I bladder cancer are often treated with transurethral resection of the bladder, during which a cutting instrument is inserted through the urethra to remove the tumor.) Cancer of the bladder is usually detected early, says Dr. Gabal, because it causes bleeding during the early stages of its growth. In this case, however, Dr. Gabal observed that during the resection she "could not find a single part of [the patient's] bladder that was free of tumor," leading her to believe that the patient's bleeding may have been going on longer than she claimed it had (L. Gabal, MD, personal communication, December 2005).

Although this patient's exact reason for forgoing follow-up visits with the first urologist was not clear (maybe she was more comfortable with a woman doctor?), she cited communication problems as her primary rationale for discontinuing follow-up treatment. In this case, fortunately, the patient's postoperative prognosis was good. However, less invasive treatment might have been possible with ongoing observation. A combination of poor patient–provider communication and the patient's lack of understanding of her condition created the potential for a darker clinical outcome.

That case is complex, but it teaches a simple lesson. Even though the woman's previous urologist, a more traditional physician in his sixties, could speak Spanish fluently, the patient was not satisfied with his answers. On the other hand, Dr. Gabal, who spoke little Spanish, managed to help the patient understand her condition simply by listening to and sympathizing with her. The clinical information that Dr. Gabal provided varied little from what the previous urologist had offered; it was her communicative style that differed.

ORAL COMMUNICATION AND LOW LITERACY

The impact of oral communication on low-health-literate patients—and that of low health literacy on the quality of patient–provider communication—is profound, as survey data suggest. Results from the National Adult Literacy Survey (NALS) of 1992 and the NAAL of 2003 are discussed at some length in chapter 1. Our concern here is what these data suggest about the relationship between having low health literacy and experiencing poor patient–provider communication. Because basic literacy skills are essential for processing information in spoken form, respondents who fell into the below basic category on the 2003 NAAL (and many who fell into the basic category as well) would be expected to have more difficulty communicating with providers about health-related information.

As we saw in chapter 1, however, generalizing about the race, sex, age, language spoken before starting high school, and educational attainment of low-literate patients is not a simple task. Thirty-seven percent of those in the below basic group on the NAAL were White, 20% were Black, 39% were Hispanic, and 4% were Asian/Pacific Islander. Although 55% finished some high school, only 23% were high-school graduates. Twenty-one percent had multiple disabilities, but 54% had no disabilities (NCES, 2005).

Despite having such varying demographics, low-literate populations do share common characteristics in terms of how they interpret and process multiple kinds of information. According to the National Cancer Institute (NCI, 1994), low-literate populations

- tend to think in concrete/immediate rather than abstract/futuristic terms
- often interpret information literally
- have insufficient language fluency needed to comprehend and apply information from written materials
- have difficulty with information processing, such as reading a menu, interpreting a bus schedule, following medical instructions, or reading a prescription label

Think of Ellen again. In any other context, she most likely knew the meaning of the word *negative*. In the context of a potential cancer diagnosis, however, with its attendant anxieties and worries, Ellen's mind became muddled at the moment the nurse phoned with the lab results. When patients with low health literacy encounter complex health information, sometimes they are afraid to veer from a literal, word-for-word understanding of what they're being told.

Imagine the older patient who interprets his doctor's brief lecture about the negative effects of a high-salt diet (and the advice to limit sodium intake) as a literal command to consume no more salt whatsoever. Taken literally, such advice might lead the patient not only to stop using a shaker to add salt to food but also to stop eating any processed or prepackaged food containing the slightest hint of sodium in its list of ingredients. Loss of appetite and weight loss can result from the total elimination of salt from the diet, creating other health problems. In the context of advice about something as precious as good health, low-literate patients become more literal than they might in other realms of life.

Needless to say, then, there is a powerful relationship between having low health literacy and experiencing problems when communicating health information. Sometimes low-literate patients are too literal, but they also have difficulty recalling health information, even immediately after leaving the physician's office. In fact, the average patient generally recalls only 50% or less of the information received during a typical office visit (Ong, Haes, Hoos, & Lammes, 1995).

And, as we have seen, low-literate patients have tremendous difficulty understanding their doctor's vocabulary (Gibbs, Gibbs, & Henrich, 1987). They have even more trouble with written materials, such as pamphlets, online information, discharge instructions, intake forms, and hospital menus. Even with oral communication, low-literate patients may have less confidence in their ability to articulate their problems (Williams et al., 2002, p. 385). Sometimes they may misrepresent the problem; other times they may say nothing at all.

Having low literacy skills along with a chronic condition can compromise patient–provider communication. Low literacy limits the effectiveness of disease management programs, for example (Rothman et al., 2004; Schillinger et al., 2003). In one study of 217 patients enrolled in a comprehensive diabetes management program, an intervention group received intensive diabetes management from a multidisciplinary team, whereas a control group received an initial management session and continued with usual care (Rothman et al., 2004). Among patients with low literacy, intervention patients were more likely than control patients to achieve goal HbA1c levels, whereas patients with high literacy had similar odds of achieving goal levels, regardless of intervention status. (To explain, A1c is a subtype of hemoglobin, the compound in red blood cells that transports oxygen. Glucose binds to hemoglobin A slowly and decomposes slowly—the more glucose in your blood, the more hemoglobin A1c in your blood. The HbA1c level in a patient's blood is an indicator of his or her average blood glucose level over approximately the previous 4 weeks.)

In the Rothman study, improvements in systolic blood pressure were similarly related to literacy status, leading the investigators to conclude that increasing access to disease management programs that address literacy could reduce health disparities between those who read and understand health information well and those who do not.

Other studies underscore the lack of communication that sometimes exists between patients and health care practitioners. In a study of 100 patients recently diagnosed with lung cancer, Quirt and colleagues (1997) found that only 64%

agreed with their provider's assessment about the extent of their disease. Most who disagreed underestimated the extent of their cancer. Furthermore, physicians often failed to recognize that their patients had such misconceptions. The investigators concluded that many of the patients could not understand their situation well enough to make truly autonomous treatment decisions. Unless lines of communication between patients and providers are clear, encouraging patients to engage in self-care may not be the most advisable approach.

In several respects, then, patients with low health literacy fare worse in the health care system than do those with average or more advanced literacy skills. Understanding this fact, we now can proceed to those approaches that work best for improving patient–provider communication.

MODELS OF EFFECTIVE ORAL COMMUNICATION

In recent years, much of the research on patient–provider communication has focused on ways to enhance communication. It is not with words alone that we communicate: body language, facial expressions, and tone of voice often provide additional clues that influence communicative effectiveness (Klein, 2005).

Mayer (2002) offers a number of recommendations for improving health care communication, from translating jargon into everyday language to asking patients to repeat health instructions. She advises sufficient interaction time and follow-up telephone calls any time that clinical instructions are "critical to the patient's well-being" (2002, p. 7). Educational materials, Mayer writes, could take the form of video- or audiotapes for low-literacy patients, especially if the materials are free of jargon, easy to understand, and illustrated clearly. However, she warns, health care providers should not come out and ask patients if they can read; such bluntness potentially could embarrass patients. Others, such as Schillinger and colleagues (2003), make similar suggestions and offer similar warnings.

In *Health Literacy: A Manual for Clinicians* (2003, p. 25), Barry Weiss, MD, synthesizes such advice by offering six easy steps to improve interpersonal communication with patients:

1. Slow down: Communication can be improved by speaking slowly and by spending just a small amount of additional time with each patient. Doing so will help foster a patient-centered approach to the clinician-patient interaction.
2. Use plain, nonmedical language: Explain things to patients as you would explain them to a family member.
3. Show or draw pictures: Visual images can improve the patient's recall of ideas.
4. Limit the amount of information provided, and repeat it: Information is best remembered when it is given in small pieces that are pertinent to the tasks at hand. Repetition further enhances recall.
5. Use the teach-back or show-me technique: Confirm that patients understand by asking them to repeat back your instructions.

6. Create a shame-free environment: Make patients feel comfortable asking questions. Enlist the aid of others (patient's family, friends) to promote understanding.

Other researchers emphasize different elements of the patient–provider encounter. Walter, Bundy, and Dornan (2005), for example, focus on the best way to begin a clinical interview. They suggest a five-step approach: (1) calling the patient to the consultation, (2) personally greeting him or her, (3) pausing for introductions, (4) making a transition to talk focused on clinical concerns, and (5) discussing next steps toward health care solutions. These five steps, they say, can help health care trainees create a context for active listening that is less prone to interruption.

Lawton and Carroll (2005) believe that effective communication calls for assessing what the patient knows about his or her illness. Cocksedge and May (2005) promote what they call the "listening loop," which emphasizes the ability of caregivers to pick up on patients' cues during face-to-face interactions. The researchers claim that these cues are often missed or ignored by providers, and they discuss several ways in which clinicians limit, block, or resist listening to their patients: these ways include reassuring them, changing the subject, interrupting them, being directive or making a plan, reducing sympathy, and using body language (Cocksedge & May, 2005).

Active listening, which calls for health care providers to give patients their utmost attention and to avoid common responses such as judging, labeling, moralizing, and prematurely evaluating, has been found to improve patient–provider communication and to empower patients in their pursuit of good care (Robertson, 2005). Providers should never sound judgmental when speaking to a patient. Neither should they use judgmental or negative language when recording information in a patient's chart. "Plenty of patients look at their medical charts and become furious at their doctors, who write that the patients 'complain' of this or that or 'refuse' rectal exams," notes Anna B. Reisman, MD, assistant professor of medicine in the Department of Internal Medicine in the Yale University School of Medicine. "These negative words don't faze [physicians or other health care providers], but to a patient, they sound insulting" (Anna B. Reisman, personal communication, December 2005).

Although no single solution to poor patient–provider communication exists, steps are being taken to improve clinical education and training of health care providers. Several models of patient–provider communication have been adopted by roughly one-third of the nation's medical schools, for example (Weiner et al., 2005). One is the SEGUE framework, a checklist of 25 essential communication tasks grouped into the following five sections: *S*etting the stage, *E*liciting information, *G*iving information, *U*nderstanding the patient's perspective, and *E*nding the encounter. According to a study by Makoul (2001), the SEGUE framework has a high degree of acceptability, can be used reliably, has evidence of validity, and is applicable in a variety of contexts. The full SEGUE checklist is available at http://www.pcm.northwestern.edu/segue/segue.pdf.

ELEMENTS OF EFFECTIVE ORAL COMMUNICATION

Clinicians can do much to jump-start effective patient–provider communication. Nonverbal factors are in play even before a health care provider opens his or her mouth to speak to a patient. The importance of smiling, a firm handshake, use of a comforting touch, and maintaining eye contact is outlined by Roter (2005). In a study by Chaplin, Phillips, Brown, Clanton, and Stein (2000), 112 participants had their hand shaken twice by trained coders. They then completed personality measures. A firm handshake was seen as a sign of the participant's extroversion and emotional expressiveness, but was observed less often among those exhibiting shyness and neuroticism. The point of the study, published in the *Journal of Personality and Social Psychology*, was to demonstrate that personality traits, assessed through self-report, can predict specific behaviors. For our purposes, such a study suggests that a caregiver's firm handshake conveys emotional expressiveness and increases the likelihood of a positive first impression.

Even the physical space in which a clinical encounter takes place is important (Roter, 2005). Are posters and handouts in the waiting room culturally appropriate, for example? Are they written at a reading level that patients can readily understand? Is the examination area sufficiently warm and private, empowering patients to be honest and to ask questions?

Weeping patients can engender feelings of inadequacy in themselves and in their doctors. However, expressing warm empathy by showing understanding and by giving support produces an atmosphere for open ventilation of feelings and, ultimately, enables patients to open up (Nyman, 1991). When patients are crying, it is advisable to respond sensitively during an interview by offering tissues or a comforting touch to soothe them, thereby encouraging them to be more expressive and to relax (Nyman, 1991). However, providers should refrain from touching patients who recoil initially. Maintaining eye contact is extremely important too, unless the patient begins to cry. In that case, the health care provider should look away until the patient regains his or her composure and then make eye contact again (Roter, 2005).

A health care provider's body language can be instructive, influencing a patient's decision about whether to ask questions or convey confusion. Try not to send nonverbal (or verbal) signals that you are too busy to elaborate on information, especially if the patient has limited health literacy skills or appears to falter when given instructions. The following anecdote, adapted from an article published in the January 1996 issue of *American Family Physician*, illustrates a typical case in which miscommunication might have led to serious health complications for the patient:

> A 68-year-old man who lived at home with family members was hospitalized with recurrent congestive heart failure and stable hypertension. At the time of the patient's discharge, a cardiologist instructed the patient to take 0.125 mg of digoxin, alternating with 0.25 mg every other day. When asked if he understood his instructions,

the patient said yes. He was offered a written instruction sheet. He looked at it and thanked the doctor. His family was later called and informed that he was being discharged, and an office appointment was made with his family physician for 1 week later to check his digoxin level.

At the follow-up visit, the patient was found to have a digoxin level well above the therapeutic range. His family physician, who had cared for him for years, asked him to show her how he was taking his medications. He indicated that he was taking both pills every day. Further questioning revealed that he hadn't asked any questions at the time of his hospital discharge because "that doctor seemed so busy that I didn't want to take up any more of his time."

The patient still had the instruction handout in his wallet, but admitted when he took it out to show his family physician that he couldn't read it. When asked why he didn't let anyone know he couldn't read it, he said, "I don't want no one to know. They'll think I'm stupid!"

The patient's family physician reviewed the proper way to take the medicine with both the patient and his daughter (who usually helps him with his medicines), and the physician and patient both demonstrated which pills should be taken on which days. The handout also was reviewed with the daughter, who was able to read and repeat the key points in the handout. Two weeks later, the patient's digoxin level was therapeutic, and he was asymptomatic (Mayeaux et al., 1996).

This patient's reticence might have proven dangerous. Elderly patients, especially those with poor kidney function or low body weight, are at the greatest risk for toxicity when digoxin levels in their blood are elevated (Marik & Fromm, 1998). Clear patient–provider communication became an even more important factor in the clinical encounter described above because it involved a patient who, because of his age, also was at high risk for having low health literacy. Health care providers should never assume that patients will read written instruction sheets, nor should they assume that low-health-literate patients will seek help from family members to comply with medical instructions they do not understand. Such patients may not realize the health implications of noncompliance.

Health care providers should respond to all questions a patient has, but should keep their responses simple. To enhance patients' understanding, as mentioned, it's best to speak in simple "living room" language, to repeat key points several times, and to avoid giving too many directives at once. Consider honing your message down to three or four critical items, leaving patients with a clear message and action plan.

Some recommend reserving direct and closed-ended questions for the end of the interview. The assumption is that the patient will already have had the opportunity to respond to any open-ended questions at the outset of the visit, when the conversation is primarily introductory and the provider is just beginning to learn about the patient's background (Myerscough & Donald, 1992). Use of nurse educators to offer one-on-one instructions in busy outpatient settings also may be beneficial, complementing physician education and enhancing patients' understanding (Mayeaux et al., 1996).

Adapted from a paper by Mayeaux and colleagues (1996), the following passage explains how to give simple oral instructions to low-literate patients who must take a prescribed medication. With a few minor adjustments, health care providers can follow this basic pattern to help patients who have trouble with any prescription:

> "This is your blood pressure medicine. It is called _____. You should take one pill two times every day. Take the pill with food." At this point, clarify that this means they should not take the medication unless they have recently eaten a meal or a snack. Then say something like this: "You can take one pill with breakfast and one pill at supper time. Take your pills every day."
>
> At this point, allow a 2- to 5-second pause so the patient can assimilate the information.
>
> Now ask, "Do you have any questions?" Allow a 5-second pause for questions and clearly answer any that come up. Look for body language that suggests confusion. If the patient merely shakes his or her head, reaffirm that it is fine to ask questions at any point during the interaction and then decide whether the patient really understands what he or she needs to know.
>
> At this point, check to see how well the patient understands the instructions by saying, "Would you tell me how you are going to take this medicine so I can be sure I've told you everything?"
>
> Finally, let the patient repeat the instructions in his or her own words or, if possible, have the patient physically demonstrate the activity.

Teach-back, used in the example above, is an effective means for improving patients' understanding. Schillinger and coworkers (2003) observed physicians in a public hospital to measure the extent to which they assessed patients' recall and comprehension of new concepts during outpatient encounters. All 74 English-speaking patients had diabetes mellitus and low functional health literacy. Patients whose physicians assessed recall or comprehension were more likely to have hemoglobin A1c levels below the mean compared to those whose physicians did not.

Two variables were independently associated with good glycemic control in the above study: higher health literacy levels and physicians' application of the interactive communication strategy. The investigators noted that primary care physicians caring for patients with diabetes mellitus and low functional health literacy rarely assessed patient recall or comprehension of new concepts. Overlooking this step in communication, they concluded, reflected a missed opportunity that could have important clinical implications.

Approaches similar to teach-back have met with success. Invite, Listen, and Summarize (ILS), which has been used at the University of Colorado School of Medicine, was developed to counter high physician-control interview techniques (i.e., a series of yes or no questions). The approach emphasizes techniques of open-ended inquiry, empathy, and engagement to gather data. It is easy to use and remember, drawing on strategies that may help achieve the three basic functions of the medical interview: creating rapport, collecting good data, and improving compliance. Although the formal curriculum is taught only in the first 2 years of training at the University of Colorado, evidence suggests that ILS improves communication skills even through the third year (Boyle, Dwinnell, & Platt, 2005).

Effective oral communication can be a powerful tool in health care, changing patients' behavior. For example, structured waiting-room interviews have been found to increase patients' participation in medical interactions (Tabak, 1988). To determine whether a print intervention could improve participation even more, Tabak (1988) randomly assigned 67 family medicine patients to receive one of two types of printed material prior to their medical visit: (1) a treatment booklet stressing the importance of recognizing information needs and encouraging patients to ask questions (the experimental group), and (2) a placebo education booklet similar in format but not in content (the control group). Patient–physician interactions were audiotaped to determine the number of questions patients asked, and a questionnaire was administered to assess patients' satisfaction.

Although the mean number of questions asked by patients was 7.46 for the experimental group and 5.63 for the control group, this difference was not statistically significant. Question asking also did not correlate with reported patient satisfaction (Tabak, 1988). These findings suggest that the use of a printed intervention to encourage additional patient involvement and increase satisfaction may be no more effective than the one-on-one oral communication approach of a structured waiting-room interview.

Even so, to be effective providers still must be attuned to patients' experiences, asking the right questions during and immediately after the office visit. In fact, simply asking patients if they have additional questions can yield positive results. In one observational study involving 477 pediatric consultations in the United Kingdom, Lloyd (2005) found that 64 further questions arose when families simply were asked if they had additional questions. Two-thirds of the families surveyed indicated that there had been what Lloyd called "suboptimal" communication during their office visit (Lloyd, 2005). We hope that, by using some of the strategies discussed so far in this chapter, health care providers can avoid such negative patient assessments in their own clinical experience.

ALTERNATIVES TO FACE-TO-FACE ORAL COMMUNICATION

Although patient education booklets meet with mixed results, multimedia approaches to patient–provider communication create real opportunities to improve the quality of patient care. Patients with cancer are known to value consultation audiotapes as an information aid, for example, and they frequently accept the offer to tape record their consultations with oncologists (Tattersall & Butow, 2002). Systematic reviews have shown that providing patients with an audiotape of their consultations increases the amount of information they ultimately remember.

In a survey of Australian doctors, many indicated a lack of enthusiasm about providing consultation audiotapes to their patients; they cited such issues as patient confidentiality and medicolegal concerns as reasons for their reluctance. But consultation audiotapes could be a valuable research tool for documenting information and for analyzing interactions between patients and providers, as Tattersall and Butow (2002) suggest.

Visual aids, such as videotapes, pictographs, cartoons, and interactive computer-based multimedia, also may be helpful for improving communication (Williams, Davis, Parker, & Weiss, 2002). Hahn and colleagues (2004) developed a multimedia program to provide a quality-of-life assessment platform acceptable to cancer patients who had a variety of literacy skills and computer experience. One item at a time was presented on a computer touch screen, followed by a recorded reading of a question. Different colors, fonts, and graphic images were used to enhance visibility, and a small icon appeared near each text element so patients could replay the sound as many times as they wanted. Evaluation questions assessed the patients' preferences. The diverse group of 126 patients reported that the talking touch screen was easy to use and that it enhanced their learning experience.

Beyond the Brochure: Alternative Approaches to Effective Health Communication (1994), a guidebook prepared by the AMC Cancer Research Center in Denver, discusses a wide variety of visual materials—everything from posters, flip charts, and talk boards to real objects and models, display boards, *fotonovelas*, and action-oriented exercises, such as role-playing, theater, songs, storytelling, and games. Use of audiotapes and radio docudramas is also featured. The guide provides resources and materials needed for production for many of the categories mentioned, and informative charts list the many benefits and limitations of each communication technology (AMC Cancer Research Center, 1994). (In chapter 9, Using Alternative Forms of Patient Communication, we examine visual forms of communication in more detail, providing several examples. However, those wishing to read the entire AMC brochure may do so by visiting http://http://www.cdc.gov/cancer/nbccedp/bccpdfs/amcbeyon.pdf.)

Instructional videos also can help clinicians. As part of its official Health Literacy Kit, for example, the American Medical Association (AMA) Foundation produced 20-minute informational and instructional videos with case studies to raise awareness about the widespread problem of low health literacy. Perhaps the best-known video, produced in 2001, is titled "Low Health Literacy: You Can't Tell by Looking." It features footage of actual office staff interacting with patients who have low health literacy (American Medical Association Foundation, 2005). For more information or to download the video, visit the AMA Foundation Web site at http://www.ama-assn.org/ama/pub/category/8035.html. The AMA Health Literacy Kit can be ordered by calling (312) 464–5355.

Health messages can be conveyed with visual aids, such as the Wong-Baker FACES Pain Rating Scale, originally designed for young children to communicate their pain (Figure 6.1). Donna Wong, RN, PhD, learned in her clinical practice that children have trouble using any scale that relies on a number concept, a ranking concept, or unfamiliar words (FACES Pain Rating Scale, 2005). Visual aids such as the Wong-Baker FACES Pain Rating Scale may help those with low health literacy and those who do not speak English convey their pain or other important health messages more clearly and accurately.

TRANSLATIONS OF WONG-BAKER FACES PAIN RATING SCALE

0–5 coding	0	1	2	3	4	5
0-10 coding	0	2	4	6	8	10
ENGLISH	No hurt	Hurts little bit	Hurts little more	Hurts even more	Hurts whole lot	Hurts worst
SPANISH	No duele	Duele un poco	Duele un poco más	Duele mucho	Duele mucho más	Duele el máximo
FRENCH	Pas mal	Un petit peu mal	Un peu plus mal	Encore plus mal	Très mal	Très très mal
ITALIAN	Non fa male	Fa male un poco	Fa male un po di piu	Fa male ancora di piu	Fa molto male	Fa maggior-mente male
PORTUGUESE	Não doi	Doi um pouco	Doi um pouco mais	Doi muito	Doi muito mais	Doi o máximo
BOSNIAN	Ne boli	Boli samo malo	Boli malo više	Boli još više	Boli puno	Boli najviše
VIETNAMESE	Không dau	Hỏi dau	Dau hòn chút	Dau nhièu hòn	Dau thât nhièu	Dau qúa dô
CHINESE	無痛	微痛	輕痛	更痛	很痛	劇痛
GREEK	Δεν Πονaΐ	Πονaΐ Λιγο	Πονaΐ Λιγο Πιο Πολν	Πονaΐ Πολν	Πονaΐ Πιο Πολν	Πονaΐ Παρα Πολν
ROMANIAN	No doare	Doare puţin	Doare un pic mai mult	Doare şi mai mult	Doare foarte tare	Doare cel mai mult

FIGURE 6.1 FACES Pain Rating Scale. *Source:* Hockenberry, M. J., Wilson, D., Winkelstein, M. L. *Wong's Essentials of Pediatric Nursing*, 7th ed. St. Louis, Mo. 2005:1259. Copyright, Mosby. Reprinted with permission.

Telephone Communication

Even now, in the age of personal computers and the Internet, the telephone remains an important lifeline for many patients. It is the primary mode of communication between physicians and patients outside the office visit; 25% of interactions between patients and physicians take place on the phone (Reisman & Brown, 2005). Health communication over the phone takes many forms: one-on-one conversations between patients and providers; conference calls involving patients, interpreters, patients' families, their primary doctors, and distant specialists; health information services; hotlines and crisis centers; telephone triage and call centers designed to assess a patient's need for services; and recorded messages to and from patients (Osborne, 2005).

Telephone medicine is but one subset of *telehealth,* which is defined as "the use of telecommunications technologies for the provision of long-distance clinical health care, patient and professional education, and health administration" (Chaffee, 1999). After-hour advice lines, for example, offer patients options for care during evenings and weekends when their primary care physicians are not available; they also offer uninsured and managed care patients a valuable service. These patients tend to comply with advice they receive on nurse lines, often choosing lower intensity care than they otherwise might (Bogdan, Green, Swanson, Gabow, & Dart, 2004). With help from an advice line, patients can learn where to find after-hours or weekend care in their community and can gain access to appropriate referrals. Most patients and providers are not aware that telephone consultation is available 24 hours a day through many clinics and community health centers (Robert Wood Johnson Foundation, 2000).

In "Preventing Communication Errors in Telephone Medicine: A Case-Based Approach," Anna B. Reisman, MD, and Karen E. Brown, MD, discuss six common situations in adult medicine in which communication errors can occur: the reporting of sensitive test results, handling requests for narcotics, treating patients who are not sick enough to be admitted to the ED, "inappropriate" late-night calls, unintelligible patients, and obtaining information from family members. To reduce communication errors in those situations, they recommend the following:

- Ensure that patients are available and can speak freely.
- Schedule follow-up appointments when test results may be sensitive.
- Use "controlled substance contracts."
- Use certain phrases to build rapport.
- Ask patients to repeat back instructions.
- Be sensitive to the patient's and your own paralanguage (i.e., tone, speech pattern, pauses, pitch).
- Allow patients time to describe their chief complaint.
- Be frank about difficulties you're having understanding the patient.
- Speak with patients directly whenever possible.

"If a doctor or nurse senses through a patient's silence, or through what sounds like some confusion, [that the patient is having trouble understanding information,] he or she might say something like, 'Many patients find medications confusing. Tell me how you understand how to take this medicine,' or 'Tell me why you're supposed to take this medicine,' or something to that effect," says Dr. Reisman, coauthor of the study. "This would give the provider a sense of whether there is a problem and will give a clue how to address it. Obviously, you want to use simple language without being offensive and avoid jargon. And you may have to consider: is it more important that the patient understands why a treatment is recommended, or is time better spent focusing on how the treatment should be taken?" (Anna B. Reisman, personal communication, December 2005)

In their study, Reisman and Brown recommend use of over-the-phone language interpretation for dealing with calls from non-English-speaking patients. Companies such as the global language services provider, Language Line Services, employ translators speaking as many as 160 different languages. Health care providers can have a trained interpreter on the phone within minutes after calling such a service. For more about Language Line Services specifically, call (800) 528–5888 or visit them online at http://www.languageline.com.

Although telephone medicine remains an important part of conventional clinical practice, only about 6% of residency programs teach anything about it

(Reisman & Brown, 2005). This is unfortunate. Health care providers report test results and schedule appointments on the phone. Patients call with questions, usually preferring the phone to newer technologies, such as e-mail or online messaging. Bergmo, Kummervold, Gammon, and Dahl (2005) found that use of a secure electronic messaging system reduced the number of office visits but not the number of phone calls patients made. Obviously the phone remains an attractive option for many patients. Much education still takes place on the phone, as patients call health information lines for advice or engage in dialogue with their caregivers during follow-up calls.

In fact, aspects of teach-back can work well on the telephone. Barenfanger and colleagues (2004) tested a program to decrease phone reporting errors by requiring recipients of critical results to repeat the message back. Of 822 outgoing calls, 29 errors were detected, for an error rate of 3.5%. The time required to ask for the message to be repeated averaged just 12.8 seconds per call, but it paid off: the repeating of messages back corrected 29 errors. In the story with which we began this chapter, having Ellen repeat back the information about her biopsy results might have helped ward off the traumatic events that followed her misunderstanding of the word *negative*.

Use of the telephone does not guarantee better communication, of course. In nearly one-third of all clinical telephone encounters, physicians and patients perceive a different reason for the call; that is, more often patients see their calls as "true emergencies," even if the physician disagrees with such an assessment (Reisman & Brown, 2005). Clinicians should not try to make definitive diagnoses on the telephone; seeing patients face-to-face is always preferable. "A basic rule," write Fatovich and colleagues, "is that diagnosis via the telephone is not possible and that the best advice is to recommend a face-to-face consultation. With common sense, the proper use of the telephone can both facilitate patient care and maximize the available human resources" (Fatovich, Jacobs, McCance, Sidney, & White, 1998, p. 146).

Knowing what to say on the phone is as critical as knowing what not to say. Bad news, such as a cancer diagnosis, should be conveyed in person whenever possible (Back, 2005). Giving a diagnosis of cancer over the phone can create problems with patients as well as their families. In one study, spouses of newly diagnosed cancer patients expressed anger and bitterness when they were called with the news. An average of 87% of those who were informed of their diagnosis by telephone reported being in "psychological crisis" by the time of their first visit (Lalos, 1997).

Disclosure of other sensitive information, such as the presence of a sexually transmitted disease, also should take place during face-to-face clinical encounters. Results of a negative HIV test in a patient with no current HIV-risk behaviors could reasonably be given on the phone, but reportable results should be given in person unless patients instruct otherwise (Anderson, 1999; Reisman & Brown, 2005).

Test results should not be given to family members without the patient's permission, nor should results be left on an answering machine (Reisman & Brown, 2005). After all, failure to respect a patient's privacy, especially when it comes to sensitive information about HIV or sexually transmitted diseases, has led to lawsuits. In 1996, patient Audrey Blazac charged Stamford Hospital with breaching her HIV-antibody testing confidentiality following a needlestick accident. Blazac claimed she pricked herself with a needle she found on the floor of the hospital. When she returned to be tested for HIV, she said, a hospital employee stated loudly, within earshot of others, that the patient was there for an HIV antibody test. Even after Blazac asked the employee to explain that she was there only because of a needlestick injury, the employee refused to do so.

The primary focus of the lawsuit was the establishment of willful misconduct, which the court defined as conduct displaying a reckless disregard for the safety and rights of others and the consequences of one's actions. The hospital succeeded in striking down one of the contested counts involving invasion of privacy, but the judge refused to dismiss four of the seven counts in the lawsuit ("Hospital loses battle," 1996).

Another area of exposure—if not to lawsuits, then to medical errors—is that of after-hour telephone answering services. In an evaluation of after-hours calls to primary care physician offices that were not forwarded to an on-call physician, for example, physician reviewers classified 50% of the calls as urgent enough to have required immediate notification of the on-call physician. The investigators concluded that all clinical patient calls should be sent to appropriately trained medical personnel for triage decisions (Hildebrandt, Westfall, & Smith, 2003).

Because low-literate patients often have trouble articulating their conditions and symptoms, they are at greater risk for encountering such obstacles when using the phone to reach providers after hours. In light of this risk, clinicians who use answering services should reexamine their policies and procedures to ensure that after-hours telephone triage services receive specific instructions in how to deal with low-literate patients. They should look for such signs as a changed speech pattern or silence as indications of poor patient understanding (Reisman & Brown, 2005).

Face-to-face clinical encounters can be compromised by the kind of "noise" described at the beginning of this chapter. Construction outside the building may distract patients or even diminish what they hear. Nervous shifting on the part of the provider, even a fly buzzing around the room, could cause the patient to lose concentration and forget or not hear parts of the conversation. Similar distractions can interfere with telephone discussions. Patients may try to listen to medical advice while children play noisily in the background. Or they may attempt to have a serious telephone exchange while cooking dinner or while driving.

A few simple steps can help eliminate distractions and increase comprehension on the phone. Advise your patients to do the following:

■ Avoid using a cell phone to discuss medical information, especially in a moving vehicle, opting for a land-based line instead.
■ Initiate important, nonemergency calls, such as those to a physician, during quiet times (e.g., when children are at school).
■ Call only when they feel refreshed, such as after a nap or a good night's sleep.

- Have a paper and pencil or a computer handy to jot down questions or to take notes.
- Turn radios and televisions off and avoid answering the door or clicking over if they have call waiting on their phone line.
- Be aware if the person on the other end, such as a busy receptionist, seems distracted, offering to call back at another time (if nothing else, this alerts the other person to cues he or she is sending and could redirect his or her focus to the call).

Office staff also should be trained in the best techniques for telephone communication. Training should include phone etiquette, policies about what information is appropriate to discuss on the phone and what is not, even logistical strategies such as having a quiet space in which to talk, having access to health-related materials to answer patients' questions, good note-taking techniques, and procedures to ensure timely follow-up and appointment rescheduling.

A major disadvantage of telephone communication, of course, is that it eliminates nonverbal elements that are essential for clear and effective communication. When talking on the telephone, in other words, we cannot make eye contact and cannot see the faces or bodies of those with whom we are conversing. Unless a Web camera is used, traditional telephone exchanges eliminate both facial and bodily cues, which could change the way we interpret the other person's intended message. Voice intonation remains, but it lacks the physical context that makes messages easier to translate.

When speaking to someone in person, by contrast, we use information from the other person's face and body to draw conclusions about his or her emotional state, as Meeren, van Heijnsbergen, and de Gelder (2005) learned in a study conducted at the Cognitive and Affective Neuroscience Laboratory of Tilburg University in the Netherlands. They found that observers judging a facial expression were influenced strongly by emotional body language. Photographs of fearful and angry faces and bodies were used to create face–body compound images, with either matched or mismatched emotional expressions. The researchers recorded electrical brain activity while the subjects attended to the face and tried to judge its emotional expression. Interestingly, when the faces and bodies conveyed conflicting information, subjects' judgment of the facial expression was hampered, becoming biased toward the emotion expressed by the body.

TELEPHONE TRIAGE

Telephone triage is more than just answering health questions. In telephone triage, health care providers are called on to assess patients' concerns without making a visual inspection or having any face-to-face interaction. Derived from the French *trier*, meaning "to sort," triage is a brief clinical assessment that determines the time and sequence in which patients should be seen. These decisions are based on a short evaluation of the patient's overall appearance, history of illness or injury, mental status, and so on (Derlet, 2004).

To be effective, triage decisions made over the phone must rely exclusively on communication skills and knowledge about disease processes and growth and development among patients of all age groups. Clinicians engaged in telephone triage must have "impeccable listening skills to pick up on the non-verbal clues the [patient] is giving regarding pain, anxiety, fear and level of comprehension" (Courson, 2005).

Most triage systems use centralized groups of nurses who talk directly to patients on the phone, directing them to EDs or urgent care centers or to see their physician at the next available opportunity. In many cases, a triage nurse will offer home health advice to patients who do not need to go to the ED. Many triage systems rely on computers with medical information databases to guide health care providers. Some systems use algorithms that closely imitate physician logic and thought patterns (Derlet, 2004). These systems offer consistency and help standardize quality.

Telephone triage plays an equally important role in private practice and the ED, with effective interpersonal communication at the center of successful patient outcomes. In one study, Fatovich and colleagues (1998) evaluated 1,682 calls received in the ED of a major hospital in Perth, Western Australia, during a 4-month period. Seventy-two percent of callers phoned because of a spontaneous illness. Advice was considered inappropriate in only 1.4% of calls. Follow-up calls were made to 1,132 people (67%), and the noncompliance rate was only 6.9%. Most calls were for pediatric problems, but the investigators found that calls also were made for other problems ranging from domestic violence and child abuse to suicide and social isolation. The researchers called the provision of telephone advice "an under-recognised function of the emergency department of which healthcare planners should be aware."

Calling the ED may be the only after-hours option of which many low-literate patients are aware. In a study that tracked more than 140,000 calls made over a 1-year period to an after-hours pediatric telephone program in Denver, 88% were for clinical illness, 5% for information or advice, 1% were duplicate calls, and 1% were for miscellaneous reasons (Belman et al., 2005). Among illness calls, 21% of callers were told to go in for urgent evaluation, 30% were told to contact their primary care physician either the next day or at a later time, and 4% were advised to contact the on-call physician. Significantly, almost half of those who called—45%—were given home care instructions (Belman et al., 2005).

Despite limited awareness of non-ED options among low-health-literate patients, effective patient education efforts can help eliminate unnecessary calls or ED visits. In a study of Head Start patients and their families, Herman and Mayer (2004) found that easy-to-read reference books written at roughly a fifth-grade level could help significantly reduce unnecessary ED visits as long as the books were provided with additional guidance and training.

Although self-care and patient education can eliminate the need for many unnecessary ED visits, often the calls patients make to the ED are made for perfectly legitimate reasons. A study by Jacobson and colleagues (2001) evaluated the nature of after-hours telephone calls made to on-call gastroenterology fellows at a major hospital in Boston. Fellows documented the length and time of roughly 100 patient-initiated calls over a 7-month period. They also recorded the issue raised by the patient, what advice the patient was given, and the sex of the patient and attending gastroenterologist.

Sixty-seven percent of patients called with specific symptoms; 30% of those were referred to the ED. Only 1 of 13 patients with procedure-related (i.e., postendoscopy) symptoms required admission immediately or within a month of calling. However, 18 of 54 patients (33%) calling with nonprocedure-related symptoms required admission to the hospital either immediately after or within a month of calling. Because a significant number of patients calling with nonprocedure-related symptoms required admission, the investigators concluded that fellowship directors should provide training to fellows in the evaluation of symptoms over the phone.

In primary care, too, telephone triage is important, even though it does not prevent all errors. In a study of first- and third-year residents, faculty, and private practitioners, Yanovski and colleagues (1992) found that roughly one-third of all residents and private practitioners reached inappropriate management decisions during a simulated phone interview with a patient, despite obtaining information that should have altered their triage decisions.

With such statistics in mind, the Accreditation Council for Graduate Medical Education (ACGME) offers a phone triage checklist that evaluators can use when assessing medical students. The checklist helps ensure that telephone interactions with patients are courteous and professional and that health care providers communicate necessary information at all times (ACGME, 2000–2005). Following are several items from the ACGME's phone triage checklist:

- Informed call recipient of nature of call (e.g., "I am calling because . . .")
- Disclosed information in an appropriate venue (e.g., setting to protect privacy, away from public earshot) and to appropriate call recipient only
- Documented phone record (e.g., patient name, date, time, content of call, signature, placed hard copy in chart)
- Determined if patient chart needed for call (e.g., hospital number, date of birth)
- Provided information in a timely (e.g., returned call) and courteous manner
- Recorded callback information appropriately, including caller name, identifier, nature of call, urgency of call, return number (including area code or extension), name and spelling (phonetic pronunciation if also necessary) of caller, organization of caller if applicable, best time to return call if needed
- Did not place caller on hold unnecessarily
- Documented phone encounter appropriately in chart (e.g., signature, time, date)

Physicians, technicians, and nurses acting as evaluators can use the form while observing either a real encounter, a simulated or standardized telephone contact with a patient, or video or audiotaped encounters between residents and their patients. Evaluators provide feedback to the residents on their performance using the checklist in a chart-stimulated recall format. Tools such as the

ACGME checklist can offer important information on resident interpersonal and communication skills, professionalism, and tact (ACGME Outcome Project, 2006).

OPTIMIZING PATIENT–PROVIDER COMMUNICATION

Assessing patient and family literacy levels is extremely important, but the means by which assessment takes place should not be chosen arbitrarily. As mentioned earlier, simply asking the patient if he or she can read may cause embarrassment, and we know that low-literate patients often feel shame about their reading skills (Parikh, Parker, Nurss, Baker, & Williams, 1996). Many feel that testing patients should be avoided for this reason. In an interview with the Center for the Advancement of Health, for example, Rima Rudd, ScD, a faculty member in the Department of Health and Social Behavior at Harvard University's School of Public Health, is emphatic in her opposition to testing. In response to the question "Should physicians find some way to test the literacy of their patients before they proceed with a consultation, to gauge their level of understanding?" Dr. Rudd responded as follows:

> I don't think I could say this strongly enough: No! . . . First, people with very good literacy skills still appreciate plain language. In a study of physician conversations with white- and blue-collar patients in the HMO setting, where the researchers compared how the physicians spoke to each group, they found that the physicians tended to use more plain and simple language with their white-collar patients. Language can be used as a cultural divide. When people are not like you, you tend to be more formal in your presentation (*Law of averages*, 2001).

In addition to Dr. Rudd's legitimate concerns, clinicians should bear in mind that such tests as the Rapid Estimate of Adult Literacy in Medicine (REALM) and the Test of Functional Health Literacy in Adults (TOFHLA) can identify patients with low literacy skills, but should never be used unless the health care provider is willing to adjust the way he or she communicates and educates patients identified by the tests as having low literacy skills (Davis, Michielutte, Askov, Williams, & Weiss, 1998). If nothing in the way the health care provider communicates with low-health-literate patients changes, the risk of shaming and embarrassing those patients has been taken for nothing. (For more information about literacy assessment tools including the REALM and the TOFHLA, see chapter 3, Assessing Patients' Literacy Levels.)

In the AMA book *Understanding Health Literacy*, Davis, Kennen, Gazmararian, and Williams (2005) discuss issues that should be considered before selecting and administering literacy tests in health care settings, including important limitations for the use of such testing in research and clinical applications. In light of these limitations, it might be more effective (and is almost certainly more sensitive to patients) to use *observation* to look for signs and clues about a patient's literacy. Does the patient regularly bring family members along to visits and look to them for clarification during the clinical encounter? Does he or she fill out intake forms incompletely or inaccurately? Does the patient often claim to have left his or her glasses at home or insist on reading forms later?

When health care providers know that a patient did not graduate from high school, they cannot conclude for certain that he or she will have low health literacy, but the odds are certainly better. As we've discussed elsewhere in this book, older patients, those for whom English is not a first language, and first-generation patients from other countries are more likely to have low literacy. In addition, nearly half of all functionally illiterate Americans live in poverty (Kirsch, Jungeblut, Jenkins, & Kolstad, 1993).

Armed with this kind of information, health care providers should involve their office staff and ancillary providers in working with low-health-literate patients. Receptionists who distribute patient information and intake forms, for example, are uniquely positioned to make initial determinations about patients' literacy levels if they have received the proper training to do so. They should know what to look for and should be prepared to deal with such patients tactfully, as we discussed in chapter 2, Creating a Patient-Friendly Environment.

DEALING WITH OTHER COMMUNICATION PROBLEMS

Some providers fear that giving patients too much access could lead to unnecessary contact, perhaps in the form of frantic 3 a.m. phone calls. In a study at the University of Pennsylvania, however, patients given their surgeon's cell phone number exercised restraint in using it (Chin, Adams, Khoury, & Zurakowski, 2005). Seventy-two percent of 201 patients surveyed also felt their surgeon was more caring as a result of having received the number. Reisman and Brown (2005) suggest that patients who make late night calls should be given an opportunity to describe their chief complaint before the provider interrupts. In fact, the proportion of "serious" symptoms tends to increase as the hour becomes later (Peters, 1994; Reisman & Brown, 2005).

Patients who continually call back asking questions pose a unique challenge to providers, who must determine whether such behavior suggests an issue of basic understanding or whether there is another personal issue at stake. Missed appointments represent yet another challenge; clinicians must determine effective ways to remind patients of their scheduled appointments. Telephone reminders are one way, of course, but Cromer, Chacko, and Phillips (1987) found that appointment compliance was related more to sociobehavioral factors, such as whether the patient owned a phone, than to the use of phone reminders per se. In a study of 339 patients treated for gonorrhea, no overall improvements in compliance with follow-up were found when attempts were made to remind patients of appointments via telephone.

In another study by Ross, Friman, and Christophersen (1993), a simple combination of a mailed reminder and a parking pass was just as effective as a telephone reminder. The most frequent reasons for missing an appointment, as Ross and colleagues explain, were waiting time, distance, transportation, parking, miscommunication about appointment date or time, and the most obvious reason: forgetting.

Patient compliance is an ongoing issue, especially with low-literate patients. Inevitably, some patients will not participate in teach-back, for example. They may nod or fail to repeat back their understanding to the provider. First, providers should determine whether the patient is actually refusing to communicate or whether some other factor may be in play, such as shyness, misunderstanding, an unusually slow response time, or even a language barrier.

"If a patient won't repeat back what you've said," says Dr. Reisman, "the problem might be that your language has been pretty incomprehensible to them, so you might want to start over and present it in a simpler way, or a shorter way" (Anna B. Reisman, personal communication, December 2005). If language does not seem to be the problem, a next step might be to evaluate the patient's emotional state, which could suggest other possible reasons for noncompliance.

Health care providers must not jump to conclusions, however, because some behaviors that stem directly from low literacy, such as noncompliance with drug regimens, can be mistaken for stubbornness. Haas and colleagues (2005) make recommendations for dealing with the "difficult patient," some of which apply here. The most important thing is to keep trying new approaches. "Ignoring the problem or exporting it to another physician does not make the difficulty disappear," they note. "Accusing the patient of being problematic may provoke patient anger and counter-blaming" (Haas et al., 2005, p. 2066).

It is a good idea to evaluate the patient's body language. Does he or she seem agitated? Frightened? Hostile? Delicately emphasize the important role that patients can play in guiding their own health care, including their responsibility for communicating confusion or problems they have in complying with advice. If possible, rephrase any questions in simpler terms, asking the patient if he or she would prefer to write down his or her concerns. It may be necessary to ask family members to be present during the clinical interview; they may be able to shed light on the patient's lack of response.

Often, though, low health literacy is the culprit. Health care providers must reinforce information that is vital. Some patients with low health literacy simply do not understand why a return visit for such conditions as hypertension is important and may take important decisions about whether to comply with instructions into their own hands. "Many patients don't understand what hypertension is, and may assume that if they're not stressed out, they don't need to take their meds or come to visits," says Anna B. Reisman, MD (personal communication, December 2005). Educating patients about their chronic conditions through teach-back, visual aids, and other low-health-literate-friendly methods can help avoid misunderstandings, ultimately improving patient compliance.

Health care providers are wise to explain to all new patients (repeating the information frequently, if necessary) that the patient–provider relationship constitutes an exceedingly strong and important bond that affects the patient's quality of life. When it comes to communicating with patients, providers ought to be up front about their needs and listen carefully to patients' responses. They should tell the patient that together they will be dealing with sensitive and critical information and that the patient is expected to express his or her wishes about how that information should be conveyed. Does the patient prefer face-to-face interactions alone or with family members? Would he or she prefer using the telephone? E-mail? Some clinicians even save the last hour of their day for call backs and additional opportunities for patient communication.

Such extra time need not be offered pro bono; billing codes exist for emergency and after-hours care, though with a few caveats. For example, clinicians who see a patient after scheduled office hours can use the current procedural terminology (CPT) code 99050, which is billed in addition to basic services (Gordy, 2001). This code should not be used if you are simply running late or if you routinely book patients into after-hours slots, however. Patients seen during those times are considered scheduled patients. If you close your office for the day or are about to do so when a patient you think you ought to see calls, however, use of CPT code 99050 is probably appropriate. Use of these billing codes offers providers incentives by optimizing reimbursement (Jorgensen, 2003–2004).

COMMUNICATING FOR INTEGRATED CARE

In our modern health care system, with its multitude of subspecialties, care must often be coordinated among more than one provider. In other words, health care providers must know how to communicate with each other, as well as with their patients. For Weiner and colleagues (2005), communication in the delivery of health care occurs along two axes: between providers and patients and among several providers. Citing the Institute of Medicine, they note that one of the aims of primary care is "whole-person care," which is provided in the context of family and community.

A second aim, though, is integrated care, which involves coordinating and combining all of the personal health care services a patient needs over an extended period, "including the provision of comprehensive, coordinated, and continuous services" (Weiner et al., 2005, p. 709).

Institutional efforts toward integrated care and improved patient–provider communication are underway. In 1999, for example, the ACGME implemented a requirement that all residency programs in the United States provide instruction in "interpersonal and communications skills that result in effective information exchange and teaming with patients, their families, and other health professionals" (Teutsch, 2003).

Similarly, the National Board of Medical Examiners, Federation of State Medical Boards, and Educational Commission for Foreign Medical Graduates proposed an examination between the third and fourth years of medical school that would require U.S. medical students to "demonstrate [that] they can gather information from patients, perform a physical examination, and communicate their findings to patients and colleagues" (Teutsch, 2003).

Clearly these are positive developments in the area of patient–provider communication. After all, a generation of physicians who know how to communicate more effectively with each other as well as with patients will be better equipped to handle clinical challenges of all kinds in the future.

REFERENCES

Accreditation Council for Graduate Medical Education (ACGME). (2000–2005). *Phone triage checklist for resident interpersonal skills, communication, and professionalism.* Retrieved December 15, 2005, from http://www.acgme.org/outcome/implement/phoneTable.pdf

ACGME Outcome Project. (2006). *Teaching and assessing the resident phone encounter.* Retrieved January 1, 2006, from http://www.acgme.org/outcome/implement/rsvpTemplate.asp?rsvpID=27

AMC Cancer Research Center. (1994). *Beyond the brochure: Alternative approaches to effective health communication.* Denver, CO: Author. Retrieved December 13, 2005, from http://www.cdc.gov/cancer/nbccedp/bccpdfs/amcbeyon.pdf

American Medical Association (AMA) Foundation. (2005). *Health literacy video.* Retrieved December 20, 2005, from http://www.ama-assn.org/ama/pub/category/8035.html

Anderson, T. J. (1999). *Revised guidelines for HIV counseling, testing, and referral. Technical expert panel review of CDC HIV Counseling, Testing, and Referral Guidelines.* Atlanta: CDC.

Back, A. (2005). Communicating with family members. *Conversations in Care Web Book* (chapter 6). Retrieved December 2, 2005, from http://www.conversationsincare.com/web_book/chapter06.html

Barenfanger, J., Sautter, R. L., Lang, D. L., Collins, S. M., Hacek, D. M., & Peterson, L. R. (2004). Improving patient safety by repeating (read-back) telephone reports of critical information. *American Journal of Clinical Pathology, 121*(6), 790–791.

Belman, S., Chandramouli, V., Schmitt, B. D., Poole, S. R., Hegarty, T., & Kempe, A. (2005). An assessment of pediatric after-hours telephone care: A 1-year experience. *Archives of Pediatric and Adolescent Medicine, 159*(2), 145–149.

Bergmo, T. S., Kummervold, P. E., Gammon, D., & Dahl, L. B. (2005). Electronic patient-provider communication: Will it offset office visits and telephone consultations in primary care? *International Journal of Medical Informatics, 74*(9), 705–710.

Bogdan, G. M., Green, J. L., Swanson, D., Gabow, P., & Dart, R. C. (2004). Evaluating patient compliance with nurse advice line recommendations and the impact on health care costs. *American Journal of Managed Care, 10*(8),534–542.

Boyle, D., Dwinnell, B., & Platt, F. (2005). Invite, listen, and summarize: A patient-centered communication technique. *Academic Medicine, 80*(1), 29–32.

Brown, J. B., Boles, M., Mullooly, J. P., & Levinson, W. (1999). Effect of clinician communication skills training on patient satisfaction. *Annals of Internal Medicine, 131*, 822–829.

Chaffee, M. (1999). A telehealth odyssey. *American Journal of Nursing, 7,* 26–32.

Chaplin, W. F., Phillips, J. B., Brown, J. D., Clanton, N. R., & Stein, J. L. (2000). Handshaking, gender, personality, and first impressions. *Journal of Personality and Social Psychology, 79*(1), 110–117.

Chapman, K., Abraham, C., Jenkins, V., & Fallowfield, L. (2003). Lay understanding of terms used in cancer consultations. *Psychooncology, 12*(6), 557–566.

Chin, K. R., Adams, S. B., Khoury, L., & Zurakowski, D. (2005). Patient behavior if given their surgeon's cellular telephone number. *Clinical Orthopaedics and Related Research, 439,* 260–268.

Cocksedge, S., & May, C. (2005). The listening loop: A model of choice about cues within primary care consultations. *Medical Education, 39*(10), 999–1005.

Collier, J. B. (n.d.). *What is health psychology?* Retrieved December 17, 2005, from http://bama.ua.edu/~jcollier/health_psych_lecture_01.htm

Courson, S. (2005). *Telephone nurse triage: PA State Nurses Association.* Retrieved December 13, 2005, from http://www.panurses.org/search1.cfm?filename=membersite/articles/profdevelop/profdev_telephonetriage.htm

Cromer, B., Chacko, M., & Phillips, S. (1987). Increasing appointment compliance through telephone reminders: Does it ring true? *Journal of Developmental and Behavioral Pediatrics, 8*(3), 133–135.

Davis, T., Kennen, E. M., Gazmararian, J. A., & Williams, M. V. (2005). Literacy testing in health care research. In J. G. Schwartzberg, J. B. VanGeest, & C. C. Wang (Eds.), *Understanding health literacy: Implications for medicine and public health* (pp. 157–179). Chicago: American Medical Association Press.

Davis, T. C., Michielutte, R., Askov, E. N., Williams, M. V., & Weiss, B. D. (1998). Practical assessment of adult literacy in health care. *Health Education and Behavior, 25*(5), 613–624.

Davis, T. C., Williams, M. V., Marin, E., Parker, R. M., & Glass, J. (2002). Health literacy and cancer communication. *CA: A Cancer Journal for Clinicians, 52*(3), 134–149.

Derlet, R. (2004). *Triage.* eMedicine Web site. Retrieved December 17, 2005, from http://www.emedicine.com/emerg/topic670.htm

DeVito, J. A. (1986). *The interpersonal communication book* (4th ed.). New York: Harper & Row.

FACES Pain Rating Scale. (2005). *Elsevier: Wong on Web.* Retrieved December 30, 2005, from http://www3.us.elsevierhealth.com/WOW/faces.html

Fatovich, D. M., Jacobs, I. G., McCance, J. P., Sidney, K. L., & White, R. J. (1998). Emergency department telephone advice. *Medical Journal of Australia, 169,* 143–146.

Gibbs, R., Gibbs, P., & Henrich, J. (1987). Patient understanding of commonly used medical vocabulary. *Journal of Family Practice, 25,* 176–178.

Gordy, T. R. (2001). *Current procedural terminology 2001.* Chicago: American Medical Association Press.

Greene, M. G., Adelman, R. D., Friedmann, E., & Charon, R. (1994). Older patient satisfaction with communication during an initial medical encounter. *Social Science and Medicine, 38*(9), 1279–1288.

Haas, L. J., Leiser, J. P., Magill, M. K., & Sanyer, O. N. (2005). Management of the difficult patient. *American Family Physician, 72,* 2063–2068.

Hahn, E. A., Cella, D., Dobrez, D., Shiomoto, G., Marcus, E., Taylor, S. G., et al. (2004). The talking touchscreen: A new approach to outcomes assessment in low literacy. *Psychooncology, 13*(2), 86–95.

Heisler, M., Bouknight, R. R., Hayward, R. A., Smith, D. M., & Kerr, E. A. (2002). The relative importance of physician communication, participatory decision making, and patient understanding in diabetes self-management. *Journal of General Internal Medicine, 17,* 243–252.

Herman, A. D., & Mayer, G. (2004). Reducing the use of emergency medical resources among Head Start families: A pilot study. *Journal of Community Health, 29*(3), 197–208.

Hildebrandt, D. E., Westfall, J. M., & Smith, P. C. (2003). After-hours telephone triage affects patient safety. *Journal of Family Practice, 52*(3), 222–227.

Hinz, C. A. (2000). *Communicating with your patients: Skills for building rapport.* Chicago: American Medical Association.

Hospital loses battle to strike suit over HIV disclosure. (1996). *AIDS Policy Law, 11*(10), 2.

Jackson, J. L., & Kroenke, K. (1999). Difficult patient encounters in the ambulatory clinic: Clinical predictors and outcomes. *Archives of Internal Medicine, 159,* 1069–1075.

Jacobson, B. C., Strate, L., Baffy, G., Huang, L., Mutinga, M., & Banks, P. A. (2001). The nature of after-hours telephone medical practice by GI fellows. *American Journal of Gastroenterology, 96*(2), 570–573.

Jorgensen, D. J. (2003–2004). *Don't miss reimbursement opportunities. Proper coding for emergencies and after hours care can optimize payment for services you provide.* Retrieved December 19, 2005, from http://www.acofp.org/member_publications/comay.htm

Kane, J. (1996). Overcoming the dreaded L-block. *Alternative Therapies in Health and Medicine, 2*(5), 111,112.

Kane, J. (2003). *How to heal: A guide for caregivers.* New York: Helios Press.

Kirsch, I., Jungeblut, A., Jenkins, L., & Kolstad, A. (1993). *Adult literacy in America: A first look at the findings of the National Adult Literacy Survey.* Washington, DC: National Center for Education Statistics.

Klein, E. R. (2005). Effective communication with patients. *Pennsylvania Nurse, 60*(4), 14–15.

Lalos, A. (1997). The impact of diagnosis on cervical and endometrial cancer patients and their spouses. *European Journal of Gynaecological Oncology, 18*(6), 513–519.

Law of averages: Casting a wide net in health literacy efforts with Rima Rudd, ScD. (2001). (2003, March). *Facts of life: Issue briefings for health reporters.* Retrieved September 12, 2005, from http://www.cfah.org/factsoflife/vol8no3.cfm#3

Lawton, S., & Carroll, D. (2005). Communication skills and district nurses: Examples in palliative care. *British Journal of Community Nursing, 10*(3), 134–136.

Levinson, W., Stiles, W. B., Inui, T. S., & Engle, R. (1993). Physician frustration in communicating with patients. *Medical Care, 31*(4), 285–295.

Lloyd, B. W. (2005). What is the yield from asking, at the end of the consultation, if there are any further questions? An observational study. *Acta Paediatrics, 94*(2), 236–238.

Makoul, G. (2001). The SEGUE framework for teaching and assessing communication skills. *Patient Education and Counseling, 45*(1), 23–24.

Marik, P. E., & Fromm, L. (1998). A case series of hospitalized patients with elevated digoxin levels. *American Journal of Medicine, 106*(4), 489.

Marvel, M. K., Epstein, R. M., Flowers, K., & Beckman, H. B. (1999). Soliciting the patient's agenda: Have we improved? *Journal of the American Medical Association, 281*(3), 283–287.

Mayeaux, E. J., Murphy, P. W., Arnold, C., Davis, T. C., Jackson, R. H., & Sentell, T. (1996). Improving patient education for patients with low literacy skills. *American Family Physician, 53*(1), 205–211.

Mayer, G. (2002, September). Physicians can improve care for low-literacy patients. *The Quality Indicator,* 6–7.

Meeren, H. K., van Heijnsbergen, C. C., & de Gelder, B. (2005). Rapid perceptual integration of facial expression and emotional body language. *Proceedings of the National Academy of Sciences USA, 102*(45), 16518–16523.

Myerscough, P. R., & Donald, A. G. (1992). *Talking with patients: A basic clinical skill.* Oxford: Oxford University Press.

National Cancer Institute (NCI). (1994). *Clear and simple: Developing effective materials for low-literate readers.* Washington, DC: U.S. Government Printing Office.

National Center for Education Statistics (NCES). (2005). *A first look at the literacy of America's adults in the 21st century* (NCES 2006-470). Washington, DC: U.S. Department of Education, Institute of Education Sciences.

National Women's Health Resource Center. (2004, October). Women & health literacy. *National Women's Health Report Online.* Retrieved December 2, 2005, from http://www.healthywomen.org/healthreport/october2004/pg2.html

Nyman, K. (1991). The weeping patient. *Australian Family Physician, 20*(4), 444–445.

Ong, L., Haes, J. D., Hoos, A., & Lammes, F. (1995). Doctor-patient communication: A review of the literature. *Social Science and Medicine, 40,* 903–918.

Osborne, H. (2001). *Overcoming communication barriers in patient education.* Gaithersburg, MD: Aspen Publishers.

Osborne, H. (2005). *Health literacy from A to Z: Practical ways to communicate your health message.* Sudbury, MA: Jones and Bartlett Publishers.

Parikh, N. S., Parker, R. M., Nurss, J. R., Baker, D. W., & Williams, M. V. (1996). Shame and health literacy: The unspoken connection. *Patient Education and Counseling, 27,* 33–39.

Peters, R. (1994). After-hours telephone calls to general and subspecialty internists: An observational study. *Journal of General Internal Medicine, 9,* 554–557.

Quirt, C. F., Mackillop, W. J., Ginsburg, A. D., Sheldon, L., Brundage, M., Dixon, P., et al. (1997). Do doctors know when their patients don't? A survey of doctor-patient communication in lung cancer. *Lung Cancer, 18*(1), 1–20.

Reisman, A. B., & Brown, K. E. (2005). Preventing communication errors in telephone medicine. *Journal of General Internal Medicine, 20*(10), 959–963.

Robertson, K. (2005). Active listening: More than just paying attention. *Australian Family Physician, 34*(12), 1053–1055.

Robert Wood Johnson Foundation. (2000, June). *Study of medically nonurgent pediatric visits to hospital emergency departments.* Retrieved January 5, 2005, from http://www.rwjf.org/reports/grr/030445s.htm

Ross, L. V., Friman, P. C., & Christophersen, E. R. (1993). An appointment-keeping improvement package for outpatient pediatrics: Systematic replication and component analysis. *Journal of Applied Behavioral Analysis, 26*(4), 461–467.

Roter, D. L. (2005). How effective is your nonverbal communication? *Conversations in Care Web Book* (chapter 2). Retrieved December 2, 2005, from http://www.conversationsincare.com/web_book/chapter02.html

Roter, D. L., Stewart, M., Putnam, S. M., Lipkin, M., Stiles, W., & Inui, T. S. (1997). Communication patterns of primary care physicians. *Journal of the American Medical Association, 277*(4), 350–356.

Rothman, R. L., DeWalt, D. A., Malone, R., Bryant, B., Shintani, A., Crigler, B., et al. (2004). Influence of patient literacy on the effectiveness of primary-care-based diabetes disease management program. *Journal of the American Medical Association, 292*(14), 1711–1716.

Safeer, R. S., & Keenan, J. (2005). Health literacy: The gap between physicians and patients. *American Family Physician, 72*(3), 387–388.

Schillinger, D., Piette, J., Grumbach, K., Wang, F., Wilson, C., Daher, C., et al. (2003). Closing the loop: Physician communication with diabetic patients who have low health literacy. *Archives of Internal Medicine, 163*(14), 1745–1746.

Street, R. L., Gordon, H. S., Ward, M. M., Krupat, E., & Kravitz, R. L. (2005). Patient participation in medical consultations: Why some patients are more involved than others. *Medical Care, 43*(10), 960–969.

Tabak, E. R. (1988). Encouraging patient question-asking: A clinical trial. *Patient Education and Counseling, 12*(1), 37–49.

Tattersall, M. H., & Butow, P. N. (2002). Consultation audio tapes: An underused cancer patient information aid and clinical research tool. *Lancet Oncology, 3*(7), 431–437.

Teutsch, C. (2003). Patient-doctor communication. *Medical Clinics of North America, 87*(5), 1115–1145.

Walter, A., Bundy, C., & Dornan, T. (2005). How should trainees be taught to open a clinical interview? *Medical Education, 39*(5), 445–447.

Weiner, S. J., Barnet, B., Cheng, T. L., & Daaleman, T. P. (2005). Processes for effective communication in primary care. *Annals of Internal Medicine, 142*, 709–714.

Weiss, B. D. (2003). *Health literacy: A manual for clinicians*. Chicago: American Medical Association Foundation and American Medical Association.

Williams, M. V., Davis, T., Parker, R. M., & Weiss, B. D. (2002). The role of health literacy in patient-physician communication. *Family Medicine, 34*(5), 383–389.

Yanovksi, S. Z., Yanovski, J. A., Malley, J. D., Brown, R. L., & Balaban, D. J. (1992). Telephone triage by primary care physicians. *Pediatrics, 89*, 701–706.

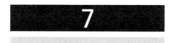

DESIGNING EASY-TO-READ PATIENT EDUCATION MATERIALS

Donovan Lowell (not his real name) is a smart, well-dressed White male in his early fifties. If you met him on the street, you would probably assume he was successful, upper middle class, holding down a respectable job, an upstanding member of his community, well liked, and a good family man. In general, you'd be correct. Donovan has an engaging smile, he never forgets a name or face, he is active in several community service volunteer agencies, and he is a wonderful father and a loving husband.

However, Donovan has two problems: he is about to be diagnosed with diabetes, and he cannot read above a fourth-grade level.

Growing up in rural Indiana, Donovan did just well enough in reading and writing to move on to the next grade. Although he dropped out of high school to go to work, from there he started his own business. His business acumen and personality have more than made up for his lack of reading skills. Although his wife knows that his reading skills are not strong, she is not aware of his exact level of illiteracy, and neither are his children.

In a cost-saving move, Donovan's company recently switched health plans, and Dr. Jeffries, Donovan's doctor for the past 10 years, is not a participating provider on the new plan. Although Donovan liked Dr. Jeffries, he decides to try someone on the new health plan, as the out-of-pocket costs to continue to see Dr. Jeffries would be considerable.

Donovan is now seeing Dr. DeGroot, who participates in the health plan. About a week ago, Donovan made an appointment with Dr. DeGroot because he had been feeling bad for several months. Dr. DeGroot had him take some tests, and now he is visiting the office for his results. During the visit, Donovan is told about his diagnosis of diabetes. He is given strict instructions on what he can and cannot eat, told he needs to lose some weight, and given a folder of materials with information about diabetes.

On his way out, the nurse hands him a newsletter. "There's a great article in here about diabetes management on page 11," she tells him as they walk down the hall, "and some dietary guidelines that Dr. DeGroot concurs with, so be sure to read it."

When Donovan gets home, he is reluctant to start sifting through all the information he has been given. He remembers how enthusiastic the nurse was about the article, but he doesn't remember what page she said it was on. He sits down with the newsletter and tries to find the article.

He looks at the first page. The headlines are long, written in all capital letters. The words look unfamiliar and difficult. He tries to read some of the words in the first story and then decides it can't be the one about diabetes. There are pictures in the newsletter, some of people smiling and playing outdoors and others of people sitting at a table talking to one another. *What does this have to do with diabetes?*, he wonders. Most of the pictures don't have any words below them, so Donovan is unsure why they are there. He continues to flip through the newsletter.

On the inside, there is an article with a drawing of a carrot, a head of broccoli, a block of cheese, and a bottle of milk. He thinks maybe this is the story the nurse was talking about. He starts to read through it. First he tries to find the word *diabetes* in the article, but as he is trying to make his way through the text, he loses his focus and his train of thought.

He starts on another article, but for some reason he keeps losing his place. It's probably because the tiny type goes all the way across the page, and he finds himself having to use his finger to keep his place in the article.

Discouraged, he finally puts the newsletter aside. *Maybe later,* he tells himself. He puts the newsletter with the pile of brochures on diabetes. For a moment, he tries to convince himself that he ought to read through the pile of materials. The thought is not very appealing.

The telephone rings and, almost with relief, he puts the materials into a drawer, where they will stay for a long time.

*   *   *

Diabetes is not Donovan's only problem; equally dispiriting is the fact that the education materials he has been given are not well suited to people on his reading level. In the case of designing *patient education* materials, the ultimate goal seems self-evident: *patient education*. We want our readers (i.e., patients) to begin to understand a concept that, before reading the materials, they did not understand.

Although this sounds like a simple, basic concept, it is one that many writers and designers of patient education materials seem to forget. There are many temptations out there that can trip up otherwise well-intentioned patient education materials:

- the desire to show off our vocabulary
- the misconception that a more formal style will fit more closely with our company's image
- the notion that more is better with respect both to the number of words and the amount of graphic elements
- the idea that if there is white space, we need to fill it

- showing off our extensive font library by using the fanciest, most outlandish type faces we have
- believing that because we *can* include more information by simply reducing the size of the type, we *should*
- using graphics that are well drawn but do not meet the needs of the low-literate reader with regard to simplicity and direct illustration of basic concepts

Unfortunately, these desires are at odds with our goal of conveying usable information in a manner in which our readers can understand and use it. Good design is clean; it does not draw attention to itself. It is often defined more by what is not there than by what is. In other words, fancy typefaces, ornate graphic design elements, and densely detailed illustrations are not helpful and are not necessarily the hallmarks of good design. They are the elements that novices use because they can, not because they should.

We should always have our end user in mind as we put together the elements of our patient education materials. After each decision you make, ask yourself these questions: Will this help or hinder the reader from understanding the underlying message? Is this element necessary to convey the information, or is it only meant to decorate?

Just as the efficient editor will take a rambling sentence, scan it for its essence, and whittle away unnecessary words, so too should we look at the patient education materials we are constructing and include only those elements that will enhance the likelihood that patients walk away informed and more able to care for themselves or their loved ones. After all, they are the clients, the customers for whom we all work, so think in terms of good customer service. Everything we do should be in support of that one effort: clear, effective communication.

BEFORE YOU BEGIN DESIGNING PATIENT EDUCATION MATERIALS

Text and graphics should be complementary elements, working together toward the same goal: clear, effective patient education. Graphics should illustrate points made in the text clearly and simply; simple labeling and captions should explain and provide reference and organizational structure to the graphics. Both should convey information in a straightforward manner.

Throughout chapter 8, Principles of Writing for Low Literacy, we offer information on writing for clarity and for communicating ideas effectively. Achieving that aim requires a thorough planning process. One excellent guide to this process, provided by the National Cancer Institute (NCI, 2003), is entitled *Clear and Simple: Developing Effective Print Materials for Low Literate Readers.* It is available online at http://www.cancer.gov/aboutnci/oc/clear-and-simple.

This chapter provides some tips on approaching the design process so that it helps meet the goal of providing clear, effective patient education. Use this information in conjunction with that presented in chapter 8 to make the best patient education materials you can. At the end of this chapter, you will find some of the resources from which this material has been drawn.

Drawing on Multiple Resources

Do not rely solely on articles and brochures about design for your inspiration; they are merely tips, guidelines, and starting points. *People* are your best resources, particularly those who will be using your materials. Don't be afraid to get input all along the way in the design process. Talk with other people; good design does not occur in a vacuum. Make use of as many resources as you can.

Tap into the resources of the community. Speak with designers at advertising agencies and public relations firms, architects, and publishers. Look to your local universities, colleges, and high schools (yes, high schools): young design students often bring fresh perspectives that you may not have considered. If you work for a nonprofit organization, you have a tremendous amount of currency in that position. Put it to use; pro bono efforts by ad agencies and public relations firms benefit everyone.

Sponsor a design contest for the graphic arts department of your local high school or college. Ask a local merchant to provide a prize for first, second, and third place. Speak with the local newspaper and arrange coverage of the prize ceremony.

Look at other patient education materials. What do you like about them? What do they do well? What do they do wrong? Keep files of existing materials and write down your ideas.

Formal and informal focus groups (discussed in more detail in chapter 8) made up of potential end users of your materials can provide invaluable information and validation of your approaches to design. Present the same materials to groups in different design formats. After participants have reviewed the materials, ask them to recall selected pieces of information. Chances are that the piece you designed more effectively will yield greater recall. (This is also a wonderful opportunity to network with academics looking for a research project that will allow them to design a study to yield statistically valid results that test and validate the text and design elements.)

The process of iterative design (i.e., test, make changes, retest) should not be limited to engineers (Bailey, 2005). The federal government's Department of Health and Human Services hosts a Web site called Usability.gov. Billing itself as "Your resource for designing usable, useful, and accessible Web sites and user interfaces," the site applies the principle of iterative design to effective Web site design. Although this chapter is not meant specifically for Web site designers, and the conventions used in a dynamic medium such as the Internet have many unique features, good ideas and good design principles are universal in many respects. Look at this Web site and in particular the article at this link—http://www.usability.gov/pubs/072005news.html—which discusses the value of usability testing and iterative design (Bailey, 2006). Can you think of any applications of this process as you design your patient education materials?

As you plan out your patient education piece, it is also important to keep in mind elements of learning theory. How do your readers learn best? Do they prefer a more visually oriented approach to learning? Do stepwise written instructions appeal more? Although you do not need a degree in education to design effective patient education materials, it is a good idea to familiarize yourself with basic concepts of how people learn best. A good resource is *Teaching Patients With Low Literacy Skills* (1996), the landmark text by Doak, Doak, and Root mentioned in various chapters throughout this book. In addition to providing an excellent review of basic learning theory, this book offers a good model for developing patient education materials and includes sections on writing and evaluating materials, using visual elements, and tips on teaching.

APPEARANCE OF MATERIALS

The goal when preparing written materials is to create a page layout that makes it easy for your intended audience to use the materials. Several elements contribute to the appearance of a written piece, including the following:

- text
- layout
- white space
- paper
- graphics

Text

The term *text* refers to the words printed on a page. To communicate successfully with the intended audience, the text in your written materials needs to be easy to read. In a number of studies conducted over a 9-year period (from 1982 to 1990), Colin Wheildon, author of *Type and Layout: Are You Communicating or Just Making Pretty Shapes?* (2005), found that more than five times as many readers were able to understand text printed in a serif font (e.g., Times New Roman, Garamond) than a sans serif font (e.g., Arial, Helvetica).

And just what is a serif? It is the small, finishing stroke you see at the ends of letters in any type family characterized as a serif font. One of the easiest letters in which to see the serif is the capital letter T. A capital T in a serif font will sport a small, downward stroke on either side of the main crossing line at the top and generally a little lateral stroke on either side of the base of the straight down line. A sans serif ("without serif") font capital T will have two lines: a vertical one, capped with a shorter horizontal one at the top—no ornaments, no little strokes, nice and clean (Figure 7.1).

If you use one of the most popular word-processing programs on your computer, Microsoft Word, try this exercise: with your Caps Lock feature on, type the alphabet in a single paragraph, with a single space in between each letter. Then, hit your Enter or Return key and repeat the exercise (or you can click your

Text Text

FIGURE 7.1 Examples of serif and sans serif fonts. The capital T on the left is set in Times New Roman, a serif font. Note the two downward details off the main top cross stroke and the two finishing details off the bottom of the main down stroke. The capital T set on the right is in Arial, a sans serif typeface. Note its lack of these finishing details.

left mouse button three times until the paragraph is highlighted, hit Control-C, then place your cursor in the next paragraph and hit Control-V to paste the same paragraph down). Next, select the first paragraph and, in your drop-down box that allows you to designate a type face, select Times New Roman. In your next paragraph, select all of the text again, but this time, format it as Arial.

Look closely at each letter and see the differences in each one. On those letters that have a straight downstroke (e.g., D, E, F, H, K, L, M, N), notice the little finishing strokes at the bottom of the line formatted in Times New Roman. Now, compare those same letters with the line formatted in Arial. You will see that there are no finishing strokes on those letters. They are sans serif, or without the serif finishing stroke (in French, *sans* means "without"). All typefaces can be categorized generally as either serif or sans serif.

Using a serif font for the majority of text in a written piece is preferable, though a sans serif font may be better for headings and subheadings unless the document is particularly short (Singer, 2002). Any font that incorporates stylized letters should be avoided because they interrupt the flow of reading and make it more difficult for your patients to receive the message. It is especially difficult to read long blocks of italic text, for example. Regardless of the font you choose, printed materials should not have more than two styles on any page (Mayer, 2003).

Write your text in upper- and lowercase letters, using the normal convention of capitalizing the first word of each sentence as well as proper nouns and acronyms (e.g., AIDS, NIH). Never write text in all capital letters for emphasis. Wheildon's (2005) studies showed that 93% of those shown a passage written in all capital letters said it was not easy to read. If you want to emphasize a portion of the text, use bolding or underlining of the word or phrase. But use these emphasis techniques sparingly, not for long passages.

The size of the text is important too. Patients should not have to strain to make out the letters in your written materials. Text size is especially important when your intended audience includes older patients and those with low health literacy. For example, Lighthouse International, a worldwide resource on vision loss and impairment, suggests that text written for older adults and the visually impaired should be at least 16 points (Arditi, 2005). For most audiences, a font that is 12 to 14 points is sufficient (Mayer, 2003). Because of space and cost limitations, you may not have the luxury of designing materials with text that large. But by striving to keep text as large as possible, you can work to optimize the readability of all your written materials.

Another typographical issue that goes hand in hand with text size is leading, or the amount of space between the lines. The term *leading* comes from the early days of manual typesetting when movable type was set by hand in lead and the space between lines was created by thin strips of lead. Wheildon's studies showed that the preferred combination of type size and leading is 11-point type over 13-point line spacing (Wheildon, 2005). However, this combination is one with which you should experiment based on the size of your finished piece, the amount and type of graphics on your page, and your choice of font. When in doubt, it is better to err on the side of larger text and more generous line spacing.

A number of rules regarding text and color are worth remembering. Wheildon's studies examined readers' comprehension when they were asked to read text that had been subjected to several different graphical treatments. When readers were given text printed in bright colors rather than black text (like you're reading now), 81% demonstrated poor comprehension. Reasons for this vary, but they include an inability to concentrate, lines of text that appear to merge together, and problems with sufficient contrast between text and paper when certain combinations were used. Some readers said they preferred reading the colored text, but when this group was actually tested, their comprehension also was much lower (Wheildon, 2005).

If colored text is difficult to comprehend, reverse text may be even worse. When they were given text that was set in reverse type—that is, white type against a black background, as opposed to the standard black text against a white background (as you are reading now)—88% of respondents showed poor comprehension. Reasons for this are fairly obvious, but think of the last time you looked at a photographic negative (an item that, in this age of digital photography, is fast becoming an artifact). Was it difficult to pinpoint and recognize all the elements you would normally be able to discern in a positive photograph? The reason is that your ability to relate the image to images you are familiar with is impeded by the reversal of expectations. We encounter black type against a white background a vast majority of the time, so that is what we expect to see. It's the norm; anything different requires our attention to reconcile the new presentation with our expectations. In other words, reversing expectations takes our concentration away, however momentarily, from the act of reading.

This brings us to a point that is covered in more detail in the upcoming section on layout: designing your patient education materials is not the time to try out new, cutting-edge design tactics. It is better to use the tried and true, meeting your readers' expectations. That way you are more likely to have the audience concentrate on—and comprehend—your message.

The overall amount of text on a page should not be so great as to be overwhelming to your intended audience. We saw this in the story of Donovan Lowell with which we opened this chapter. The diabetes article he attempted to read was intimidating, causing him to lose his focus and concentration. Having too much text on a page makes it difficult for readers to find important points. It also increases the odds that patients will not read the material at all. Even those patients who read such text will have difficulty identifying its critical message. A good rule of thumb is to have no more than 5 inches of type running horizontally across the page (Mayer, 2003). Try using bulleted lists to cut down on the amount of text and to highlight important ideas.

Layout

In general, layout refers to the way text and graphics are arranged on the page. It includes the spacing between lines of text, the spatial relationship between text and graphics (including the directional flow of text as it is influenced by the presence of graphics), and the width of columns of text (and whether you use columns at all). It is, in effect, the final product of the decisions you make while "building" the page.

Layout also includes navigational decisions your reader must make to read and process information you present. In large measure, your decisions will determine whether navigation is an easy, intuitive task or a difficult, convoluted one. Your decisions also affect comprehension of the material—the reason your patient education materials exist in the first place.

In Western culture, in which we read a language of a Latin-based alphabet, we are trained and accustomed to reading in a certain pattern and direction: across the page from left to right, then down to the next line, and again from left to right. This pattern is intuitive and natural for readers of virtually any skill level. But when designers violate this basic rule of what Wheildon (2005) calls "reading gravity," we force our readers to start making conscious decisions that they normally do not need to make. This detracts from the normal concentration efforts and can wreak havoc with comprehension. Therefore, we need to consider some basic rules on flow, eye movement, and how we want our readers to proceed through our document.

In general, given a page filled completely with nothing but plain, uninterrupted, unindented, single-column type, readers will start in the upper left corner, read across, and work their way down to the bottom of the page, starting each line at the left margin of text. Then they will read across and return to the left margin to start the next line down, and so on, until they have finished (assuming, of course, you can actually induce someone to read such an imposing block of plain text).

This is the natural flow, and any time we violate this pattern, we throw up a road block to our readers. In effect, we ask them to multitask or to do something other than concentrate on the task at hand (which, in our case, is to read and comprehend our patient education materials). Asking them to accommodate our poor design decisions results in diminished comprehension. Is the tradeoff worth it?

Keeping it simple in layout is, at its most basic level, a show of respect for our readers. We are saying that their time is valuable, that we wish to help them in their goal of reading information to acquire knowledge, and that such a goal is more important than any other. Once we have accepted this goal, we can then proceed with designing effective patient education pieces.

If we are following the basic rules of reading gravity, we will start with our graphic at or very near the top and follow it with a short, informative headline. Our text will follow below this headline. There are many variations on this layout, but as long as we keep in mind the natural tendency of the eye when reading materials—left to right, then down and back to the left margin, then left to right again—and we ensure that our combination of text and graphics supports this movement, we should be on the right track.

Arranging text in columns is generally a good idea. Columns provide structure for the reader, making it easier for them to keep a mental note of where they are while reading. In addition, columns respect the left-to-right rule and, perhaps most important, make the horizontal "jump" the eye must make from the end of one line to the beginning of the next a much shorter jump. This helps readers keep their place as they read.

Suggestions on line length vary, from no more than 5 inches of type across any given column (Mayer, 2003) to no fewer than 20 and no more than 60 characters across (Wheildon, 2005). Characters are defined as letters and spaces and include punctuation.

It is a good idea to indent the first line of each paragraph. This is a recognizable and accepted formatting practice, and it provides a place for readers to "take a breath," reset, and brace themselves for another idea (the basic building block of a well-written paragraph). Indented paragraphs also provide visual breaks in the text that make it less intimidating and provide additional white space on the page. They serve as navigational tools too, providing readers with another placeholder or guide to remind them where they are in the text.

In longer pieces, subheads help organize the text and prepare the reader for what comes next. Subheads should be short—just a few words, and no more than one line or two at the most—and can be set in bold type to draw attention and provide another visual break and navigational aid for readers. The type size should be no more than one or two points larger than the text; subheads the same size as the main body text are acceptable.

Wheildon's studies showed that readers prefer that type be set in a range from 10 to 14 points. At least one point of line spacing, and preferably two, should be used (Wheildon, 2005). Although Wheildon acknowledges that different typefaces vary in size within a set point size, the overwhelming choice (98% percent) in his studies of type size and line spacing is 11 point with 13 line spacing. (If you wish to achieve a specific line spacing in Microsoft Word, select your type, then go to the Format dropdown menu, select Paragraph, then select the Indents and Spacing tab. In the Spacing section, select Exactly from the Line Spacing dropdown menu, and the specific number you want from the "At:" menu adjacent to that. Type size is chosen from the Format menu under Font.)

If you are designing patient education materials for the visually impaired rather than for low-literate patients, however, there is a different set of recommendations. Lighthouse International, a nonprofit service organization for those with visual impairments, provides resources on designing for the visually impaired. Visit their Web site at http://www.lighthouse.org and type "designing" in the search engine for references. Major departures from the recommendations for low-literate patients include a preference for reversed-out type, larger-than-usual type size, and ragged right-set type over justified.

Another decision must be made on the justification of type. No, this does not mean providing a rationale for using an alphabet. Justification refers to the alignment of the left and right sides of the column. When each line begins flush with the left margin and ends indiscriminately on the right in roughly the same area, depending on how long or short the last word is, that is called *ragged right* (also referred to as *flush left* or *left justified*). Conversely, text that meets flush on the right side of the column but does not match up on the left is called *ragged left*. Text that is a uniform length from left to right margin (first line indent notwithstanding) is called *justified text*.

Wheildon's studies showed that using ragged right or left text justification is not a good idea. Comprehension was judged at three levels: good, fair, and poor. Good comprehension levels for justified type came in at 67% (19% fair, 14% poor). When type was set ragged right, good comprehension dropped to 38% (22% fair, 40% poor). When type was set ragged left (a much more unconventional and unfamiliar type justification), good comprehension plummeted to an abysmal 10% (18% fair and 72% poor; Wheildon, 2005). The message is clear: justified columns are the clear favorite.

Does this mean that we should never, ever set our type in any style other than justified? No. Like anything else, thinking in absolutes is generally not a good plan. In some word-processing programs when certain fonts are used, justified type results in awkward, uneven spacing between words, leaving big holes and uneven spacing in the lines. In these cases, justified type forces the eye to jump over a space to get to the next word. In shorter sections, ragged right type generally can be used without a devastating effect.

White Space

To make your patient education materials look more inviting, include ample white space (i.e., space without printing on it). There is some temptation to cram as much information as you can into the space you have to save money. However, materials for low-literate patients are not the place to be budget conscious. In fact, the more white space you can incorporate, the better. Try using extra-wide margins and widely spaced sections of text.

A generous amount of white space makes a page look less intimidating. Two pages of densely packed text will appear much harder to read than four pages of the same text with generous white space. The psychological barrier of the dense two-page document may be enough to keep readers from even trying to get through all the information.

Plenty of white space also allows for more contrast for your graphic elements. Try this simple experiment. Find two black jellybeans (or any dark-colored objects about the same size). Next, cut out an 8 1/2″ by 11″ sheet from a newspaper with mostly text, not ads. Set this sheet next to a plain, unlined sheet of white bond paper, the kind you put in a laser printer or use in a photocopier.

Now, place one jellybean anywhere on each page. Stand about 3 feet away. On which sheet does the jellybean stand out more? On the newspaper sheet, it is just one more graphic element lost in the gray sea of type. It has much less contrast. On the plain sheet of paper, however, your attention is diverted immediately to the jellybean. Why? Because of all the white space. The contrast between the jellybean and the white space is powerful. Contrast is what allows us to appreciate the difference between the plain paper and the jellybean.

Think of it another way. If all you ever ate were jelly donuts, then all you would have experience tasting would be the sensation of sweet. You would have no appreciation for what sweet really was, because you would have nothing with which to contrast it. However, if you ate the sweet jelly donut after drinking a cup of bitter espresso, the sweetness would stand out in contrast to the bitter taste. The espresso allows you to make a value judgment, a clear distinction, between the two. Similarly, contrast on the page allows readers to pay more attention, making it more likely that they will notice the graphical elements.

Paper

The color and finish of the paper you choose for your written materials are important. Strive for the highest possible contrast between your paper and your type. Using black letters on white paper is a good standard for written materials (Sanner, 2003). As for finish, a matte (dull) finish is generally preferable to glossy paper. A gloss finish can create a glare, which can be distracting, especially to older patients (Sanner, 2003). Rudd (2005) recommends not using a shaded or patterned background. Printing your text on a background with shading or a pattern reduces the amount of contrast and violates the general rule against clutter. Placing type on a pattern creates a fight for attention, which is the last thing you want to create when you are trying to present a message clearly to readers.

It is a good idea to work with your printer ahead of time when making decisions about what type of paper to use. Discuss how people are going to use the materials because the most appropriate size depends on its use. Is it going to be kept in a purse and used on a daily basis? Is it going to be taped to the refrigerator door? Are you expecting that the patient will write on it? Will it be folded up and kept in someone's back pocket, brought out time and time again for reference purposes?

The answers to all of these questions will provide you with guidance on the size and type of paper you should ultimately choose. For instance, if you provide space on your education piece for patients to write something (such as the number of times they've taken their medication that day, a food diary, or their blood pressure or blood sugar level), you need to be sure that the paper can take pencil or pen marks without smearing. You will definitely want to choose an uncoated stock.

If you expect that the piece is going to be carried around and referred to over and over again, then you want it printed on a sturdier stock, and you may wish to consider a coated stock. Talk to the printer and ask for a low-gloss finish that resists glare and will wear well. It is important to know whether a finish will fade, smear, run, or become illegible if it gets wet or become stained if food is dropped on it.

Will the pages be folded over and over again? Certain types of paper will crack and split at the seams when folded and unfolded many times. Does the piece need to be in a booklet format? If so, consider how it will be used. Some booklets are designed to open and lay flat naturally, making it easier to refer to if your hands are full (for instance, if the piece is providing instructions on how to do something, such as give yourself a shot, which requires the use of both hands). Others have a tendency to close back up and require the user to crease them or put something on each page to keep it open. Choosing the right type of binding, or method of holding all the pages together, will be helpful here. A comb or ring binding will help allow pages to lay flat. One money-saving method of binding is a simple staple. When larger sheets of paper are folded in the middle and stapled along the fold to keep them together, it is referred to as a stitch (or, more frequently, a saddle stitch).

Think through the way the piece will be distributed, used, kept, and stored, and make your decisions with your printer based on this information. If possible, ask patients how they would use such materials or how they have used similar materials in the past. You can use their experience as a guide to your decisions.

Graphics

Tables, charts, photos, and illustrations can help make complex information easier to understand. Any graphics you include in written materials should complement your text. It should be clear to readers exactly what a particular illustration is intended to portray. If you are not sure what you are supposed to be looking at in a given illustration, it is not working. Ideally, the illustrations used in materials intended for low-literate patients should be simple line drawings. This type of drawing allows such patients to focus on the important information the illustration is meant to convey. The texts and illustrations in Figures 7.2 and 7.3, reproduced from the Institute for Healthcare Advancement's (IHA's) easy-to-read book *What To Do When Your Child Gets Sick* (2001), exemplify this practice, with simple line drawings that reinforce messages written at or below a fifth-grade reading level (Mayer & Kuklierus, 2001).

Illustrations are most successful when they match the experience of the target audience. Photographs, says Sanner (2003), should depict people who appear to be roughly the same age as the intended audience, who resemble the intended audience, and who wear the same type of clothing as the intended audience. Make sure originals are well lit with good contrast. They should show clearly the concept to be explained, without a lot of unnecessary detail. If you use photographs, be sure to evaluate how they will appear in the final printed piece. If you are photocopying the piece, photographs tend to become muddy and more difficult to see.

Aracely Rosales, president of Plain Language and Culture, Inc., and former director of the Latino Health Project, offered an excellent example of how

Fever

- Check your child's temperature every 4 hours during the day. Check it more often if your child looks or acts sick.

- If your child is fussy or is not eating and drinking, give your child Tylenol every 4–6 hours if fever is over 101 degrees F (oral). Read the label to find out how much medicine to give, or ask your doctor or nurse.

- **Do not give aspirin to anyone younger than 21 years.** Aspirin can make a child very sick.

- Take your child's temperature 30 minutes after giving Tylenol. If the fever is still over 102 degrees (oral) or 103 degrees (rectal), sponge your child with lukewarm water.

- This is how to sponge your child. Put your child in three inches of lukewarm water. Sponge your child with a wash cloth for 10–15 minutes. Stop the sponge bath if your child starts to shiver. Shivering increases fever.

- Do not put rubbing alcohol in the sponge bath water.

When do I call the doctor or nurse?

- Your baby is younger than 2 months and has a fever of 100.2 degrees F (rectal) or higher.

- Your baby is between 2 and 6 months old and has a fever of 101 degrees F (rectal) or higher.

- Your child is older than 6 months and has a fever of 103 degrees F (rectal) or higher.

FIGURE 7.2 Sample illustration and text from *What To Do When Your Child Gets Sick* (p. 15). Note how the illustration supports the text immediately next to it, showing a graphic illustration of the instructions on how to provide a sponge bath for a baby with a fever.

important illustrations and photographs can be during her presentation at an annual conference hosted by IHA in May 2005. She told how, during the development of a bilingual education piece for women cancer survivors, *Celebramos el Mañana: Latinas que Sobreviven el Cancer del Seno* ("We Celebrate Tomorrow: Latinas Living Beyond Breast Cancer"), information from focus groups resulted in the cover being redesigned three times. The issue, she explained, was that the women wanted to see photos that included the important people in their

CPR (Cardiopulmonary Resuscitation)

What can I do for a baby (younger than 1 year)?

1. Try to wake the baby up. If baby does not wake up, yell for help. Tell someone to **call 911.**

2. Lay baby on something hard like the floor or a table. Put the baby on his or her back.

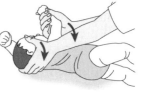

3. Tilt baby's head back by lifting the chin with one hand and pushing the forehead back with the other hand. Do not close the baby's mouth.

4. Look at baby's chest to see if it's moving. Listen for sounds of air going in and out. Put your cheek next to baby's mouth and see if you feel air on your cheek.

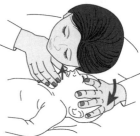

5. If baby is not breathing, start mouth-to-mouth breathing. Open your mouth and take a breath. Cover baby's nose and mouth with your mouth. Make a tight seal.

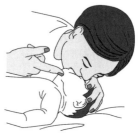

6. Give 2 slow breaths into the baby. The breaths should be about 1½–2 seconds long. Take a breath yourself between breaths into the baby. Look at baby's chest to see if it goes up and down. Keep baby's head tilted back with the mouth open.

FIGURE 7.3 Sample illustrations and text from *What To Do When Your Child Gets Sick* (p. 156). Illustrations also can visually demonstrate a stepwise process, as in this series showing how to turn the baby over onto his or her back, tilt baby's head back by lifting on the chin, listen for air coming in or out of the baby's mouth, and provide mouth-to-mouth breathing. Each illustration shows one or two related concepts. The illustrations are close to the text describing them and show only what is necessary, with no excess details or background.

Raw meat, raw poultry, raw seafood, and raw eggs can make you sick. Cook them until they are done.

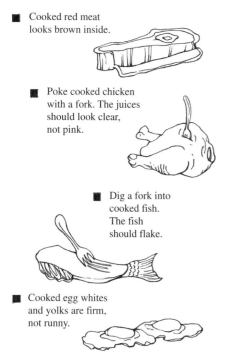

■ Cooked red meat looks brown inside.

■ Poke cooked chicken with a fork. The juices should look clear, not pink.

■ Dig a fork into cooked fish. The fish should flake.

■ Cooked egg whites and yolks are firm, not runny.

FIGURE 7.4 "Keep Your Food Safe." This graphic demonstrates several features of reader-friendly visuals discussed throughout chapter 7. *Source:* National Cancer Institute (NCI). 1994. *Clear and Simple: Developing Effective Materials for Low-Literate Readers.* Washington, DC: U.S. Government Printing Office.

lives—especially men—who were excluded from early versions of the piece's cover. In other words, these women wanted the pictures to more accurately depict them and their experience with breast cancer, including support from family (Rosales, 2005).

All charts or tables included in materials created for patient use should be simple and easily understood. The charts and tables you would use in a professional presentation are probably not appropriate for your patient population (Sanner, 2003). See Figures 7.4 and 7.5, which are taken from the Web site of the National Cancer Institute (2003) and represent the effective use of illustrations and accompanying text.

What type of picture should you use in your text? The picture ought to complement and help explain the text; pictures used in this way enhance learning. Pictures that are merely decorative in nature (i.e., that are pleasant to look at but bear little or no relation to the text) do nothing to enhance learning and should be avoided (Carney & Levin, 2002). Unfortunately, some novice designers turn to these ornamental elements to spruce up the page or to make their materials look, in their minds, more attractive. This effort rarely succeeds.

Doak and colleagues (1996) strongly warn against using stylized or abstract images, which require readers to make inferences and jumps in logic. Poor readers, they note, tend to be more literal in their interpretation of graphic

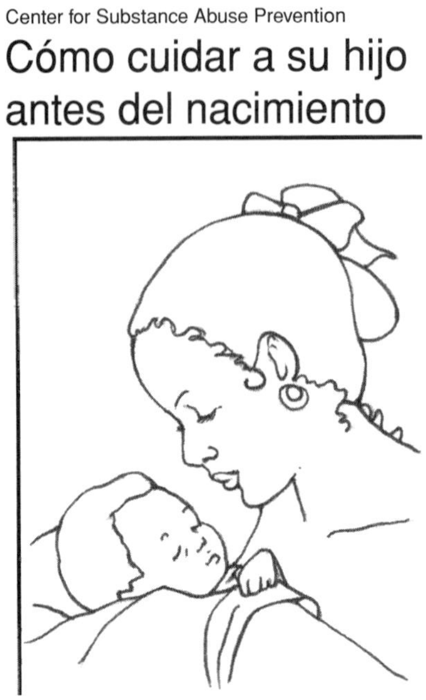

Center for Substance Abuse Prevention

Cómo cuidar a su hijo antes del nacimiento

FIGURE 7.5 *Cómo cuidar a su hijo antes del nacimiento* ["How to Take Care of Your Child Before Birth"]. *Source:* National Cancer Institute (NCI). 1994. *Clear and Simple: Developing Effective Materials for Low-Literate Readers.* Washington, DC: U.S. Government Printing Office.

elements. The authors give an example of a graphic used in a diabetes education piece showing a dump truck delivering "energy" to body cells. They warn that the imagery is likely lost on the poor reader because it requires some logical maneuvering to tie together the concept of delivering energy (as in a dump truck) to a body process (energy in the bloodstream). If this connection is not made, the intended result of using this graphic is lost and only confusion is delivered.

Graphics should be action oriented and delivered in usable chunks, according to Doak and colleagues (1996). Again, those developing patient materials should not try to cram all the information they want to convey on one page. Chunking information into more accessible, "digestible" clusters of information is more likely to produce a successful result. If you are trying to teach a procedure or process, such as how to take a medication, use graphics to help tell a story. *Fotonovelas,* discussed in chapter 9, are a good way to present this information. Simple line drawings showing a task (such as taking a pill at specific times during the day) can be provided in linear fashion.

For instance, if you want to impart the instructions to take a pill three times a day with meals and once at bedtime with a snack, a four-panel line drawing could be used. In the first panel, show the person swallowing the pill. Reinforce the message with a meal in front of the person, a clock on the wall reading 9 a.m., and the sun on the left. The next drawing shows the same thing, only the clock shows 1 and the sun is midway through the sky. The third illustration repeats the main elements of the person taking the pill with a meal on the table, but this time the clock shows 5 and the sun is nearly set, on the right. The final drawing shows the same person, but perhaps in pajamas; the clock shows 9 again (p.m. this time), the sky outside is dark except for a crescent moon and a star, and a glass of milk is on the table.

Each illustration used should serve a purpose for the reader. Carney and Levin (2002) discuss three types of illustrations and their uses: illustrating a concept or element (*representational* illustration), providing a structural framework or stepwise explanation of an idea (*organizational* illustration), or showing a difficult concept in terms of another, easy-to-understand concept, such as showing the heart (literally) as a mechanical, metal pump *(interpretational* illustrations).

Figure 7.4 offers some representational illustrations. The graphics provide a pictorial representation of the message conveyed in the text. Notice how they enhance the potential for learning by providing a visual counterpoint to the text: they make the idea more concrete and thereby provide a means for the learner to "see" what the text is saying.

The graphics also complement the text well and in some ways even work on their own without the text. They show the object to which they are referring (in this case, the food itself) and the tools described in the text (the fork piercing the chicken and flaking the fish). By using easy-to-read and easy-to-understand text as well as simple graphics that work with the text, each element helps explain the other, thereby providing a stronger message that increases the likelihood of its comprehension by the reader.

The example also illustrates how graphics can be appropriate to the age of the intended audience (the drawings are simple but not childish), free from clutter, and appropriately located close to the text that they explain. Graphics should always be accompanied by text that is short, to the point, written at an easy-to-read level, and strictly applicable to the graphics. Those developing materials should use arrows to refer to specific areas of the illustrations and use boldface type or underlining to emphasize more important words or phrases.

Doak and colleagues (1996) note that poor readers do not approach printed material in the same manner as skilled readers. Poor readers use a more random approach than do skilled readers, who scan the page, find the important or central concept through identifying key words or graphics, cull the important facts from the supporting details, and interpret the information to arrive at the meaning of the message. The poor reader, by contrast, tends to skip over important features to focus on a less important but more engaging detail (remember the pretty but useless ornamental illustrations we discussed earlier?), thus missing the central message. Such readers may work on interpreting words literally, one at a time, and may or may not focus on the key message the materials are trying to convey.

This is why it is important to place suitable illustrations close to the text of key messages. Poor readers are more likely to zero in on engaging illustrations, and they are more likely to be rewarded for their efforts. Because it does take more effort on the part of the poor reader to process information, clustering key messages with appropriate, complementary, and explanatory graphics is crucial. Keep it simple; keep it close together.

The illustration in Figure 7.5 is taken from a brochure on newborn care designed for Hispanic mothers. Like the previous example, it is also simple but appropriate to adult readers. It uses images that look like the intended audience (in this case, Hispanic women), and the title—*Cómo cuidar a su hijo antes del nacimiento,* or "How to Take Care of Your Child Before Birth"—clearly identifies the information covered in the brochure.

A PARTING THOUGHT: KNOW YOUR AUDIENCE

Those who design patient education materials, especially if the average patient receiving them has low health literacy, should have a very clear idea about their audience before beginning the design and development process. Will the pieces be distributed in an urban or rural area? Do patients range in age from preteens to the elderly, or is a particular age group disproportionately represented? What are the patients' most common diseases or conditions? Do they use complementary and alternative therapies? What language or languages do they speak?

It pays to know a thing or two about your patients' cultural backgrounds. Health care providers who work in a primarily Asian or Hispanic clinic should use photos or illustrations that show people of a similar background or ethnicity. Doing so helps patients identify more closely with the characters in the graphics and makes the message seem more personalized.

It does not make sense to intentionally use representational graphics that do not occur in the reader's daily life. For instance, if your audience is primarily low income or working class, you wouldn't show a woman in a fur coat stepping out of a chauffeured limousine. Similarly, if your audience is primarily middle class, showing a person who is a manual laborer is less likely to engender feelings of identification.

REFERENCES

Arditi, A. (2005). *Making text legible: Designing for people with partial sight.* Retrieved December 10, 2005, from http://www.lighthouse.org/print_leg.htm

Bailey, B. (2005). *The value of iterative design.* Retrieved March 12, 2006, from http://usability.gov/pubs/072005news.html

Bailey, B. (2006). *Getting the complete picture with usability testing.* Retrieved March 12, 2006, from http://www.usability.gov/pubs/030106news.html

Carney, R. N., & Levin, J. R. (2002). Pictorial illustrations still improve students' learning from text. *Educational Psychology Review, 14*(1), 5–26.

Doak, L. G., Doak, C. C., & Root, J. H. (1996). *Teaching patients with low literacy skills* (2nd ed.). Philadelphia: J.B. Lippincott.

Mayer, G. (2003, May). *Writing easy to read, easy to use health information.* Paper presented at Organizational Solutions to Low Health Literacy, Institute for Healthcare Advancement Second Annual Health Literacy Conference, Anaheim, CA.

Mayer, G., & Kuklierus, A. (2001). *What to do when your child gets sick.* Whittier, CA: Institute for Healthcare Advancement.

National Cancer Institute (NCI). (2003). *Clear and simple: Developing effective print materials for low-literate readers.* Retrieved December 5, 2005, from http://www.cancer.gov/cancerinformation/clearandsimple

Rosales, A. (2005, May). *Cross cultural communications: Identifying challenges and finding solutions.* Paper presented at Culture, Language, and Clinical Issues: Operational Solutions to Low Health Literacy, Institute for Healthcare Advancement Fourth Annual Health Literacy Conference, Irvine, CA.

Rudd, R. E. (2005). *How to create and assess print materials.* Retrieved March 12, 2005, from the Harvard School of Public Health, Health Literacy Web site: http://www.hsph.harvard.edu/healthliteracy/materials.html

Sanner, B. M. (2003, July/August). Are your written materials missing the mark? *Journal of Active Aging,* 18–24.

Singer, D. (2002). *Ten steps to good document design.* Retrieved December 29, 2005, from http://www.uah.edu/colleges/liberal/english/shared/doc_des_singer.htm

Wheildon, C. (2005). *Type and layout: Are you communicating or just making pretty shapes?* Berkeley, CA: Strathmore Press.

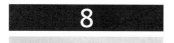

8

PRINCIPLES OF WRITING FOR LOW LITERACY

Look around the reception areas and waiting rooms of the health care offices where you work or visit as a patient. Odds are good that they are well stocked with literature on a variety of health topics ranging from arthritis to nutrition. The abundance of health-related written materials is no surprise when you consider that health care is largely about communicating information. Consequently, health care professionals can spend a good deal of time developing written materials. These materials may be brochures on starting a fitness program, informational pamphlets on diabetes, or posters detailing how to administer cardiopulmonary resuscitation.

At the core of the health care system is the assumption that it is the responsibility of patients to ask for and obtain professional advice and then to comply with recommended treatment plans. In many cases, doing so involves patients reading written materials, understanding the messages of those materials, and remembering those messages. But if patients are expected to absorb complex clinical information, it is the responsibility of the health care community to make that task easier by providing materials that are easy to read, understand, and remember.

We expect that the materials provided by health care professionals are thoroughly researched and present the most up-to-date information on the topics covered. But, to be useful, written materials also must be well matched to patients' reading and comprehension levels. In addition to concentrating on the accuracy of the information they are presenting, those writing health-related materials must pay attention to the communicative aspect of those materials. That is, they must take steps to ensure that the materials are written in a manner that enables patients to read, understand, and remember them. Unfortunately, materials that have been carefully researched and edited often fail to communicate effectively.

Health care professionals who are charged with the task of writing materials for patients have several good reasons to focus on the communication aspect of those materials. There is convincing evidence to support the idea that easy-to-read materials increase patients' compliance, for example (Davis, Williams, Marin, Parker, & Glass, 2002; Dreger & Tremback, 2002; Safeer & Keenan, 2005). In fact, such an effect was recognized more than 30 years ago: Bradshaw, Ley, and Kincey (1975) reported that patients have a higher rate of compliance, remember better, and make fewer mistakes when materials are easy to read. More recently, Davis and colleagues (1994) found that people at various income and education levels prefer simpler materials. The researchers showed that patients' comprehension of materials went up when the materials were simple and easy to read and suggested that materials written at a third- or fourth-grade level may be best for patients (Davis et al., 1994).

The vast majority of patients are willing and able to learn. They have the intelligence to use written materials to gain information and guidance regarding their health care—provided that those materials are suited to their abilities. Therefore, the onus is on health care providers to improve written instructions to allow that to happen. The good news is that there are steps you can take to make sure that your written materials are a good match with the abilities of your patients.

PLANNING YOUR WRITING

Good written materials begin with a good plan. Without a doubt, planning can be the most time-consuming part of the entire writing process. The planning phase focuses on the following questions:

- Why create this material?
- Who is the intended audience?
- What is the reading level of the intended audience?
- What is the desired patient behavior?
- What information should be included?
- What can I learn from the patients themselves?
- What can I learn from existing materials?

Why Create This Material?

The first step in planning an educational piece for patients is to define the purpose of the material. That is, you need to have a clear understanding of why you are creating the piece. This may seem simple, but it can be a fairly complicated exercise.

Materials are generally created in response to an observed or anticipated need. Identify as specifically as possible what that need is. What spurred the creation of the material? What are you trying to accomplish with it? What result are you trying to achieve? Before you start to write, you also should consider whether new material really needs to be created. Can existing materials accomplish your goal? Or could some existing materials accomplish your goal if they simply were rewritten?

Who Is the Intended Audience?

Once you know why you are creating the material and what you want to accomplish with it, you need to consider who will use the material. Be as specific as possible when defining your intended audience. Brigid Sanner (2003), communications and marketing consultant for the Active for Life national program and a consultant to the Robert Wood Johnson Foundation, offers the following suggestions for learning about your intended audience:

- Consider the attributes that define your audience as a group. For example, are the patients who will use your written materials part of a particular age group? Do they share the same ethnic background? Do they have special physical abilities or challenges? What is their average socioeconomic status and educational background? Is there any other characteristic that these patients have in common?
- Use available population and demographic research to understand the audience better.
- If possible, use focus group research to gain insight into the beliefs and values of the patients who will use this material.

What Is the Reading Level of the Intended Audience?

Reading level is one of the most important characteristics you can find out about your intended audience. If you want to be sure that the materials you create will be understandable to your patients, you must ensure that the information is written at their reading and comprehension level. This is not always easy: the National Assessment of Adult Literacy (NAAL) of 2003 estimates that 14% of American adults have below basic prose literacy, or "no more than the most simple and concrete literacy skills," whereas another 29% have only basic prose literacy, defined as having the "skills necessary to perform simple and everyday literacy activities" (National Center for Education Statistics, 2003).

Determining patients' literacy levels can be tricky, as we have seen. Low literacy is typically difficult to identify through casual interaction with patients. Patients with low literacy skills are not likely to volunteer the fact that they have trouble reading, and they generally do not ask for help. In fact, they tend to cover up their literacy challenges by avoiding situations that might reveal the problem. They make excuses to keep from having to read. Health care providers cannot make assumptions about an individual patient's literacy level. Knowing his or her level of education does not amount to knowing his or her literacy level. As Baker, Parker, Williams, Clark, and Nurss point out,

> The most important factor in analyzing the relationship between education and health is educational attainment: not merely the number of years of schooling but, rather, what was learned during those years. Reading level averages four grades below number of years of schooling, and functional literacy varies widely among people who have completed high school. If low educational attainment directly affects health, then literacy should be a better predictor of health outcomes than number of years completed (Baker et al., 1997, p. 1027).

What Is the Desired Patient Behavior?

In the health care environment, patient education materials are often created to convince patients to modify their behavior. Some materials may urge them to make better food choices, for example. Others may encourage sedentary patients to begin exercising. Still others may instruct them on how to take a particular medication. By focusing on the behavior you want your materials to elicit, you will be able to make strategic decisions about those materials.

In *Clear and Simple: Developing Effective Print Materials for Low-Literate Readers* (2003), the National Cancer Institute (NCI) explains that the objectives of written materials should focus on concrete action, rather than being purely informational. The NCI document (2003) provides the following examples of possible behavioral objectives for written materials designed to promote mammography among low-literate women:

- The reader will ask the clinic or doctor about mammography at her next visit.
- The reader will make an appointment for a mammogram.
- The reader will call us to discuss her options.

Such objectives, the NCI explains, are more effective than something like, "The reader will understand why mammography is important to her health," because they help communicate action-oriented messages, which is what low-literate readers need (NCI, 2003).

For materials designed to influence patients' behavior, the measure of the success of the material is obvious: whether the patient's behavior has changed. Of course, to get an accurate picture of the impact of a specific written piece, you must be able to compare patients' behavior after reading the material to their behavior before reading the material. This means that you must test and evaluate patients' behavior twice. And that means testing should be incorporated into your planning.

What Information Should Be Included?

Once you have determined why you are writing the material, for whom you are writing, and what impact you hope the materials will have on patients' behavior, you will need to identify what information should be included in the written material. To figure out what should be included, you'll need to answer two questions:

1. What does the intended audience already know about the topic?
2. What information is essential?

By identifying what your intended audience already knows about the topic, you will be able to identify what they *do not* know. And once you have pinpointed the holes in your patients' knowledge, you can provide the necessary information. It seems simple. However, determining the scope of your audience's knowledge is not always straightforward.

To some extent, the question of what your audience knows and needs to know will be answered by defining as precisely as possible who will use the materials. But there will be areas in which the extent of your audience's knowledge will be unknown. In these cases, it would be helpful to enlist the aid of representative members of the intended audience, either through formal focus groups or through more informal interviews.

Armed with information on your intended audience's existing knowledge, you can move on to the question of what information is essential. At first glance, this might seem the same as asking what the audience does not yet know. But it isn't. Though closely related, the question of what information is essential differs from the question of what the audience doesn't know. Essential information is information that must be provided to give patients a foundation or framework on which an understanding of the message can be built. What information do you need to provide to ensure that your intended audience can understand the message?

The next step—limiting the concepts included in your written material to only those that are absolutely necessary—can be even more difficult than identifying the intended audience's knowledge level. But planning the scope of the materials is time and effort well spent. Limiting objectives only to those that are required increases patients' compliance. Barbara Van Horn, MEd, codirector of the Institute for the Study of Adult Literacy at Pennsylvania State University, advises writers to address no more than three to five concepts in a single document (Sanner, 2003).

"Limiting the number of concepts in a written piece is especially important when material is being developed for older adults," says Van Horn. "It is not that older people cannot comprehend more than three to five concepts at one time," she explains, "but it often takes [them] more time to integrate new information with prior knowledge, resulting in reduced comprehension of the entire piece" (Sanner, 2003, p. 22).

Of course, there are many multifaceted and complicated topics in health care. A discussion of colon cancer, for example, could easily fill hundreds of pages. You might have sections on causes, prevention, symptoms, diagnoses, tests and procedures, stages, and treatment. Any one of these sections could be presented as a separate printed piece—and perhaps it should be. With such complicated topics, it is generally more effective to cover the various topics in separate, short, written pieces rather than in one large piece that appears difficult to read because of its large size.

You should recognize that the effects of planning your written materials are cumulative. If you take the time to explore *why* you are writing a particular piece and defining the specific effect you want it to have, you will have an easier time figuring out what information belongs and what can safely be excluded.

What Can I Learn From the Patients Themselves?

When you are designing materials for use by a particular group, who better to ask for input than members of that group? Patients are usually happy to help by answering questions or offering suggestions, and their input can be invaluable.

In some cases, you may be able to put together a formal focus group to help in the planning stage of a project. At those times when you're lucky enough to have this kind of resource, give samples of possible choices and carefully consider the choice of the group. Ask questions that focus on what you honestly wish to find out and then listen, listen, listen. In fact, listen far more than you talk. Listen for certain vocabulary. If participants say "shots" when they're talking about injections, consider using that term in written materials. It would be a great idea to record the focus group's discussions for later use and review. If that isn't possible, try to get someone to take notes—or do it yourself. Remember, you are not obligated to act on the input you receive, but you should at least consider it and evaluate its intrinsic strengths and weaknesses.

If getting a focus group together is not possible, you may still be able to get feedback from individual members of your target audience. Doak, Doak, and Root (1996) report that some nurses have successfully used feedback gathered from individual hospital patients. Even this kind of informal research can yield valuable information. The insight of just one or two patients could be just what you need to plan and write exceptional written materials.

What Can I Learn From Existing Materials?

Numerous written pieces for patients have been designed and produced already. Many are used regularly by health care professionals to educate, instruct, and persuade their patients. Others exist but don't get much use. Some of the existing materials look great but don't seem to produce the desired effect. Some, though, work very well: they communicate the intended message accurately and effectively—and in a manner that matches the abilities of the patients for whom they are written.

When you are faced with a problem that you intend to address through writing, it is a good idea to take a look at what materials exist already. Either by yourself or with your work group, critique each piece. What are the strengths and weaknesses of each piece? What is the intended message? Can you define the intended audience? Does the piece succeed at its perceived goal? Why or why not? Can you pinpoint precisely what makes one pamphlet effective while another is not? Can you compare different types of materials (e.g., brochures, instructions, and forms) and determine which attributes the successful pieces have in common? What do you like about the piece? What works about it? What doesn't?

WRITING HEALTH-RELATED PATIENT MATERIALS

Not every patient or group of patients will have the same needs when it comes to written materials. Consequently, there is no magic formula for writing effective patient education materials. The trick is to match your writing to the particular constellation of needs that your intended audience exhibits, keeping your materials either at or below the audience's reading level. Although there is no one right way to write for every patient, you can work to address your patients' needs by concentrating on a few specific attributes of your writing.

Once you have gathered as much information as you can about the characteristics and knowledge base of your intended audience and planned exactly what you will cover in your written piece, you can begin to write. Writing patient materials is more than just sitting down at a computer and typing out the information your intended audience needs to know. Writing involves managing a number of variables such as the following:

- writing style
- appeal
- appearance
- organization

Writing Style

The actual text in material designed for patients' use is extremely important. The challenge is to write text that is accurate, contains all of the necessary information, conveys the importance or complexity of the topic, and does all of this in language that is accessible and comprehensible by your intended audience.

A number of factors play a role in determining the writing style of a given selection of text. However, there are things you can do to help ensure that the text you write for patients is written in a style that is appropriate for that audience. Following are some suggestions:

- Write the way you talk.
- Use common words.
- Use short sentences.
- Give examples to explain hard words.
- Choose words carefully.

Write the Way You Talk

Several positive things happen to your writing when you—quite literally—write the way you talk. First of all, the readability grade level of the information drops, often by as many as five or six grade levels (Bailey, 1996). This is a welcome effect because, as we have established, most patient materials are written at reading levels above those of the intended audience. In addition to becoming easier to read, patient materials also become easier to understand when you write the way you talk. This is largely because we tend to use more words to explain something when we talk, and some of those words serve to reiterate or clarify an idea. These extra or redundant words can serve as informal (and even unintentional) definitions of terms or concepts, thereby giving readers (or patients, in this case) more opportunities to comprehend the message of the material.

Finally, writing the way you speak makes written materials more inviting and interesting, which increases the odds that patients will actually read them. And, ultimately, no matter how accurate a piece of written material is, no matter how well researched and well reviewed, patients can only understand the message if they actually read it.

TABLE 8.1 COMPARISON OF ACTIVE VOICE WITH PASSIVE VOICE

Active Voice	Passive Voice
Take this medicine with food.	This medicine should be taken with food.
Elevate your feet.	Your feet should be elevated.
Grasp your fist with your other hand and press into the victim's upper abdomen with a quick upward thrust.	Your fist should be grasped with your other hand and pressed into the victim's upper abdomen with a quick upward thrust.

Some specific suggestions for simplifying your writing are as follows:

Use Pronouns

More than any other technique for writing the way you talk, using the word *you* speaks directly to your intended audience. It makes the text important and relevant to the reader. Remember that even though your material may be relevant to thousands of people, it speaks to just one reader at a time. Similarly, using *we* to refer to your health care group or organization makes your materials friendlier. It also helps keep your sentences short (Interagency Committee on Government Information, 2005).

Keep It Simple

Using the present tense helps keep writing from becoming cluttered with compound verbs. Keeping subjects and objects close to their verbs also cuts down on confusion (e.g., "Babies drink milk" is easier to understand than "Milk is something that babies like to drink"). Placing modifiers such as "only" or "always" next to the word they modify promotes clarity (e.g., "Always floss your teeth" versus "Floss your teeth always"). Positioning long conditions after the main clause helps patients understand better (e.g., "Call your doctor if you feel very sick or have a headache" rather than "if you feel very sick or have a headache, call your doctor"; Interagency Committee on Government Information, 2005).

Use the Active Voice

One thing that happens when you strive to write the way you talk is that you begin to use the active rather than the passive voice. When you write in the active voice, the subject of the sentence is also the "doer" of the action of the sentence. In general, active voice is easier to understand than passive voice. It also has the advantage of clearly identifying who is responsible for what action (Interagency Committee on Government Information, 2005), which can be especially important when you are trying to affect patient behavior in some way.

Table 8.1 presents examples of messages presented in both active and passive voice. Compare the effect of the active-voice versions with their passive-voice counterparts. You can tell when a piece of writing is in the passive voice because it includes some form of the verb "to be." Such writing usually includes the word "by" and, often, a helping verb. You may wonder what difference this makes. If the message is the same, it shouldn't matter if the writing is in the active voice or the passive voice, right?

Wrong. Messages written in the active voice are more likely to be understood by your intended audience (Rudd, 2002; Weiss, 2003). And if members of your intended audience understand the message, they will find it easier to act on that message.

Use Terms Consistently

If you use a word to identify a specific thought or object, you should use that same word to refer to that thought or object throughout your written material. For example, do not use "review" in the beginning of a document and "evaluate" toward the end of the document. Even though the terms are technically interchangeable, switching from one to the other can confuse your intended audience. Choose one term and stick with it.

Use Contractions

Contractions like *don't* and *wouldn't* are less formal (and more accessible) than writing out "do not" and "would not." Your intended audience is used to hearing contractions, so when they see "should not" in writing, they mentally turn it into "shouldn't" anyway. Therefore, using the contraction to begin with quickens the reading process (Doak et al., 1996). It also aids in accurately communicating your message because some readers will miss the second word (i.e., the "not") and take the exact opposite meaning (Doak et al., 1996).

There are, of course, some exceptions to using contractions. If the culture of your intended audience makes slightly more formal writing preferable, you might want to forgo contractions. In addition, in cases where you need to send a more emphatic message, the two-word form may be more appropriate. "Do NOT drink alcohol while taking this medication" is a stronger message than "Don't drink alcohol while taking this medication."

Use Common Words

What are common words? Which words are easily understood by patients and which should be avoided? Here is where all the planning you did before you started writing will come in handy. If you have accurately and thoroughly defined who constitutes your intended audience, you will be better able to determine which words will be familiar to them and which will not.

In general, the language best suited for patient materials will be the kind you would use if talking to a nontechnical friend. It should be living room language or layman's terms, rather than the specialized jargon of health care professionals. For example, when talking to friends at home you'd probably say "high blood pressure" rather than "hypertension" and "swelling" rather than "edema," so the simpler words would be the better choice.

Legal language also poses a problem in materials written for patients. Medicare Beneficiary Services, for example, recognized that the language used in an already short letter to the public could be made even clearer through the use of plain language. Take a look at the difference between the "before" and "after" samples presented below:

Before:

Investigators at the contractor will review the facts in your case and decide the most appropriate course of action. The first step taken with most Medicare health care providers is to reeducate them about Medicare regulations and policies. If the practice continues, the contractor may conduct special audits of the provider's medical records. Often, the contractor recovers overpayments to health care providers this way. If there is sufficient evidence to show that the provider is consistently violating Medicare policies, the contractor will document the violations and ask the Office of the Inspector General to prosecute the case. This can lead to expulsion from the Medicare program, civil monetary penalties, and imprisonment.

After:

We will take two steps to look at this matter: We will find out if it was an error or fraud. We will let you know the result (PlainLanguage.gov, 2005).

Clearly, the revised version is shorter. Although it does not include the same information as the original version, it can be argued that the revised letter does contain all of the information that was necessary *at the time it was sent.* Presumably, more specific information (including information on penalties and follow-up action) could be communicated once investigators determined whether the provider in question committed fraud.

In some situations, the use of confusing legalese can directly affect patient care. The most obvious example is the language of advance directives. These forms, intended to give patients a tool for communicating their wishes regarding end-of-life care, can be loaded with legal language. As the American Association of Critical-Care Nurses notes, the use of complex terminology that is misunderstood by patients and advocates is one of several limitations that affect those who wish to develop effective advance directives of their own (Westphal & Wavra, 2005).

Some efforts have been undertaken to eliminate this legalese. In the aftermath of the Terri Schiavo tragedy—the high-profile case in which a woman who had been in a persistent vegetative state for 15 years became the subject of a national debate about medical decision making—the Institute for Healthcare Advancement (IHA) placed an easy-to-read advance directive written in English, Spanish, and Chinese on its Web site. Designed by Rebecca Sudore, MD, of the University of California, San Francisco, the simple, fill-in-the-blank document uses a bullet-point style and features helpful illustrations.

It is divided into three parts: (1) choose a health care agent who can make medical decisions for you if you are too sick to make them yourself; (2) make your own health care choices now so those who care for you won't have to guess what you want if you are too sick to tell them yourself; and (3) necessary signatures that make the document legally binding (Institute for Healthcare Advancement, 2005). To download the form, visit http://www.iha4health.org. (Note: though the form complies with California law, readers are cautioned to consult with a legal authority to verify its applicability in their own state before they attempt to use it with patients.)

Having an advance directive written in plain language is helpful for patients with reading difficulties. In fact, in a randomized trial of 204 patients older than 50 years, an easy-to-read advance directive written at a fifth-grade level and containing culturally appropriate graphics was rated easier to complete (80% vs. 62%) and easier to understand (83% vs. 58%) than a standard California Advance Health Care Directive form. Study participants randomized to a group that used the easier form reported greater self-efficacy and greater confidence with their treatment decisions. The easier form was preferred overwhelmingly by subjects with high and low literacy and by both English and Spanish speakers (Sudore & Mayer, 2006).

One advantage of the Sudore form is that it avoids using too many multisyllabic terms. Sanner (2003) points out that the more syllables there are in a word, the more difficult it is for people to understand. The word *shots* is typically more widely understood than the word *inoculations,* for example, and more patients probably know "heart" than know "cardiovascular." The general public—and low-health-literate individuals in particular—may be unfamiliar with terms that refer, say, to physiology. You might therefore be better off using the longer phrase "the large muscles on the front of your thighs" instead of "quadriceps" and "kneecap" instead of "patella." Therefore, whereas occasionally you may find it necessary to use words with three or more syllables, using shorter words and phrases with the same meanings is preferable when you are writing easy-to-read patient materials.

However, the number of syllables in a word is not the only element that influences a person's understanding of it. There are some words that, despite being short, can be troublesome in patient materials. These troublesome words are terms that communicate concepts (general or abstract ideas), categories (groups of things), and value judgments (subjective measurements; often thresholds for action). The problem with such terms is that they can and do mean different things to different people (Doak et al., 1996).

The problems associated with such words can be avoided by using more specific terms. Instead of instructing patients not to lift anything heavy, for instance, you can tell them exactly how much weight to avoid lifting: "Do not lift anything over 25 pounds." And although the recommendation to get adequate rest may be interpreted differently by different patients, the instruction to "get at least 8 hours of sleep each night" is less likely to be misunderstood.

Use Short Sentences

Just as short words are generally easier to understand than longer ones, shorter sentences are easier to understand than those containing more words. Shorter sentences are better for communicating complex information than long ones because they present the information in smaller, easier-to-digest chunks (Interagency Committee on Government Information, 2005). Your cut-off point should be roughly 15 words (Doak et al., 1996). Keeping sentences under 10 words long is even better. If you find yourself writing long sentences loaded with dependent clauses, try breaking each sentence into its various parts. Make each part the subject of its own sentence.

However, sentence length should not take precedence over conversational style. Although short sentences are easier to read, do not let a focus on keeping sentences short lead to "choppy" writing (Mayer, 2003). That means that if it is more natural for you to express an idea in a longer sentence, you should do so. In such cases, using examples and explanations can make the ideas contained in the longer sentence easier to understand (Doak et al., 1996).

Give Examples to Explain Hard Words

No matter how hard you work at using common words, avoiding jargon, and writing the way you talk, at some point you will want or have to use a term that the majority of your patients may not understand. In such cases, the best course of action is to follow the unfamiliar term with an example. A pamphlet encouraging patients to eat a low-fat diet probably cannot avoid using the word *cholesterol,* for example. Still, if the document explains that cholesterol is a type of fat produced by the body that is also in animal products and then provides examples of high-cholesterol foods, it could go a long way toward clearing up any confusion.

Choose Words Carefully

In addition to choosing words that your intended audience can easily understand, you need to be sensitive to their probable reaction to certain words. For example, in research conducted as part of its Active for Life physical activity initiative, the American Association of Retired Persons, a nonprofit membership organization for adults aged 50 years and older, found that people in its membership age range responded positively to the phrase "physical activity" but negatively to "exercise" (Sanner, 2003).

Word choice also can affect the tone of your materials, which can affect the degree to which your patients accept your message (Interagency Committee on Government Information, 2005). Choose your words carefully based on the tone you want to present. In large part, the proper tone for your materials will be determined by the characteristics of your intended audience, but it will be influenced as well by your subject matter and the nature of the relationship between the patient and the organization or individual provider.

Appeal

Overall appeal is an important consideration when you are developing written materials for use by patients. If you have done your homework with respect to planning the material, you should have a good sense of exactly who is your intended patient audience. You should have a sense of their ethnic background, sex, and age. You might know a bit about their lifestyles and habits, their beliefs and attitudes, and their background and education. And if you know all that about the patients for whom you are writing, you can take that information and allow it to influence your decisions about the materials you are creating.

Materials that match the experiences of your patients are more appealing than those that are outside their frame of reference. And appeal is extremely important. Seth Godin, in his acclaimed bestseller on business and marketing, *Purple Cow* (2003), laments how difficult it is for today's marketers to attract consumers' attention. Consumers, says Godin, have less time and inclination nowadays to listen to messages they have not sought out (Godin, 2003).

So what does marketing have to do with health care? Actually, marketing material and written health care materials have a lot in common. Health care materials, like marketing materials, must deliver a message to the intended audience. To receive the message, the audience must be paying attention. Yet quite often, as Godin notes above, the intended audience is not paying attention. Good health care materials, like good marketing, catch the attention of the audience. They are appealing and engaging.

Appeal does not mean that the message of the written material must be something the audience happily accepts. A handout on the dangers of drinking alcohol while pregnant may not be embraced by mothers-to-be who enjoy imbibing on a Saturday night, for example. But that doesn't mean the handout can't be appealing on other levels. If the material is age appropriate and culturally relevant to the intended audience, there is a greater chance the message will be consciously understood and accepted. Combining strategies that invite interaction—questions, quizzes, suggestions, and so on—increases the odds that the intended audience will pay more attention to the message in your written materials.

Appearance

As we discussed in chapter 7, Designing Easy-to-Read Patient Education Materials, the goal when considering the appearance of written materials is to create a page layout that makes it easy for your intended audience to use the materials. Text, layout, white space, paper, and graphics are examples of important elements that contribute to the appearance of a written piece. For a full discussion of these elements and their role in the creation of effective patient education materials, see chapter 7.

Organization

Effective organization of information in written materials is crucial. When you are designing materials for use by patients, ask yourself if the way the materials are organized will aid patients in receiving and understanding the message. According to the U.S. Government's Plain Language Initiative Web site (http://www.plainlanguage.gov), in general, people read documents to find answers. You need to organize your materials in ways that make it easy for your patients to find the answers they seek. Analyze your written materials carefully. Does the organization of each piece make it easier for patients to find what they need?

Your analysis of the organization of written materials should include a consideration of the following elements:

- cover
- sequence of information
- important information
- organizational elements

Cover

The cover of a brochure or pamphlet should be more than just a pretty picture. It should indicate both the core content of the material and its intended audience. Look at the graphics used on the covers of your written materials. Are they germane to the topic? Do they evoke an attitude consistent with the message of the material? What about the title? Does it make clear the focus of the material? Will members of the target audience know that the material is intended for them?

Sequence of Information

The sequence of information in written materials should be logical. It should mirror the mental processes that readers need to work through to understand the message of the material. Instructions, for example, should be presented in the order in which the reader is supposed to complete them. Presenting steps out of order could seriously compromise the effectiveness of those instructions. A parallel can be drawn with other written materials. If the information is presented in an order that does not reflect a logical movement from one point to the next, the effectiveness of the written material might be diminished.

To help ensure that your written materials are organized in a logical order, put yourself in the place of your patients. Try to imagine what questions your patients are likely to ask when presented with the information and then answer those questions. You might even use a question-and-answer format for your material.

Important Information

Effective written materials stress the "need to know" information while leaving out extraneous details. Too much information can detract from the core message. Do the materials you are creating present three to four main points and no more? After reading these materials, will your patients understand what you want them to do? Does the writing clearly define the desired behavior and clearly explain why your patients should adopt it?

Organizational Elements

Using organizational elements allows you to provide your intended audience with levels of organization, quick and easy navigational tools, and message repetition. Below are some particularly useful organizational elements.

Headings

Headings can highlight important information. There are three types: question headings, statement headings, and topic headings (Interagency Committee on Government Information, 2005). Question headings usually take the form of a rhetorical question, asking the question your intended audience most likely needs answered (e.g., What Is Colon Cancer?). In other words, the information that follows a question heading answers that question. This type of heading is the most useful because it anticipates your audience's questions and poses them as your audience would (Interagency Committee on Government Information, 2005). Statement headings are the next best choice: they use a noun and a verb and are specific enough to communicate information to the intended audience (e.g., "Nurses Can Help With Your Medicine"). Topic headings are the most formal. They use a single word or a short phrase (e.g., "Best Treatments").

Vertical Lists

Vertical lists call attention to a series of pieces of information, such as specific steps patients need to take or possible symptoms they should look for. They are visually appealing and easier to read than running text (Interagency Committee on Government Information, 2005). When you use lists, it is generally best to use solid round or square bullets because more ornate or unusual bullets can distract from the information. In some cases, numbering a list can aid in communicating your message (e.g., to highlight the order of steps in a process).

Remember these points when using a vertical list:

- Introduce the list with a sentence that explains what you are listing.
- Indent the list.
- Use left justification so that your bullets or numbers line up directly under one another.

Section Summaries

Summarizing the important points covered in each section at the end of that section is a great way to help your intended audience identify what information they should take away from that section.

Use of Boldface, Italics, and Color

Any one of these text-level techniques—or any combination of them—can be used to make important concepts stand out. However, using underlining or writing in all capital letters is not recommended. Although these techniques may attract attention, they actually make the text more difficult to read.

Get your appointment for a Pap test today!

1. **Could I have cancer of the cervix and not know it?**

   Yes–often there is no pain.
   And this kind of cancer kills many women every year.

2. **What does that mean for me?**

   It means get a Pap test.
   A Pap test can find cancer early.
   If it's found early, it's easier to cure.

3. **How often should I get a Pap test?**

   Get a Pap test every year.

4. **How is the Pap test done?**

   The nurse or doctor wipes a swab on the cervix in your vagina. This takes only a few seconds.

5. **Where do I get a Pap test?**

   ▶ **Family doctor**
   ▶ **OB/GYN**
   ▶ **Medical clinic**
   ▶ **Local health department**

6. **Who needs to have a Pap test?**

   You do if:
   ▶ **You are over 18; or**
   ▶ **You are 18 or under and have sex**

   There is no upper age limit for the Pap test. Even women who have gone through the change of life (menopause) need a Pap test every year.

7. **Why is a Pap test important to me?**

   Because it can tell if you have cancer of the cervix early–while it's still easier to cure.

   It can save your life!

For more information on the Pap test, call the National Cancer Institute's toll-free Cancer Information Service at 1-800-422-6237.

☎ **Turn Page** ➡

FIGURE 8.1 Excerpt from NCI brochure, *The Pap Test: It Can Save Your Life! Source*: National Cancer Institute (NCI). 2003. *Clear and Simple: Developing Effective Materials for Low-Literate Readers.* Washington, DC: U.S. Government Printing Office.

The example from the brochure *The Pap Test: It Can Save Your Life!* illustrates a number of the suggestions that have been made in this chapter (Figure 8.1). First of all, it provides an excellent example of the use of question headings. It also shows how a careful consideration of white space makes text look easy to read. Its use of color and bold type highlights important material and aids readers in finding specific information. And the size of the type (14 point in the actual printed piece) makes it easy to read (NCI, 2003).

Examine the materials you are currently using with patients or those you are in the process of creating. Do they take advantage of the opportunity to highlight or restate your intended message?

TESTING AND REVISING MATERIALS

It's tempting to think that your work of creating written materials is finished once you have a complete draft of your document. But, ideally, you should use that draft to move on to the next step in the process, which is to ensure that your written materials communicate effectively with your intended audience. After all, it is the ability of the materials to communicate with their intended audience that matters most. Low health literacy among patients makes this a challenge.

Gauging the Reading Level of Your Written Materials

Even the most well-written pamphlet or set of instructions will be ineffective if the patients who are supposed to use it cannot understand it. Therefore, an important part of communicating a message to your intended audience via written materials is matching the readability levels of those materials to the abilities of your audience. It seems obvious: if you want your patients to use your written materials, make sure they are written at a level your patients can understand. Yet many of the materials created for use by patients fail to do that.

At what grade level do your patients read? For adult patients, an eighth-grade reading level is generally assumed, but a large number actually read below that level (Institute of Medicine, 2004; Weiss & Coyne, 1997). Yet most health-related patient materials are written at a 10th-grade level (Safeer & Keenan, 2005). To accommodate low-literate individuals, it is a good idea to target a sixth-grade reading level or lower for your written materials (Safeer & Keenan, 2005).

Although such targeting initially may seem difficult to accomplish, there are materials available that successfully present adequate information written at the suggested reading levels. For example, IHA has developed the "What To Do for Health" series of self-help books, which are written at or below a fifth-grade reading level. (Sample text and illustrations from the first book in the series, *What To Do When Your Child Gets Sick* [Mayer & Kuklierus, 2001], appear in chapter 7, Designing Easy-to-Read Patient Education Materials.)

Informal surveys and several reports (e.g., a progress report commissioned by the Dwyer Family Foundation, independent surveys by Molina Healthcare of California and by Northwest New Jersey Maternal and Child Health Network) have suggested that parents trained in the use of IHA's *What To Do When Your Child Gets Sick* refer to it often, avoiding unnecessary worry and cutting down on trips to the doctor or ED (Molina Healthcare, 2002; Northwest New Jersey Maternal and Child Health Network, 2002; Population Empowerment Project, 2002). A pilot study by Herman and Mayer (2004) found that parents enrolled in Head Start were highly satisfied with the book; overall ED visits were reduced by 48% and clinic visits by 37% after parents received the easy-to-read reference book along with training in how to navigate it properly.

The impact of writing materials at lower reading levels becomes evident when you contrast the selections below. The following text is written at a ninth-grade level:

> One of your doctor's primary roles is to prescribe and monitor the use of your asthma medicines. Medications, when taken correctly and combined with appropriate lifestyle changes, can effectively control your asthma.

Compare the same information presented at a fourth-grade level:

> Both you and your doctor will check on how your medicines are working. When you take the right medicine in the right way, you can control your asthma. Of course you will also need to deal with the things in your life that bring on the asthma.

Note that the message has not been altered from the first text selection to the second. It is simply presented in language that is more familiar to most people. By changing "monitor" to "check on," for example, the second selection makes clearer exactly what the physician will be looking for. And by splitting the more complex second sentence into two distinct sentences, the fourth-grade version actually emphasizes the importance of lifestyle in controlling asthma.

Determining the readability of written materials is not difficult. There are several easy-to-use tools available. Some of the most popular include the following:

Flesch-Kincaid

This U.S. Department of Defense standard test actually encompasses two tests:

1. The Flesch-Kincaid Reading Ease scores text on a scale of 0 to 100. The higher the score, the easier the text is to read. For text to be considered an eighth-grade level, it must score 60 or higher on this test.
2. The Flesch-Kincaid Grade Level Formula translates the Reading Ease test into a U.S. grade level.

You can automatically calculate the Flesch-Kincaid grade level of your writing by using the Microsoft Word software. Simply follow these steps:

1. Click on "Tools" on the Microsoft Word toolbar and choose "Options." (On Macintosh versions of Microsoft Word, "options" appears under the Spelling & Grammar tab on the Tools pull-down menu.)
2. Click on the Spelling & Grammar tab.
3. In the grammar section, locate the "Show Readability Statistics" box and make sure that it is checked.
4. Click "Okay" at the bottom of the menu.
5. Click on "Tools" on the Microsoft Word toolbar again.
6. Click on "Grammar" or "Spelling and Grammar." The software will conduct a spelling and grammar check of your entire document and then display a Readability Statistics box. Look in the Readability section for both the Flesch Reading Ease and Flesch-Kincaid Grade Level results.

Unfortunately, there is some controversy surrounding this tool. For example, Mark Hochhauser, PhD, a readability consultant who specializes in written health care materials, believes that the version of the Flesch-Kincaid formula found in Microsoft Word is flawed. He points out that the original formula scores up to grade 16 or 17, but that the Microsoft version only reports scores up to grade 12 (Hochhauser, 2004).

More important, there is some question of the accuracy of this tool even when working with writing at lower grade levels. Pfizer Inc., the global pharmaceutical company, has developed a handbook aimed at promoting clear communication in the health care environment. Titled *Pfizer Principles for Clear Health Communication* and developed by leading health literacy experts Leonard and Cecilia Doak in partnership with Pfizer Inc., the document includes the following warning: "In particular, the Flesch-Kincaid readability formula tends to give artificially low scores. Moreover, there are specific techniques necessary to prepare a document before using a computerized program. Most people omit this step and get inaccurate results" (Doak & Doak, 2003). Among such techniques for preparing a document is to remove the periods in abbreviations because the program assumes that each period it sees represents the beginning of a new sentence.

McLaughlin SMOG (Simple Measure of Gobbledygook) Readability Formula

This quick, consistent, easy-to-use tool allows you to gauge the readability levels of written materials. However, it is not considered as accurate as other methods for assessing texts written at lower grade levels (i.e., under sixth grade). The steps are simple:

1. Select three samples of 10 consecutive sentences (at least 100 words total). Each sample should be from a different section of the text.
2. Count the words that have three or more syllables in the 30 sentences.
3. Refer to the conversion table at http://uuhsc.utah.edu/pated/authors/ readability.html (adapted from McLaughlin, 1969) to find the grade-level equivalent.

Fry Formula

Although some people find this tool tedious to use, it is helpful for assessing materials written at lower reading levels. To use it, complete the following steps:

1. Select three 100-word passages from the text (omit headings). If you are testing a very short written piece, you can select a single 100-word sample. Because readability levels may vary from section to section, choose samples from different sections of the document.
2. Count the number of sentences in each 100-word sample.
3. Estimate the fractional length of the last sentence to the nearest 1/10 (e.g., if the 100th word is the fifth word of a 15-word sentence, the fraction of the sentence is 5/15 or 1/3 or 0.3).
4. Count the syllables in each 100-word passage.
5. Calculate the average number of sentences and the average number of syllables from the three passages.
6. Visit http://www.clearhealthcommunication.com/public-health-professionals/fry-testing.html and use the Fry graph to find the grade-level equivalent of the text.

SAM (Suitability Assessment of Materials)

Created by Cecilia and Leonard Doak, this tool assesses not only readability but also usability and suitability. According to the SAM, grade-level readability is just one of a number of factors that contribute to the overall readability of materials. The SAM scores materials in six categories: content, literacy demand, graphics, layout and typography, learning stimulation, and cultural appropriateness. It yields a percentage score that falls into one of three categories: superior, adequate, or not suitable.

This tool can help you identify specific shortcomings of your written materials. To learn how to apply the SAM to your materials, see Doak and colleagues' *Teaching Patients With Low Literacy Skills* (1996).

CONDUCTING FOCUS GROUPS

Representative members of your intended audience can be a tremendous help when you are testing the effectiveness of written materials. They can offer you invaluable feedback that you can incorporate into your materials before they are finalized. Focus groups are an excellent addition to your repertoire of testing materials in progress. They are aimed at getting people to share their thoughts and feelings on a subject or a document (Cruzalegui, 2003). As such, focus groups have the potential to give you information about the material that formal tests like those for readability cannot, such as the following:

- complexity of the ideas
- logical order of the content
- appropriate vocabulary for your audience
- any gender, class, or cultural biases
- design that is attractive and helps or hinders the readers
- information that is easy to read in form and typestyle

A focus group, composed of 8 to 12 representatives of the target audience, engages in discussions led by a facilitator for 1- to 2-hour sessions (Cruzalegui, 2003). An advantage of using a focus group is that it requires fewer audience representatives than other research methods. Focus groups are faster and can be less expensive than formal surveys, and the information they provide goes beyond numerical data. Participants in focus groups have the opportunity to discuss the materials and explain why they are responding to the materials in a particular way.

There are disadvantages to focus groups, too. The findings gathered from focus groups cannot be projected to the population as a whole. For a focus group to be effective, those conducting the discussion and gathering, reporting, and applying the results must be trained to do so appropriately. They must identify people who are appropriate for participation and then motivate them to take part in the group. This becomes increasingly difficult as the target audience for the recruitment effort becomes narrower. In addition, with some ethnic groups there is the additional complication of having to structure focus groups in accordance with those groups' gender dynamics (Cruzalegui, 2003).

When putting together a focus group, you may find it helpful to develop a discussion guide. A typical guide might include the following elements:

- moderator introduction and greeting
- instructions
- participant introduction
- other relevant details (e.g., guidelines for interaction, expectations, disclaimers)

You also will want to take care when selecting the facility in which to conduct the focus group. Consider whether you will hold one focus group at a single location or several groups at multiple locations. Factors such as cost, additional services required (e.g., audio, video), and the possible need for bilingual speakers ought to be figured into your planning.

As for the focus group moderator, he or she should be able to establish a good rapport with the participants while remaining impartial. Ideally, the facilitator should share some characteristics with the target audience. His or her job is not so much to lead the discussion as to ensure that it remains focused on the topic. The moderator should understand the topic well enough to explain it to the participants without leading them or imposing his or her opinions on the group. Ideally, moderators should listen more than they talk (Cruzalegui, 2003).

The moderator should answer questions with questions whenever possible to facilitate the discussion. He or she needs to have a thorough understanding of the reason for the study and the objectives. That way, the moderator will be able to recognize when the discussion is approaching important issues and can encourage that line of conversation. After the focus group ends, the moderator should participate in the debriefing. He or she should be encouraged to suggest adjustments to the discussion guide or to the process (Cruzalegui, 2003).

Finally, the results of the focus group should be formally analyzed and reported. The report should contain an explanation of the background and methodology of the focus group. It should then present key findings and use those findings to draw reasonable conclusions and to make relevant recommendations. Remember that all results are worth noting; no news is news (Cruzalegui, 2003). The report should not contain percentages, but it can include the results of a show of hands. It can also contain the moderator's impression of participants (e.g., were they what you expected?) and their nonverbal responses (Cruzalegui, 2003).

OTHER APPROACHES THAT INVOLVE THE END USER

As useful as formal focus groups can be, they are often beyond the budget of those creating written patient materials. For example, Beth Leber of the New York branding agency, Siegel and Gale, estimated the cost of running a two-evening focus group session at $11,640 (in 1998 dollars)—a figure that excluded some staff costs but did include many other expenses: $2,400 to $2,800 for a high-end moderator ("I included the cost of a moderator from the top of the estimated range since it really pays to get a good moderator for your focus groups," Leber notes [Nielsen, 1997]), $20 to $45 for observer meals, $12 for each respondent's meal, a $100 per person recruiter incentive, $800 for the room rental, $300 for stationary video, $300 for computer rental, and $400 for an oversized monitor (Nielsen, 1997).

This estimate for a two-evening focus group assumes 10 people recruited for each group and a total of 5 observers. Admittedly, though, it is an estimate for New York City, which is one of the most expensive areas of the country; in many other regions of the United States it would be considerably cheaper to conduct a focus group. According to the Dallas Marketing Group (DMG, 2006), $4,000 to $4,500 per group is a national average.

In the example above, reducing the number of observers and the cost of incentives, plus scaling back on some of the audiovisual equipment, could save hundreds or thousands of dollars. But the main point is that even a bare-bones focus group includes significant costs and requires thoughtful planning. However, even if the costs of running a focus group are prohibitive, you need not miss out completely on the information that your end users can offer. One simple yet effective informal testing method is to interview representative readers to assess their understanding of the material. An alternative would be to consult with experts who know the needs and characteristics of your intended audience. Regardless of whether you use representative readers or experts, such "protocol testing" requires one-on-one interviews. Generally, three to nine readers should be interviewed to determine what each sentence in the written material means to them. Their answers can yield in-depth information about which words or sentences are potentially confusing. Conducting such interviews is, however, relatively time and labor intensive.

You may want to consider conducting a Knowledge, Attitudes, and Practices (KAP) survey. KAP surveys measure respondents' knowledge, attitudes, and practices on a specific topic. They can be conducted by telephone, by mail, or face-to-face with representative members of the target audience. Unlike focus groups, these surveys can provide information that is representative of the total population. The information they yield is generally highly targeted and relevant to the materials in question. On the other hand, conducting KAP surveys and other kinds of representative surveys requires time, statistical expertise, and resources. There must be a mechanism for locating and reaching large numbers of the target audience.

Revising Materials Based on Feedback, Focus Groups, and New Information

No matter how you obtain feedback from your intended audience, once you have it you must make some decisions about how to use it. As the writer of patient materials, you must decide what information and advice should be incorporated into the final version.

WRITING IN ANOTHER LANGUAGE

Writing materials that will appear in a different language (e.g., a pamphlet that will be produced in both English and Spanish) poses unique challenges. One issue is whether the material should be written in English first and then translated into the second, target language, or whether the material should be written from the beginning in the target language by someone who is fluent in that language.

Most often, difficulties in translation result from the failure to recognize the meanings of words or phrases peculiar to a particular context in the mind of the reader (Sobero & Giraldo, 2004). Good translators must take into account cultural, idiosyncratic (i.e., those having to do with the peculiarities of the original author's lexicon), physical, and lexical contexts of the original material. They must do their best to communicate the same meaning from the source to the target language in order to evoke the same response in the reader (Sobero & Giraldo, 2004).

Handing a translation project over to a professional service is one option that may avoid common errors made by amateur translators, but such services can be costly. Typically, translators working for professional services take several steps to ensure that the document will be translated correctly. They begin by clarifying any unclear text and sometimes ensuring that the written text is at an appropriate reading level for the target audience (Roat, 2005). One professional, usually a native speaker of the language into which the document is being translated, translates the document, and then a second professional (usually a native English speaker) edits and proofreads it.

One of the problems of translation is that a word or saying that is commonly understood in one language may not have a counterpart in another language. Literal translations of English idioms, for example, often do not make sense. A translator faced with the phrase "out of the frying pan and into the fire" would do well to avoid a literal translation into Spanish because such a translation would likely confuse readers. Instead, he or she might write *salir de Guatemala y meterse en guatepeor,* which literally means "to leave Guatemala and arrive in worse cornstalks." Not every Spanish reader would understand the phrase (just as some English-language idioms are not known to all English-speaking readers), but using an equivalent idiom conveys the message's intent more clearly to native speakers of another language.

Writing in English and translating into the other language may be problematic if the original document contains too many idioms. Even when a term or phrase has an equivalent in the target language, a good translation may not convey quite the same meaning. In addition, even if the definition of a word or phrase is the same in both the original/source language and the translated/target language, the connotation may be different. Employing an experienced translator who understands English idioms and can find equivalents in the target language is one possible solution. Another is to have a native speaker compose the document in the other language.

One useful exercise for ensuring accuracy when written materials are translated from one language to another is back-translation. Just like it sounds, *back-translation* is the practice of translating back into the original language text that has been translated into a second language. Ideally, the original translation and the back-translation should be completed by different translators. (The same translator may be biased by his or her original translation, altering the back-translation accordingly.)

Because translation is often more art than science, however, one should not expect the back-translation to match the language of the original text exactly. In fact, some professional translators disagree about whether back-translation is truly effective for verifying the quality of a translation. Translator Fuad M. Yahya explains,

> Because of the nature of human language, there will always be differences between the original text and the back-translation. It is entirely unrealistic to expect the back-translation to be identical or even nearly identical to the wording of the original text. What is hoped for is a text that, to the mind of the client, conveys a meaning that is essentially identical to the meaning of the original text. In a sense, the back-translation will itself be a "translation," in the sense of being a restatement of the original text in possibly different words, albeit in the same language as the original text. Only the client can determine whether the differences between the original text and the back-translation represent a real [semantic] shift or merely a difference in the choice of words, and whether remediation is called for.
>
> The purpose of identifying trouble spots is not to embarrass the translator by petty fault-finding, but to help the translator fine-tune the translation in these specific spots so as to maximize the accuracy and readability of the translation, or to help the client modify the text in a manner that makes it more amenable to translation. Rarely does an author write a text with potential translation pitfalls in mind. As back-translation brings the pitfalls to light, some pitfalls may be corrected by modifying the translation, but others may be best managed by reworking the original text itself (Yahya, 2002–2004).

Software programs that perform translations from one language to another can be used to get the gist of a foreign-language text, but they should never be used as translation tools (Roat, 2005; Sobero & Giraldo, 2004). When accuracy matters, human translation is always preferable to machine translation. The following example from the California Academy of Family Physicians' document, *Assessing Language Access Issues in Your Practice: A Toolkit for Physicians and Their Staff Members* (2005), shows what happened when a text from a standard medical consent form written in English was run through the "Free Text Translator" on the Web site FreeTranslation.com. Here's the original:

> I consent to the administration of anesthesia by my attending physician, by an anesthesiologist, or other qualified party under the direction of a physician as may be deemed necessary. I understand that anesthetics involve risks of complications and serious possible damage to vital organs such as the brain, heart, lung, liver and kidney that in some cases may result in paralysis, cardiac arrest, and/or brain death from both known and unknown causes.

After being translated into Spanish, the passage was back-translated on the site as follows:

> I spoil the administration of anesthesia by me is doctor that helps, by an anesthesiologist, or by another qualified game under the direction of a doctor can be believed necessary. I understand that all [word in English] implies the risks of complications and grave possible damage to essential organs such as the brain, the heart, the lung, the liver and the kidney that in some cases can result in paralysis, the heart being arrested (by the police), and/or death of the brain of both of the (two) known and unknown causes (Roat, 2005, p. 16).

When selecting a translator, health care providers should look for someone who translates into his or her dominant language, learned the receptor language at different times (preferably in two different cultures), and is college educated in the receptor language. Good translators often have college certification in translation, some background in the areas in which they translate (such as health or marketing), and serve a majority of their customers in their field of expertise. At least 5 years of experience is recommended (Sobero & Giraldo, 2004).

To learn more about professional translator services or to locate translators in your area, visit the American Translators Association's (ATA's) Web site at http://www.atanet.org. Founded in 1959, the ATA is the largest professional association of translators and interpreters in the United States, with more than 8,500 members in over 60 countries (ATA, 2006).

REFERENCES

American Translators Association (ATA). (2006). *ATA Web site*. Retrieved January 2, 2006, from http://www.atanet.org

Bailey, E. P. (1996). *Plain English at work: A guide to business writing and speaking*. New York: Oxford University Press.

Baker, D. W., Parker, R. M., Williams, M. V., Clark, W. S., & Nurss, J. (1997). The relationship of patient reading ability to self-reported health and use of health services. *American Journal of Public Health, 87*(6), 1027–1030.

Before-and-after comparisons: Medicare fraud letter. (2005). Retrieved December 22, 2005, from http://www.plainlanguage.gov/examples/before_after/medicarefraudltr.cfm

Bradshaw, P. W., Ley, P., & Kincey, J. A. (1975). Recall of medical advice: Comprehensibility and specificity. *British Journal of Social and Clinical Psychology, 14*(1), 55–62.

Cruzalegui, A. R. (2003, May). *Understanding and conducting focus groups*. Paper presented at Organizational Solutions to Low Health Literacy, Institute for Healthcare Advancement Second Annual Health Literacy Conference, Anaheim, CA.

Dallas Marketing Group (DMG). (2006). *Focus groups*. Retrieved February 7, 2006, from http://www.dallasmarketinggroup.com/pages/focus.html

Davis, T. C., Bocchini, J. A., Fredrickson, D., Mayeaux, A. C., Murphy, P. W., Jackson, R. H., et al. (1994). Parent comprehension of polio vaccine information pamphlets. *Pediatrics, 97*(6 pt 1), 804–810.

Davis, T. C., Williams, M. V., Marin, E., Parker, R. M., & Glass, J. (2002). Health literacy and cancer communication. *CA: A Cancer Journal for Clinicians, 52*(3), 130–133.

Doak, L. G., & Doak, C. C. (Eds.). (2003). *Pfizer principles for clear health communication: Chapter 6, Using readability formulas.* Retrieved January 10, 2006, from http://www.pfizerhealthliteracy.org/pdfs/Using_Readability_Formulas_v2.pdf

Doak, L. G., Doak, C. C., & Root, J. H. (1996). *Teaching patients with low literacy skills* (2nd ed.). Philadelphia: J.B. Lippincott.

Dreger, V., & Tremback, T. (2002). Optimize patient health by treating literacy and language barriers. *AORN Journal, 75*(2), 280–285, 287, 289–293.

Godin, S. (2003). *Purple cow: Transform your business by being remarkable.* New York: Portfolio Hardcover.

Herman, A. D., & Mayer, G. (2004). Reducing the use of emergency medical resources among Head Start families: A pilot study. *Journal of Community Health, 29*(3), 197–208.

Hochhauser, M. (2004). Plain language is ethical language. *Consulting Success Newsletter.* Retrieved April 17, 2004, from http://www.consultingsuccess.org/publications/consultingsuccess/feature_art/plain_language_is_ethical_language

Interagency Committee on Government Information (ICGI). (2005). *How to/tools.* Retrieved December 20, 2005, from http://www.plainlanguage.gov/howto/index.cfm

Institute for Healthcare Advancement (IHA). (2005, April 18). *Document for making your health care wishes known available from IHA for 90 million low-literate Americans* [press release]. Retrieved January 8, 2006, from http://www.iha4health.org/index.cfm/act/newsletter.cfm/category/Press%20Releases/menuitemid/112/MenuGroup/Home/NewsLetterID/55/startrow/2.htm

Institute of Medicine (IOM) of the National Academies. (2004). *Health literacy: A prescription to end confusion.* Washington, DC: The National Academies Press.

Mayer, G. (2003, May). *Writing easy to read, easy to use health information.* Paper presented at Organizational Solutions to Low Health Literacy, Institute for Healthcare Advancement Second Annual Health Literacy Conference, Anaheim, CA.

Mayer, G., & Kuklierus, A. (2001). *What to do when your child gets sick.* Whittier, CA: Institute for Healthcare Advancement.

McLaughlin, G. (1969). SMOG grading: A new readability formula. *Journal of Reading, 12*(8), 639–646.

Molina Healthcare, Inc. (2002). *Decreasing inappropriate ER utilization: Internal quality improvement project.* Long Beach, CA: Author.

National Cancer Institute (NCI). (2003). *Clear and simple: Developing effective materials for low-literate readers.* Washington, DC: U.S. Government Printing Office.

National Center for Education Statistics (NCES). (2005). *A first look at the literacy of America's adults in the 21st century* (NCES 2006-470). Washington, DC: U.S. Department of Education, Institute of Education Sciences.

Nielsen, J. (1997). *Estimated cost of running a focus group.* Retrieved January 3, 2006, from http://www.useit.com/papers/focusgroupcost.html

Northwest New Jersey Maternal and Child Health Network. (2002, March). *Programs progress report for the Dwyer Family Foundation.*

Population Empowerment Project. (2002). *Participant survey results.* Long Beach, CA: Coalition of Orange County Community Clinics.

Roat, C. E. (2005). *Addressing language access issues in your practice: A toolkit for physicians and their staff members.* San Francisco: California Academy of Family Physicians.

Rudd, R. E. (2002). *Health literacy overview presentation.* Retrieved August 27, 2005, from the Harvard School of Public Health, Health Literacy Studies Web site: http://www.hsph.harvard.edu/healthliteracy

Safeer, R. S., & Keenan, J. (2005). Health literacy: The gap between physicians and patients. *American Family Physician, 72*(3), 387–388.

Sanner, B. M. (2003, August). Are your written materials missing the mark? *Journal of Active Aging,* 18–24.

Sobero, R., & Giraldo, G. P. (2004, May). *Beyond translations: Culturally adapting and developing low-literacy materials.* Presented at Clinical and Educational Solutions to Low Health Literacy, Institute for Healthcare Advancement Third Annual Health Literacy Conference, Anaheim, CA.

Sudore, R. S., & Mayer, G. (2006). Advance directives designed for low-literate patients. *Group Practice Journal, 55*(2), 24–26.

Weiss, B. D. (2003). *Health literacy: A manual for clinicians.* Chicago: American Medical Association Foundation and American Medical Association.

Weiss, B. D., & Coyne, C. (1997). Communicating with patients who cannot read. *New England Journal of Medicine, 337*(4), 272–274.

Westphal, C., & Wavra, T. (2005, September). *Acute and critical care choices guide to advance directives.* Retrieved December 10, 2005, from http://www.aacn.org/AACN/ practice.nsf/Files/cchoices/$file/Acute%20and%20Critical%20Care%20Choices% 20to%20Advance%20Directives.pdf#search='westphal%20wavra%20advance% 20directive%20AACN'

Yahya, F. M. (2002–2004). Back translation. *Arabic Freelance: The translation office of Fuad M. Yahya.* Retrieved February 11, 2006, from http://www.arabicfreelance.com/back. html

9

USING ALTERNATIVE FORMS OF PATIENT COMMUNICATION

We live in an age of information and communication, of full disclosure and informed consent. We live in an age of technology, too, at a time when advances in hardware and software constantly offer us new options for connecting with others. Yet still we are plagued by our inability to reach all people at all times. It is an unavoidable characteristic of communication that our messages must be packaged differently for different audiences to be fully understood by them.

For those in the health care community, the plethora of communication options combined with the strides that are regularly made in knowledge about health, disease, prevention, and treatment result in even greater expectations with respect to patient communication. In particular, advances in communicative media hold promise for providers who are dedicated to conveying accurate and meaningful health care messages to their low-literate patients.

To reap the benefits of all this choice in communicative technology, however, health care providers must make informed decisions about how to present their messages. With so much information to convey and so many different groups to reach, providers are called on to understand how these groups receive and understand information and how the medium affects the message.

VERBAL COMMUNICATION

Human beings are hard-wired to learn through listening. It is the way children learn, at least initially. It is the way learning took place for thousands of years before writing systems were invented. And it is the way many adults still learn best. Verbally explaining a diagnosis or giving instructions has some advantages over presenting the same information in writing. Tone of voice, for example, can highlight important points and add to the compelling nature of the information, providing cues for patients to give certain information their full attention. Therefore, face-to-face consultations with patients appear to be the ideal context in which health care communication takes place.

In fact, face-to-face interactions between patients and providers form the very foundation of medical care. Seeing patients in person offers health care professionals the chance to gauge how well they understand diagnoses, treatment options, and medical instructions. Face-to-face consultations are usually required for health care providers to make accurate diagnoses. But what happens afterward? How can health care providers and their patients take advantage of the benefits of speech when they're not in proximity to one another?

Telephone

The telephone is one way. As McBride and Rimer pointed out back in 1999,

> The technology for using the telephone to deliver interventions to improve health behavior and health care has expanded dramatically, and exciting innovations continue to emerge. These developments enable the telephone to be used to deliver individualized services to a broad cross section of target groups, while minimizing logistic and system barriers, and cost.

More than just a tool for making appointments or scheduling tests, the telephone has been shown in a number of studies to have the potential for affecting patient care and health—and, in some cases, even the well-being of patients' family members.

Telephone contact can serve as an appropriate means of follow-up care, for example. Wylie, Allen, and Hallam-Jones (2005) evaluated the effect of the introduction of telephone follow-up with men who had been prescribed erectogenic agents. The phone consultations were well received, with 91.9% of participants reporting that they found them more convenient than traditional follow-up because they did away with the need to travel to see a doctor and spend time in a waiting room (Wylie et al., 2005).

There is also some evidence that the telephone can be a useful tool in counseling patients. Research by Helmes, Culver, and Bowen (2006), for example, examined the appropriateness and usefulness of telephone interventions for women interested in obtaining genetic counseling for breast cancer risk. The study of 340 women indicated that both in-person and telephone counseling decreased women's cancer worry, risk perceptions, and intentions to pursue genetic testing (Helmes et al., 2006). The authors point out that the results have implications for telephone use and, in particular, that telephone use may increase the reach of counseling to better serve women in remote areas (Helmes et al., 2006).

Badger, Segrin, Meek, Lopez, and Bonham (2004) also looked at the potential for telephone use in counseling. They conducted a case study of telephone interpersonal counseling for a woman diagnosed with breast cancer and her partner and noted,

> Substantial evidence exists that face-to-face psychosocial interventions improve psychological adjustment and health-related quality of life for patients with cancer. Yet psychosocial interventions are not offered routinely, and many patients with cancer do not use face-to-face counseling mechanisms (Badger et al., 2004).

The authors reason that the phone might offer some assistance in delivering much-needed counseling. As a result of the telephone-delivered counseling, this patient and her partner reported substantial positive changes in symptoms such as depression and anxiety and in the nature of their relationship with each other and with their children. The authors noted that, although the intervention required additional training of nurses, some techniques of the intervention could be used by all nurses, regardless of their specialty training (Badger et al., 2004).

A study by Hardyman, Hardy, Brodie, and Stephens (2005) suggests that patients who contacted a cancer telephone helpline were less likely to request factual information but more likely to request information on sensitive topics than patients who accessed a cancer Web site. This study provides valuable information about the types of health information people seek from different sources. It also indicates that telephone contact can play a significant role in complementing other information sources.

Finally, advances in technology and service create new uses for the telephone in the context of health care. Oslin and coworkers (2006) looked at a telephone-based systematic clinical assessment service, the Behavioral Health Laboratory (BHL), and its feasibility in primary care. The BHL provides primary care providers with a summary of patients' mental health and substance abuse symptoms and with treatment decision support (e.g., triage to specialty mental health and substance abuse services). The system was implemented to assist in evaluating patients in whom physicians detected symptoms of depression.

The implementation of BHL resulted in an apparent change in clinical practice. The researchers found an association between BHL use and an increase in the proportion of patients screened for depression in primary care (Oslin et al., 2006). The BHL successfully provided a comprehensive assessment for 78% of those referred. The broad-based approach of the system led to the identification of significant comorbidity of depression with alcohol misuse, illicit drug use, and suicidal thoughts, symptoms likely to have been missed in routine practice. The authors believe that the BHL offers a practical means for assessing and monitoring patients identified as having mental health and substance abuse problems and for assisting in treatment planning for those individuals (Oslin et al., 2006).

There is also significant support in the literature for the use of videophones in health care. Savenstedt, Zingmark, and Sandman (2003) investigated the potential role of videophones in the care of elderly patients. They conducted and analyzed interviews with family members and nursing staff regarding their experiences of communicating with elderly people via videophone. The results suggested that it is possible for elderly patients with cognitive impairment to engage in remote communication when certain conditions are met. In addition, the researchers found that videophone interaction occasionally increased the attention and focus of elderly subjects (Savenstedt et al., 2003).

Similarly, Oakley, Duffill, and Reeve (1998) assessed an interactive telemedicine service used to conduct dermatology consultations, finding that the system resulted in savings in time and money for patients. Only about 20% of the consultations with new patients resulted in another face-to-face appointment, and most patients found the telelink acceptable (Oakley et al., 1998).

Audiotaped Messages

Another option for reaping the benefits of speech when health care providers cannot personally meet with patients—whether because of time constraints or distance—is to use audiotaped messages. Although many health care providers see the advantage of using audiotapes when teaching patients about disease prevention and overall health promotion, Doak, Doak, and Root (1996) note that the medium has additional potential. These researchers claim that providers who receive as little as 1 hour of training in the development and use of such materials can produce effective audiotaped instructions (Doak et al., 1996). What's more, they say, a little training tends to create a great deal of enthusiasm for audiotaped instructions on the part of both health care providers and patients (Doak et al., 1996).

Research already has shown that audiotapes have applications in health care. A study of smoking cessation and long-term smoking abstinence rates in patients using guided imagery audiotapes revealed that those patients who used the audiotapes in addition to educational and counseling sessions had higher smoking abstinence rates at 24 months after intervention than those who did not use the audiotapes (Wynd, 2005).

Millions of adults in the United States are functionally illiterate, as studies such as the National Adult Literacy Survey (NALS) of 1992 and the National Assessment of Adult Literacy (NAAL) of 2003 have amply demonstrated. For such individuals, audiotaped messages are one of the few ways that health care providers can communicate important information or instructions. This segment of the population either cannot read printed materials or has a difficult time doing so; pamphlets and instruction sheets simply aren't effective for them. One-on-one communication is an option, of course, but it can be time consuming. In addition, information communicated in such a way is not consistently retained. Audiotaped messages can bridge this gap.

VISUAL COMMUNICATION

In addition to the media discussed above, there are options for communicating with low-literate patients that use visuals as the primary means of communicating a message. These visuals are not the complicated graphs and charts of technical presentations, but rather are clear and simple pictorial images. There are good reasons to incorporate visuals into the communication of health-related messages, as Doak and colleagues (1996) suggest. Human memory systems favor visual storage, and complex concepts are understood more easily when presented visually. Visuals tend to stir emotions too. As a result, people respond quickly to what they see (Doak et al., 1996).

These are compelling arguments for incorporating visuals into health care messages, regardless of the intended audience. But when the target audience has low literacy or low health literacy levels, visually dominant forms of communication may be particularly appropriate.

Pictographs

Pictographs (also called *pictograms*) are clear, simple symbols that convey meaning without the use of words. Think of the nearly universal symbol for restrooms. Wherever you go, that pictograph easily conveys the intended message concerning the location of public toilets. Other examples of pictographs that we encounter on a regular basis include the U.S. Department of Transportation signs pointing the way to airports and train stations, escalators, and elevators. Laundry care symbols are pictographs, too, as are the pictures on chemical hazard labels.

Clearly, using pictographs or simple line drawings as a communicative medium is not a new concept; their use dates back to cave paintings. Still, the examples above illustrate how useful and effective pictographs can be in the present day. Their pervasiveness highlights the potential for using them in other, more important contexts, such as the health care environment.

Pictographs have been used in nonliterate societies to aid individuals in remembering spoken instructions. Some suggest that they should be used today to help nonliterate patients remember verbal instructions (Houts et al., 1998). In one study, 60 low-literate patients were given either a patient information leaflet that included pictographs plus text or one that included text only. The inclusion of pictographs in the informational material was shown to improve patients' comprehension of more complex information (Mansoor & Dowse, 2003).

A study by Houts and colleagues (1998) found that patients' recall of verbal medical instructions averaged 14%, but that figure rose to 85% when spoken instructions were supported with pictographs. A follow-up study showed that low-literate patients can recall large amounts of medical information for significant periods of time when pictographs are used (Houts et al., 2001). The authors point out, however, that the ultimate impact of such visuals on patients' quality of life has not yet been determined (Houts et al., 2001).

Dowse and Ehlers (2005) found that pictographs positively influence both patients' understanding of instructions and adherence. Eighty-seven patients who had been prescribed a short course of antibiotics were given either text-only labels or labels that incorporated pictographs with the text. Follow-up home visits were conducted after 3 to 5 days to assess patients' understanding of instructions and adherence to those instructions. The researchers found that 54% of the patients who had received the instructions with pictographs had an adherence rate of greater than 90%, whereas only 2% of those who had received text-only instructions had such high rates of adherence. Average percentages for understanding in the text-only group and the text-with-pictograph group were 70 and 95%, respectively; average adherence was 72 and 90%, respectively (Dowse & Ehlers, 2005).

Clearly, then, there is evidence that pictographs contribute positively to understanding and adherence among literacy-challenged patients. However, Knapp, Raynor, Jebar, and Price (2005) caution that the size of pictographs is important and that making them small to fit into conventional written formats could negatively affect patients' understanding.

Pictographs are most likely to be encountered in pharmacies and on the bottles of prescription and other medications. The U.S. Pharmacopeia (USP) is the official public standards-setting authority for all prescription and over-the-counter medicines, dietary supplements, and other health care products manufactured and sold in the United States. As an independent public health organization, the USP does not itself regulate medicines, but federal law dictates that prescription and over-the-counter medicines available in the United States must meet the standards set by USP, where such standards exist. This agency offers a library of 81 pictographs designed to help ensure safe drug practices and good pharmaceutical care for patients (USP, 2006). (For samples of the USP pictographs, see Figure 9.1a–f. To view them all, visit http://www.usp.org/audiences/consumers/pictograms/form.html.)

The USP pictographs use standardized, widely understood images to convey medication instructions, precautions, and warnings to patients. Health care providers and those tasked with providing patient information can use the USP pictographs free of charge to reinforce printed or verbal instructions. Low-health-literate patients stand to benefit from their use. According to USP (2006), "pictograms are particularly helpful in passing on important information to patients with a lower level reading ability and patients who use English as a second language."

The USP takes steps to ensure that the pictographs it provides to the health care industry are understandable to patients of various backgrounds and experiences. In fact, it tests the images it uses with representative groups from various segments of the population to determine whether the pictographs are communicating the desired message successfully.

The USP's first condition for granting a license to use its pictographs is that they not be used as the sole means of communicating medical information because there is always the potential for misinterpretation (USP, 2006). In other words, pictographs are designed to be used as a supplement to and not as a replacement for other instructions, whether printed or verbal. They are meant to serve as a reminder to patients of the proper way to take and to store their medications, for example. Nevertheless, the original instructions should be communicated in some other medium as well.

Fotonovelas

Another option for communicating with low-literate patients that has a minimal reliance on text and a maximum use of visuals is the *fotonovela*. These materials are comic-book-like printed materials that tell a story using photographs and dialogue bubbles to indicate which of the characters pictured is speaking. According to the Public Broadcasting Service (PBS, 2006), *fotonovelas* have been used for a long time in Mexico and Latin America and in Latino and Chicano communities in the United States. In this format, these communities have a vehicle through which they can address social concerns using innovative and highly visual means. "Activists and religious groups," notes PBS, "have also turned to the form as an organizational tool for outreach, education and proselytizing" (PBS, 2006).

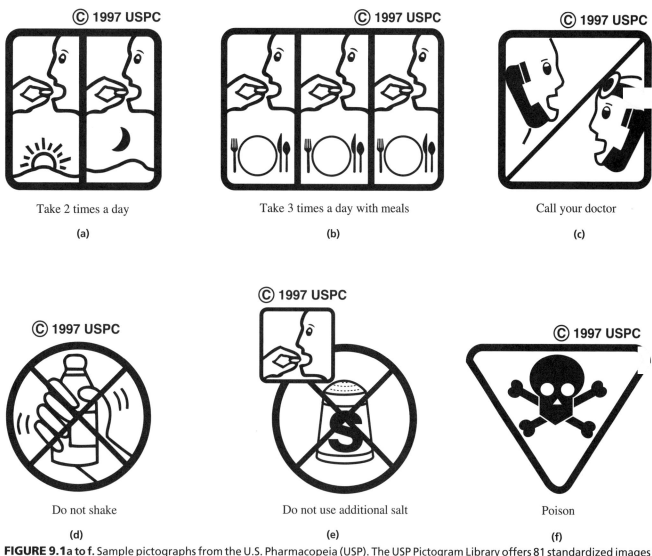

Take 2 times a day

(a)

Take 3 times a day with meals

(b)

Call your doctor

(c)

Do not shake

(d)

Do not use additional salt

(e)

Poison

(f)

FIGURE 9.1a to f. Sample pictographs from the U.S. Pharmacopeia (USP). The USP Pictogram Library offers 81 standardized images to convey medication instructions, precautions, and warnings to patients and consumers. Pictographs (also called pictograms) are helpful for conveying important information to patients with low literacy and those for whom English is a second language. They are free for professionals and patient information providers to reinforce printed or oral instructions. Source: USP. 2006. *USP Pictograms*. Available at: http://www.usp.org/audiences/consumers/pictograms/form.html

A guidebook developed by the AMC Cancer Research Center in Denver, entitled *Beyond the Brochure: Alternative Approaches to Effective Health Communication* (1994), describes the potential benefits for using *fotonovelas* in the health care community:

> With its conversational approach, a *fotonovela* can be a good low-literacy educational medium if dialogue is written at a low reading level. The story is told through a realistic, entertaining and educational plot.... *Fotonovelas* are generally most effective in communities that are familiar with the medium (AMC Cancer Research Center, 2004, p. 33).

A number of organizations have recognized the potential for *fotonovelas* to reach certain segments of the low-literate patient population in a meaningful way. Studies published in the 1990s revealed a gap between the reading levels of the majority of U.S. adults and the reading levels required to read and understand most health education pamphlets and informed consent documents (Doak, Doak, Friedell, & Meade, 1998; Dollahite, Thompson, & McNew, 1996; Hearth-Holmes et al., 1997). Since then, numerous health care providers and government agencies have explored alternative means of communication with low-literate patients. As a result, much of the health-related information that previously was available only in text form has been repackaged in formats—including the *fotonovela*—that aid in patient understanding (Wilson, 2000).

For example, in 2000 the California Department of Health Services and Managed Risk Medical Insurance Board introduced two Spanish-language *fotonovelas* to help educate and raise awareness among the Latino community of the two child health care coverage programs offered by the state (Healthy Families, 2000). Called *Historias de la Vida,* these outreach tools detail the realistic experiences and concerns of Latino families in their attempts to secure health care for their children. These concerns include the cost of programs, eligibility, income levels, and immigration status.

The Rural Women's Health Project (RWHP) also has made extensive use of *fotonovelas*. An organization that has worked with women farm workers and their families since 1992, the RWHP created *fotonovelas* to present health messages, document its work within communities, and improve individual and community well-being. Some of the health-related topics addressed by the RWHP's *fotonovelas* include HIV/AIDS prevention, condom use, tobacco awareness, eye injury prevention, and health insurance (Rural Women's Health Project, n.d.). For more information, visit the organization's Web site at http://www.rwhp.org/nov_ed/fotonov.html.

Despite the promise of the *fotonovela* as a communication tool, research suggests that, even within populations expected to be receptive to their use, the medium should probably not be used as the only form of communication for health-related messages. In fact, in a study of the perceived credibility of channels and sources of AIDS information among Hispanics, Marin and Marin (1990) found that *fotonovelas* were not considered particularly credible. Among the 460 Hispanic adults interviewed over the phone regarding the credibility they assigned to various channels of AIDS information dissemination, *fotonovelas* received the lowest ratings. An AIDS hotline and printed information (e.g., books, pamphlets) received the highest ratings (Marin & Marin, 1990).

Of course, these respondents' preference could be a matter of habit: conventional written texts have long been seen by members of literate societies as authoritative—as the gold standard against which other modes of communication should be measured—sometimes to the detriment of other forms of communication such as oral language (Ong, 1982). In the study above, patients assigned high levels of credibility to oral language when it was used on the telephone, but predictably saw certain forms of written communication as more preferable and authoritative.

INCORPORATING BOTH SPEECH AND VISUALS

Some media, of course, incorporate speech and visuals together. When done well, these materials can have numerous points of connection with the patients who use them. By appealing to two different learning sensory pathways, the materials created in these media can capture patients' attention more fully and communicate a health care message more completely.

Video Messages

Video messages are one way that creators of health care messages can appeal to patients using both speech and visuals. Such messages can be conveyed on VHS, DVD, CD, portable players such as the iPod, and other formats. Video messages on a variety of health care topics are currently available, and thanks to the many private and government agencies producing health care materials, the number is constantly growing.

Many videos are available for a small fee or even free on loan from various government and private agencies, including libraries. Some materials are available as monthly rentals for about a quarter of the purchase price. This option might be preferable for health care providers who offer the information in a one-time presentation or informational series. For those providers in areas that serve a large number of patients from a particular ethnic group, videotaped messages designed particularly for those groups may be available from various local sources. Because the production costs of these materials can be quite low—particularly with recent advances in taping, editing, and production—their purchase prices are often low as well.

Each of the various formats of videotaped messages has its advantages and disadvantages. VHS tapes may be the cheapest to produce and to purchase, and there are a great variety of topics and titles from which to choose. However, using a VCR can be time consuming and inefficient. To set up a section of the tape or to review previously viewed scenes, users must forward or rewind the tape. Still, VHS may be the only option for patients who do not own DVD players or computers. The catch, however, which you know if you've been to your neighborhood video store lately, is that VHS tapes are becoming extinct; DVDs are now the norm.

There are good reasons why DVDs have supplanted VHS tapes. One reason is that DVDs offer superior access to particular sections of the video, eliminating the need for forwarding and rewinding. This feature allows users to more quickly find, access, and view the information they want to study or review.

The CD-ROM format offers users similar control. Like DVDs, CD-ROMs are easy to navigate. Users can skip quickly and easily to the information they need to know. Of course, to use a CD-ROM, users must own or at least have access to a computer. In addition, they must be somewhat computer literate because using a CD-ROM requires users to know how to load and run the CD, as well as how to use a computer mouse or keyboard to move through the information contained on the CD.

Videotaped materials can be an economical way to increase patients' understanding and compliance with medical advice. A randomized controlled trial comparing videotape instruction with personal instruction by a physical therapist on exercise following arthroscopic full-thickness rotator cuff repair surgery, for instance, revealed that patients who used the videotape had self-reported outcomes equal to patients instructed in their home program by a physical therapist (Roddey, Olson, Gartsman, Hanten, & Cook, 2002). However, it should be noted that a therapist was available to answer questions for patients who used the videotape. The study suggests that resources such as the expertise of physical therapists might be supplemented and maximized through use of technologies like videotapes.

Many other studies support the efficacy of videotaped information in the health care environment. Smith, Koehler, Moore, Blanchard, and Ellerbeck (2005) tested a videotape intervention designed to improve patients' self-management of heart failure. The video content followed national, scientifically validated guidelines for heart failure home management. The study tested patients' knowledge, symptom reporting, and functional status. The data indicated that participants had a clinically relevant improvement in heart failure knowledge and improved or maintained health status. None of the patients were rehospitalized during the 60-day follow-up period, and one patient contacted his physician to report weight gain, as prompted by the videotapes (Smith et al., 2005).

A study by Jean Wiese and colleagues (2005) on the use of a videotape designed to enhance patients' understanding of obstructive sleep apnea and of the purpose, logistics, and benefits of treatment suggested that videotapes can positively affect compliance. Specifically, viewing of a patient education video at the initial visit was found to significantly improve the rate of return for the follow-up visit (Jean Wiese et al., 2005).

Research suggests that videotapes can be a highly effective method for communicating health care information. A study by So and colleagues (2003) on the influence of videotapes on patients' compliance with silicone gel sheeting and their subsequent burn scar outcomes revealed that the use of detailed videotapes for patient education improved compliance with the therapy and resulted in better scar outcomes. May and colleagues (2003) report that video presentations can be an effective way to convey information about nicotine replacement treatment to smokers.

Like audiotaped messages, videotaped information can be particularly helpful in communicating with patients who function at the lowest literacy levels. A study comparing the effectiveness of a printed message about polio vaccinations with the same message converted into a production of animated cartoons using marketing and advertising techniques showed that the animated cartoons were more effective (Leiner, Handal, & Williams, 2004). Such techniques can be both helpful and attractive to low-literate patients.

A study of different approaches to violence prevention among adolescents revealed that children of the video age respond well to visual material (Tucker et al., 1999). The investigators encourage the use of multimedia presentations in violence prevention programs aimed at adolescents. Their study measures middle-school students' recall of a program presented in four parts: a rap music video created by violence prevention staff, a facilitated discussion about dealing with anger, a video of an emergency department trauma resuscitation, and a commercial video of a teenage boy paralyzed after a gunshot wound.

One month after presentation, the students' retention, problem identification, and impact were highest for the commercial video and rap music video. However, the audience ranked the program as a whole higher than any of the individual parts when measured by success at problem identification and impact. This suggests that using a variety of methods in combination works well for this population (Tucker et al., 1999).

A study on the effects of a videotape designed to increase the use of poison control centers (PCCs) by low-income and Spanish-speaking families similarly revealed that videotape intervention was highly effective in changing the knowledge, attitudes, behaviors, and behavioral intentions concerning PCCs within this population (Kelly, Huffman, Mendoza, & Robinson, 2003).

Research shows that patients also are receptive to video presentations of materials. A study of patients' responses to a patient-information DVD in a surgical oncology department revealed that 71% of the 108 patients who watched it considered that viewing the DVD had been positive and encouraging; 83% recommended its use (Evrard et al., 2005). Another study compared three methods of conducting the preanesthetic visit: a preanesthetic interview, a brochure plus an interview, or a documentary video plus an interview. Researchers found that those patients in the video-plus-interview group scored highest for satisfaction and information gain (Snyder-Ramos et al., 2005).

In addition, a study by Stanton and colleagues (2005) offered some evidence that a peer-modeling videotape (i.e., a videotape that demonstrated positive ways study participants might cope with their disease, such as seeking social support, as modeled by the behavior of peers in very similar circumstances) could accelerate the recovery of energy during the reentry phase (i.e., following completion of cancer therapy and the resumption of everyday life) in women treated for breast cancer, particularly among those who felt less prepared for this stage.

Evidence suggests that videotapes may be particularly useful when addressing sensitive topics. For example, one study assessed a videotape intervention for sexual counseling after myocardial infarction. Sexual integrity, quality of life, and stress and coping were key concepts underpinning the intervention. In addition to the usual written and verbal instructions they received while hospitalized, patients in the study were given the videotape to view in the privacy of their homes. Study results indicate that the use of such a tool in the home setting provides an additional method of patient education that appears ideal for this sensitive topic (Steinke, 2002).

Web-Based Alternatives

Web-based tools and their applications offer health care providers an ever-increasing number of options for communicating with patients. These options rely to varying degrees on speech and visuals. However, the jury is still out on whether the Internet will help or hurt the health care industry's efforts to communicate more successfully with low-literate patients. To date, this technology mostly has been used simply to repackage existing printed materials. The result of such repackaging is merely to make printed materials—whether useful or not—available to a wider range of patients whenever they want them.

In addition, a number of recent studies have documented barriers faced by minority and low-health-literate patients as they attempt to use the Internet to access health information (Birru et al., 2004; Fogel, 2003; Zarcadoolas, Blanco, Boyer, & Pleasant, 2002). Among these barriers is the reading level of the average Web site, which is several grade levels higher than the average user's reading level, making them no easier to read than standard print materials (Birru et al., 2004).

Although making materials available to a larger number of patients is itself a worthwhile goal, such a goal fails to acknowledge the true potential of the Web, which is a multimedia environment. Numerous health care researchers and technology practitioners are convinced that Web-based applications can offer something truly new and meaningful to the patient population—even if those applications have yet to be developed.

Many computer-based technologies already are helping improve health care outcomes. For example, Rogers and colleagues (2005) found that the use of audio computer-assisted interviewing may encourage patients to share more information than they do in interviews conducted by health care providers. In the study, 1,350 patients were assigned to complete a behavioral survey on sexual risk practices, previous sexually transmitted infections and symptoms, condom use, and drug and alcohol use. Some of the patients used an audio computer program to answer the questions; others were interviewed by health care providers. The researchers found that the patients who used the computer were more likely to report engaging in recent risky behaviors, such as sex without a condom in the past 24 hours, anal sex, and one or more new partners in the past 6 months, compared to those who were interviewed by a health care provider.

One problem with using the Internet as a health care resource is that much of the material generated by patients' Internet searches lacks adequate quality, according to the research. Wallace, Turner, Ballard, Keenum, and Weiss (2005) found this to be true in their assessment of the osteoporosis material obtained using search strategies typical of many patients' searches. The same kind of results were reported by Bichakjian and colleagues (2005), who assessed melanoma information generated by entering the term *melanoma* into the search fields of eight search engines. They evaluated 74 Web sites in the study. The researchers found that the medical information retrieved was likely to lack complete basic melanoma information. In addition, 14% of the sites contained errors (Bichakjian et al., 2005).

It therefore appears that health care professionals are missing the mark not only when it comes to producing information that is appropriate to patients' reading levels but also in providing complete and accurate information via the Internet. The problem is that patients do not have a reliable way to separate the accurate information from the inaccurate.

Purchasing Existing Materials Versus Creating Your Own

The first step in creating anything new is to determine whether it is truly needed. Before you take on the task of developing a solution to a perceived need related to health care communication, take some time to research what already exists. Is there already a video that addresses the special needs of your patient population? Are there audiotapes or interactive Web-based solutions? Using existing materials obviously has a financial advantage for health care providers because they do not have to dedicate the time and money to produce something new.

However, saving development costs is not a good reason to settle for using materials that do not successfully address the problem that you observe or that otherwise miss the mark. So, although there are plenty of useful, effective materials available to patients and providers alike, you may find yourself in the position of having to revise or repackage some of those materials or even having to create something brand new.

GUIDELINES FOR DEVELOPING ALTERNATIVE MATERIALS

The guidelines for developing nontext-based sources of information for low-literate patients do not differ much from guidelines for developing print materials for that segment of the population. Alternative methods of communication addressed throughout this chapter do not (with the possible exception of Web-based tools) require consideration of such elements as white space or text length. However, guidelines discussed in chapter 8 dealing with tone, word choice, cultural relevance, and so on also apply to the communication tools addressed in this chapter.

Rather than reiterating those rules (refer to the previous chapter to refresh your memory), we make three suggestions for nonprint-based materials aimed at low-health-literate patients. The first is to make the materials interactive wherever it is appropriate to do so. All of the forms of communication discussed in this chapter have the potential for interaction. Doak and colleagues (1996) explain the strategic nature of using interaction to lend emphasis to key points. Using visuals that ask for patients to respond, they say, highlights the point being made by implanting the message in the patient's memory. Other researchers have found that high-quality participatory videos can enhance health care providers' interpersonal skills to effectively communicate messages to their patients (Uccellani & Rosales, 1992).

Some of the communicative tools that have been described above are, by their very nature, interactive. The pictographs used on prescription bottles, for example, are simply requests that the patient mirror the depicted behavior. And telephone interventions rely on interaction with the patient to be effective. Although other alternative means of communication are not as intrinsically interactive, there are opportunities to build useful interactive qualities into them. Developers of audio- or videotapes can incorporate interaction into the material by asking patients to give a verbal response or to write down their ideas or answer questions on a printed supplement. Web-based tools have the potential to be very interactive. A game or survey on a Web site can help ensure that important information sticks with patients.

The second suggestion is that the materials—whether audio, video, Web-based, or printed visuals—be action oriented. Regardless of the medium chosen, the materials should serve as a call to action. The message should be clear; patients should be able to recognize and understand the objective of the material.

Finally, the materials should focus on behaviors. What do you want patients to do? How do you want them to do it? Tell patients exactly what behaviors they should target. If the materials are clear about the habits or activities patients need to add or modify, there is a better chance they will actually achieve the goal.

Choosing the Appropriate Medium

Clearly, there are many good choices when it comes to deciding which media to use to convey health care messages. And although there is no overall "best" choice, there are probably one or two very good choices for any given health care communication and scenario. To discover what those choices might be, health care providers should consider the message they want to send and the environment into which they will be sending it.

What Is the Message?

The first thing to consider when choosing a medium for your message is the message itself. What are your objectives in crafting and disseminating this message? Most likely, you are developing materials in response to an existing or anticipated need. Consider exactly what that need is, and define for yourself clearly and specifically what you want to achieve with your communication. Although you may believe that the need for and objectives of the materials are obvious, you should spell these things out for yourself before you decide on the best way to package your message.

Who Is the Audience?

When you have pinned down what need you are addressing with the materials and what you want to accomplish, you should ask yourself who will use them. Knowing your audience is key to making appropriate, strategic decisions when it comes to choosing the kinds of language and visuals you will use. Ultimately, your audience can have a great influence on your choice of medium to deliver your message.

Suggestions offered in chapter 8 regarding learning about your intended audience when creating print materials are equally applicable to the development of audio- and videotapes, telephone interventions, interactive Web-based tools, and other forms of health care communication. Consider the age, ethnic background, socioeconomic status, and educational experience of the individuals who make up your target audience. What do these factors tell you about them and their beliefs and interests? Use the available research to find out more about your audience. If possible, employ focus groups to gain further insight (Sanner, 2003).

What Other Materials Are Available?

You may be the first person to develop patient materials on your particular subject, but more than likely there already are some materials available. It's a good idea to explore exactly what those materials are and how successful they have been in communicating health care messages. Identifying which ones work and why, as well as which ones do not work and why, will help you see what kinds of strategies are effective for your audience. Despite the fact that you may develop materials using a different medium, understanding what has been successful with your target audience will give you insight into the kind of finished product you should be shooting for. It also may keep you from reinventing the wheel. That is, if you know there is a highly effective videotape on your subject, you don't have to create another one.

For example, those looking for a video on the general problem of health literacy and its impact on public health and medicine need go no further than the Web site of the Harvard School of Public Health, where they will find a downloadable electronic version of *In Plain Language* (2006), the educational video produced by Drs. Rima Rudd and William DeJong. Also available on VHS and DVD, the video includes testimonials from adult learners about meeting literacy demands in the health care setting. According to its developers, *In Plain Language* can be used as a starting point for courses, workshops, or conferences addressing health communication issues. If such a video suits your needs, you might be able to use money budgeted for the project to produce material that supplements it, such as an interactive Web site or a telephone intervention.

Additional characteristics of existing materials that you will want to assess include reading level and cultural appropriateness. Even when you create materials that are not dependent on text, you should ensure that any text used is geared toward the reading level of your target audience. A *fotonovela*, for instance, may not contain much text and may rely heavily on pictures. But if the little text it does contain is written at a level above that of your intended audience, the message of the piece may not be conveyed accurately. There are a number of tools that you can use to assess the reading level of texts; they are explained in detail in chapter 3, Assessing Patients' Literacy Levels.

Although it is not strictly a tool that measures reading level, the Suitability Assessment of Materials (SAM), developed by Doak and colleagues (1996), may be a particularly good choice for evaluating nontext-based materials. The SAM was designed for use with print materials and illustrations, but it has been used successfully to assess audiotapes and videotapes as well (Doak et al., 1996; Rudd, 2005). One of the evaluation criteria used by the SAM is cultural appropriateness. The tool measures how well the logic, language, and experience of the material being assessed matches the logic, language, and experience of the intended audience (Doak et al., 1996).

Another good idea for evaluating existing patient materials is to have a third party review them. That person might be an expert who verifies the accuracy of the information presented in the materials or a representative of your target audience who can tell you which parts of the materials work from a cultural or a persuasive standpoint. Either way, with a third-party review of your material, you can gain important insight. A study by Meade (1996) showed that assessment and inclusion of target audience members throughout the development process of cancer education videotapes helped ensure that the content met learners' needs.

One final point on which to evaluate existing materials is the degree to which they achieve their educational objectives. You also can assess the degree to which the materials might support the objective you have designed for your own planned product.

Which Medium Best Fits My Patients' Needs?

When choosing a medium for your health care message, consider how closely that medium fits the needs of the target audience. Cost is a major concern when you are developing materials for patients. You should be aware of your development budget for the project, of course, but also you must be conscious of the cost of the final materials to your patients. If health care materials are cost prohibitive for them, use and compliance will be negatively affected. Having a clear picture of your target audience can help you be more sensitive to the impact that the cost of your final materials will have on your patients.

You also should ensure that the message you want to send is consistent with that of the medium. Are interactive touch screens in a public setting the best way to screen patients about sexually transmitted diseases, for example? And would a *fotonovela* with accompanying text designed to educate patients about their diabetes be more effective than a CD-ROM or a video? This is especially important when you are choosing from among the numerous existing materials available. But it is also important when developing your own materials. As the above examples illustrate, some messages are conveyed and received better when a particular medium is used. Consider the problem you want to address and the objectives you want to achieve, and then consult the research to see if other initiatives suggest that one medium might be particularly well suited to that goal.

Data from evidence-based approaches are important to consider when evaluating the effectiveness of different media. In the health care community, more and more studies are being published on community-based interventions with culturally diverse groups. These results are important for our efforts to address health literacy and to take patients' health literacy levels into account when developing new materials (Institute of Medicine, 2004).

It is also a good idea to do your own assessment of existing materials to determine whether they are effective and what characteristics make them so.

Imitation is the sincerest form of flattery. Go ahead and see what other people have done and which forms of media have been successful in achieving objectives similar to yours. Then, when you have a working version of the materials you are developing (but before you get to a final version), assess your own work to make sure the medium you have chosen works as well as you thought it would.

BARRIERS TO MEDIA USAGE

There are a number of significant challenges to using alternative communication media to reach low-literate patient populations. One of those challenges is access. Not all patients have access to a CD or audiotape player. Nor does everyone have a DVD player. And as difficult as it may be to believe for those of us who depend on Internet-based technology such as e-mail to plan our daily schedules, many individuals still do not have Internet access.

In fact, data from the Pew Internet and American Life Project, a nonprofit research group that regularly conducts surveys on Internet use, indicate that 27% of American adults live in a household that does not have an Internet connection (Fox, 2005). Some of these people have Internet access at work, school, or some other location, but for most of these 27%, lack of Internet access means that they cannot get information from the Internet even if they wanted to.

And whether they actually want to retrieve information from the Internet is open to debate. A full 32% of American adults—about 65 million people—do not go online (Fox, 2005). Of these, 32% say they are simply not interested in connecting to the Internet (Fox, 2005). This suggests a barrier to Internet access that is different from the more predictable barriers like high cost, not having a computer, and not knowing how to use the technology. Clearly, lack of interest or desire is a significant barrier to Internet access for quite a few people.

A number of other barriers should be considered when developing patient materials that make use of alternative media. One of those is lack of technical skills necessary to use the tools. In addition to their literacy skills—or lack thereof—patients who wish to make use of electronic technologies to gain health information also are affected by their level of technological proficiency. Before you send a patient home with a DVD, be sure he or she has access to a DVD player and knows how to use it. Before you schedule a videophone consultation with a patient, be sure he or she has access to the technology and can operate the video camera. Before you direct a patient to a health care Web site, be sure that he or she not only has access to a computer but also knows how to connect to the Internet.

It's not just the patient who needs to know how to use the technology, however. Health care providers must be familiar with the medium as well. If patients have specific technology questions to which they need answers before they can use the materials you provide them, you should be able to answer them—or at least be able to put patients in touch with someone who can. It might be appropriate to conduct an in-office evaluation of patients' technology skills before you provide them with nontext materials. If you find that patients are having difficulties with a DVD player, cell phone, computer, or other technology, you should be able to offer a quick tutorial that will enable them to successfully use the materials you are offering. Or, on the other hand, the results of the in-office evaluation might help you decide not to use a technology-based education approach with a particular patient.

Several additional barriers to information are specific to Web-based tools. Cynthia E. Baur, PhD, health communication and e-health adviser to the Office of Disease Prevention and Health Promotion, explains that even within the realm of Internet access, patients must have a variety of abilities to use the technology effectively:

> Individuals must make decisions about what kinds of technology are appropriate for gaining access to the types of information they want. They must learn how to operate different technologies by typing in queries, touching screens, moving a mouse, and opening a Web browser. There are also the conventions of Web pages—scrolling and using radio buttons, hyperlinks, and search boxes—that require users to move around a space and make multiple decisions, including where to focus their attention, the relevance of the information that appears, and the relationships among the information on a screen (Baur, 2005, p. 144).

Before they can concern themselves with the content of Web-based health care materials, patients must be able to access that material. Baur (2005) cites research supporting the idea that, for many patients, what is needed is practice with the technology used to access the materials. This includes more than just practice with the mechanical steps necessary to navigate the Internet: patients need practice with the necessary cognitive steps as well. The Internet invites patients to seek out information on their conditions and treatment options, on disease prevention, and on healthy lifestyles. It holds the promise of a multitude of informative materials. These materials are indeed available, but finding them can prove more challenging than patients expect.

Studies indicate that patients seeking health-related information on the Internet typically do not employ sophisticated search strategies. A common approach is to type one or two words into the Search box of an Internet search engine. The problem with this strategy is that it can result in an overwhelmingly long list of results, often in the millions. There is no doubt that accurate information is buried somewhere in that list, but research shows that Internet searchers only look at an average of 10 results per search session (Jansen & Pooch, 2001). Another study showed that searchers tend to look only at the first page of results without realizing that many are paid placements (Marable, 2003). Add to this the fact that there are no generally accepted labels or standards to help Internet users identify quality information, and you end up with patients coming up short when they search for useful and accurate information online.

Even when the top search results are reliable sources, patients seeking to access health information on the Internet may have to work through multiple layers and links to find information related to their original questions. Navigating through page after page of electronic text can be confusing for anyone, and the challenge that such nonlinear organization of materials presents is amplified when the searchers have limited literacy skills.

After problems of access and technical competence are addressed, low-health-literate patients still face enormous challenges in using Web-based health care materials. Despite the possibilities that the medium offers to those who wish to access health-related information, the preferred means of presenting information via the Internet remains text based. Whether it is the associated development cost or the limitations of technology that keeps information providers from producing nontext messages for the Internet, the result of this continued reliance on text is the same: the needs of low-literate patients are not met.

By definition, low-literate patients find that their reading challenges affect their ability to obtain useful health care information from the Internet when it is presented in text form. It doesn't matter whether the information is printed on paper or posted on the Internet; patients are equally derailed in their efforts to understand the information if it is presented in unfamiliar language or in an intimidating, text-heavy format.

To aid in patients' understanding, text materials presented via Web-based technologies should follow the same guidelines for readability and appeal that govern the creation of printed materials—several of which are explained in chapter 8, Principles of Writing for Low Literacy. But today, much of the material on the Internet tends to be merely electronic versions of the printed brochures, books, and flyers available in your local waiting room. In other words, the literacy challenges inherent in print materials have not been dealt with adequately simply by placing them on the Internet. They've just been transferred to another medium.

More than one study has been conducted to evaluate the readability of health care information on the Internet, and the results are overwhelmingly disappointing. An evaluation of Web-based osteoporosis educational materials, for example, revealed that most of the materials obtained in the first 30 Web sites listed after entering the term *osteoporosis* into the search fields of the Google, Yahoo, and Microsoft Network (MSN) search engines were written above the reading level of most adults (Wallace et al., 2005).

In fact, most Internet health education materials are written at a 10th-grade level or higher (Birru et al., 2004). Every one of the English-language health sites examined in a 2001 study (and 86% of the Spanish sites) required at least a high-school reading proficiency level (Berland et al., 2001; Fogel, 2003). Another study found that only 10 of 1,000 Web sites studied contained writing and content that were accessible to low-literate adults in the United States (Lazarus & Mora, 2000).

EVALUATING PATIENT LEARNING AND OUTCOMES

Once you have developed new materials and introduced them to your patient population, you must determine whether they are working properly. The first step is to define your objectives for patient learning. This is actually an activity that was begun during the development of your materials, back when you endeavored to make them action-based and focused on behaviors. For purposes of evaluating the materials, you should define those objectives clearly. Decide exactly what your patients should learn by listening to your audiotapes, watching your video, or otherwise using the materials you've created.

It is critical, though, that the objectives be measurable. That is, you should be able to measure some patient behavior to determine how well your materials achieve the objectives you've identified. How will you measure the success of your materials? Will you ask patients to fill out a questionnaire? Will you track adherence to a treatment plan? Whatever the approach, you should be able to compare postintervention data with preintervention data. In other words, you must be able to apply your measurement tool to your patient population (or a representative sample) before and after the participants make use of your newly created materials.

Finally, you will want to draw some conclusion from the data you collect. Do you see the kinds of results you expected when you designed the new materials? If not, why not? In some cases, an examination of the materials will yield information that could make your materials more effective. There are numerous tools and suggestions available from experts in nonhealth care industries that can be useful for evaluating the patient materials you have created and for making decisions regarding them.

For example, Jakob Nielsen, PhD, a well-known business consultant and expert on increasing the usability of company Web sites, has written numerous books, articles, and interviews that may be useful when assessing your own health care Web site, even though his writing is focused primarily on business Web sites. As we discussed in chapter 8, the marketing of health care and of nonhealth care materials has much in common.

A variety of nontext media are available that health care providers can use to meet the needs of their diverse patient populations. And every day, it seems, new technologies emerge. These developments place the locus of responsibility for accurate and effective patient communication on health care providers themselves. But that responsibility needn't be a burden. With a logical approach to the design and production of health-related materials, health care professionals have better opportunities than ever to reach all segments of their patient populations and to effect positive change in their patients' clinical outcomes.

REFERENCES

AMC Cancer Research Center. (1994). *Beyond the brochure: Alternative approaches to effective health communication.* Denver, CO: Author. Retrieved January 29, 2006, from http://www.cdc.gov/cancer/nbccedp/bccpdfs/amcbeyon.pdf

Badger, T., Segrin, C., Meek, P., Lopez, A. M., & Bonham, E. (2004). A case study of telephone interpersonal counseling for women with breast cancer and their partners. *Oncology Nursing Forum, 31*(5), 997–1003.

Baur, C. E. (2005). Using the Internet to move beyond the brochure and improve health literacy. In J. G. Schwartzberg, J. B. VanGeest, & C. C. Wang (Eds.), *Understanding health literacy: Implications for medicine and public health* (pp. 141–154). Chicago: American Medical Association Press.

Berland, G. K., Elliott, M. N., Morales, L. S., Algazy, J. I., Kravitz, R. L., Broder, M. S., et al. (2001). Health information on the Internet: Accessibility, quality, and readability in English and Spanish. *Journal of the American Medical Association, 285*(20), 2612–2621.

Bichakjian, C. K., Schwartz, J. L., Wang, T. S., Hall, J. M., Johnson, T. M., & Biermann, J. S. (2005). Melanoma information on the Internet: Often incomplete—a public health opportunity? *Journal of Clinical Oncology, 20*(1), 134–141.

Birru, M. S., Monaco, V. M., Charles, L., Drew, H., Njie, V., Bierria, T., et al. (2004). Internet usage by low-literacy adults seeking health information: An observational analysis. *Journal of Medical Internet Research, 6*(3), e25. Retrieved January 3, 2006, from http://www.jmir.org/2004/3/e25

Doak, C. C., Doak, L. G., Friedell, G. H., & Meade, C. D. (1998). Improving comprehension for cancer patients with low literacy skills: Strategies for clinicians. *CA—A Cancer Journal for Clinicians, 48*, 151–162.

Doak, L. G., Doak, C. C., & Root, J. H. (1996). *Teaching patients with low literacy skills* (2nd ed.). Philadelphia: J.B. Lippincott.

Dollahite, J., Thompson, C., & McNew, R. (1996). Readability of printed sources of diet and health information. *Patient Education and Counseling, 27*, 123–134.

Dowse, R., & Ehlers, M. (2005). Medicine labels incorporating pictograms: Do they influence understanding and adherence? *Patient Education and Counseling, 58*(1), 63–70.

Evrard, S., Mathoulin-Pelissier, S., Larrue, C., Lapouge, P., Bussieres, E., & Tunon De Lara, C. (2005). Evaluation of a preoperative multimedia information program in surgical oncology. *European Journal of Surgical Oncology, 31*(1), 106–110.

Fogel, J. (2003). Internet use for cancer information among racial/ethnic populations and low literacy groups. *Cancer Control, 10*(5), S45–S51.

Fox, S. (2005, October 5). *Digital divisions: There are clear differences among those with broadband connections, dial-up connections, and no connections at all to the Internet.* Washington, DC: Pew Internet & American Life Project. Retrieved January 3, 2006, from http://www.pewinternet.org/pdfs/PIP_Digital_Divisions_Oct_5_2005.pdf

Hardyman, R., Hardy, P., Brodie, J., & Stephens, R. (2005). It's good to talk: Comparison of a telephone helpline and website for cancer information. *Patient Education and Counseling, 57*(3), 315–320.

Healthy Families Medi-Cal for Children. (2000, December). *Information.* Retrieved January 29, 2006, from http://www.healthyfamilies.ca.gov

Hearth-Holmes, M., Murphy, P. W., Davis, T. C., Nandy, I., Elder, C. G., Broadwell, L. H., et al. (1997). Literacy in patients with chronic disease: Systematic lupus erythematosus and the reading level of patient education materials. *Journal of Rheumatology, 24*(12), 2335–2339.

Helmes, A. W., Culver, J. O., & Bowen, D. J. (2006). Results of a randomized study of telephone versus in-person breast cancer risk counseling. *Patient Education and Counseling, 64*(1–3), 96–103. [Epub 2006, Jan 19.]

Houts, P. S., Bachrach, R., Witmer, J. T., Tringali, C. A., Bucher, J. A., & Localio, R. A. (1998). Using pictographs to enhance recall of spoken medical instructions. *Patient Education and Counseling, 35*, 83–88.

Houts, P. S., Witmer, J. T., Egeth, H. E., Loscalzo, M. J., & Zabora, J. R. (2001). Using pictographs to enhance recall of spoken medical instructions. *Patient Education and Counseling, 43*, 231–242.

Institute of Medicine (IOM) of the National Academies. (2004). *Health literacy: A prescription to end confusion.* Washington, DC: National Academies Press.

Jansen, B. J., & Pooch, U. (2001). A review of Web searching studies and a framework for future research. *Journal of the American Society for Information Science Technology, 52*(3), 235–246. Retrieved January 17, 2006, from http://jimjansen.tripod.com/academic/pubs/wus.pdf

Jean Wiese, H., Boethel, C., Phillips, B., Wilson, J. F., Peters, J., & Viggiano, T. (2005). CPAP compliance: Video education may help! *Sleep Medicine, 6*(2), 171–174.

Kelly, N. R., Huffman, L. C., Mendoza, F. S., & Robinson, T. N. (2003). Effects of a videotape to increase use of poison control centers by low-income and Spanish-speaking families: A randomized, controlled trial. *Pediatrics, 111*(1), 21–26.

Knapp, P., Raynor, D. K., Jebar, A. H., & Price, S. J. (2005). Interpretation of medication pictograms by adults in the UK. *Annals of Pharmacotherapy, 39*(7–8), 1227–1233.

Lazarus, W., & Mora, F. (2000). *Online content for low-income and underserved Americans: The digital divide's new frontier: A strategic audit of activities and opportunities.* Retrieved February 10, 2006, from http://wwww.childrenspartnership.org

Leiner, M., Handal, G., & Williams, D. (2004). Patient communication: A multidisciplinary approach using animated cartoons. *Health Education Research, 19*(5), 591–595.

Mansoor, L. E., & Dowse, R. (2003). Effect of pictograms on readability of patient information materials. *Annals of Pharmacotherapy, 37*, 1003–1009.

Marable, L. (2003). False oracles: Consumer reaction to learning the truth about how search engines work. *Consumer Web Watch.* Retrieved January 23, 2006, from http://64.78.25.46/dynamic/search-report-false-oracles.cfm#tips

Marin, G., & Marin, B. V. (1990). Perceived credibility of channels and sources of AIDS information among Hispanics. *AIDS Education and Prevention, 2*(2), 154–161.

May, S., West, R., Hajek, P., Nilsson, F., Foulds, J., & Meadow, A. (2003). The use of videos to inform smokers about different nicotine replacement products. *Patient Education and Counseling, 51*(2), 143–147.

McBride, C. M., & Rimer, B. K. (1999). Using the telephone to improve health behavior and health service delivery. *Patient Education and Counseling, 37*(1), 3–18.

Meade, C. D. (1996). Producing videotapes for cancer education: Methods and examples. *Oncology Nursing Forum, 23*(5), 837–846.

Oakley, A. M., Duffill, M. B., & Reeve, P. (1998). Practising dermatology via telemedicine. *New Zealand Medical Journal, 111*(1071), 296–299.

Ong, W. J. (1982). *Orality and literacy: The technologizing of the word.* New York: Methuen.

Oslin, D. W., Ross, J., Sayers, S., Murphy, J., Kane, V., & Katz, I. R. (2006). Screening, assessment, and management of depression in VA primary care clinics. The Behavioral Health Laboratory. *Journal of General Internal Medicine, 21*(1), 46–50.

Public Broadcasting Service (PBS). (2006). *What is a foto-novella?* Retrieved January 29, 2006, from http://www.pbs.org/independentlens/fotonovelas2/what.html

Roddey, T. S., Olson, S. L., Gartsman, G. M., Hanten, W. P., & Cook, K. F. (2002). A randomized controlled trial comparing 2 instructional approaches to home exercise instruction following arthroscopic full-thickness rotator cuff repair surgery. *Journal of Orthopaedics and Sports Physical Therapy, 32*(11), 548–559.

Rogers, S. M., Willis, G., Al-Tayyib, A., Villarroel, M. A., Turner, C. F., Ganapathi, L., et al. (2005). Audio computer assisted interviewing to measure HIV risk behaviours in a clinic population. *Sexually Transmitted Infections, 81*(6), 501–507.

Rudd, R. E. (2005). *How to create and assess print materials.* Retrieved March 11, 2006, from the Harvard School of Public Health, Health Literacy Web site: http://www.hsph.harvard.edu/healthliteracy/materials.html

Rudd, R., & DeJong, W. (2006). *In plain language video.* Retrieved February 8, 2006, from the Harvard School of Public Health, Health Literacy Studies Web site: http://www.hsph.harvard.edu/healthliteracy/overview.html#Two

Rural Women's Health Project. (n.d.) *Novelas.* Retrieved January 20, 2006, from http://www.rwhp.org/novelas.html

Sanner, B. M. (2003, August). Are your written materials missing the mark? *Journal of Active Aging,* 18–24.

Savenstedt, S., Zingmark, K., & Sandman, P. O. (2003). Video-phone communication with cognitively impaired elderly patients. *Journal of Telemedicine and Telecare, 9*(suppl 2), S52–S54.

Smith, C. E., Koehler, J., Moore, J. M., Blanchard, E., & Ellerbeck, E. (2005). Testing videotape education for heart failure. *Clinical Nursing Research, 14*(2), 191–205.

Snyder-Ramos, S. A., Seintsch, H., Bottiger, B. W., Motsch, J., Martin, E., & Bauer, M. (2005). Patient satisfaction and information gain after the preanesthetic visit: A comparison of face-to-face interview, brochure, and video. *Anesthesia and Analgesia, 100*(6), 1753–1758.

So, K., Umraw, N., Scott, J., Campbell, K., Musgrave, M., & Cartotto, R. (2003). Effects of enhanced patient education on compliance with silicone gel sheeting and burn scar outcome: A randomized prospective study. *Journal of Burn Care and Rehabilitation, 24*(6), 411–417.

Stanton, A. L., Ganz, P. A., Kwan, L., Meyerowitz, B. E., Bower, J. E., Krupnick, J. L., et al. (2005). Outcomes from the Moving Beyond Cancer psychoeducational, randomized, controlled trial with breast cancer patients. *Journal of Clinical Oncology, 23*(25), 6009–6018.

Steinke, E. E. (2002). A videotape intervention for sexual counseling after myocardial infarction. *Heart and Lung, 31*(5), 348–354.

Tucker, J. B., Barone, J. E., Stewart, J., Hogan, R. J., Sarnelle, J. A., & Blackwood, M. M. (1999). Violence prevention: Reaching adolescents with the message. *Pediatric Emergency Care, 15*(6), 436–439.

Uccellani, V., & Rosales, M. C. (1992). Training videos: The next best thing to being there? *Development Communication Report, 77,* 12–13.

U.S. Pharmacopeia (USP). (2006). *USP pictograms.* Retrieved January 22, 2006, from http://www.usp.org/audiences/consumers/pictograms/form.html

Wallace, L. S., Turner, L. W., Ballard, J. E., Keenum, A. J., & Weiss, B. D. (2005). Evaluation of web-based osteoporosis educational materials. *Journal of Women's Health (Larchmont), 14*(10), 936–945.

Wilson, F. L. (2000, February). Are patient information materials too difficult to read? *Home Healthcare Nurse, 18*(2), 107–115.

Wylie, K., Allen, P., & Hallam-Jones, R. (2005). An evaluation of a telephone follow-up clinic in urology. *Journal of Sexual Medicine, 2*(5), 641–644.

Wynd, C. (2005). Guided health imagery for smoking cessation and long-term abstinence. *Journal of Nursing Scholarship, 37*(3), 245–250.

Zarcadoolas, C., Blanco, M., Boyer, J. F., & Pleasant, A. (2002). Unweaving the Web: An exploratory study of low-literate adults' navigation skills on the World Wide Web. *Journal of Health Communication, 7*(4), 309–324.

INTERPRETERS AND THEIR ROLE IN THE HEALTH CARE SETTING

It's probably happened to you before, but not necessarily in a hospital or in a doctor's office. You speak to a stranger when you're out for a walk or running errands. Maybe you've just asked for directions or simply commented on the weather. For a brief moment the stranger stares at you, unwilling or unable to respond. You look into his or her eyes, and there you see no trace of recognition, no hint that your words have been understood. Perhaps you pause for a second or two, unsure how to proceed. You repeat yourself and then attempt to pantomime like you're playing charades, hoping you might communicate your message clearly with some hastily chosen gestures and facial expressions.

But it doesn't work. Finally you just nod and smile or perhaps say something like, "Oh, I see. You don't speak English." This much is certain: unless an interpreter is standing by at the ready or unless you can miraculously learn a handful of useful phrases in this other person's language, a mutually enlightening exchange is not likely to occur.

Such moments occasionally border on the comic, demonstrating how desperately we need culturally competent, mutually understandable, expert interpreting services when we encounter those who don't speak our language. Consider a scene from the film *Lost in Translation* (2003), in which Bill Murray plays Bob Harris, an aging American movie star visiting Tokyo to shoot a commercial for Suntory whiskey. Although Harris does not relish the job, he has been paid a considerable sum to be there, as his agent reminds him during a brief cell phone conversation. So he relents: dressed in a stiff-looking tuxedo and seated in a leather chair on an austere set beneath studio lights, the jet-lagged actor patiently awaits his instructions.

A stylish young Japanese director approaches, intense and serious, pacing back and forth as he rants to Harris entirely in Japanese for what seems like a long time. Ms. Kawasaki, Harris's exceedingly polite interpreter, crouches down next to him and translates into English.

"He want you to turn . . . look in camera. Okay?"

"That's all he said?" Harris asks, befuddled.

"Yes," she responds. "Turn to camera."

Amused at this, Harris asks whether the director wants him to turn from the right or from the left. Ms. Kawasaki, behaving deferentially toward the young director, appears to ask him Harris's question, but uses considerably more Japanese than Harris had used English. The director responds again, pointing to his watch and speaking directly to Harris for several moments more. The word *camera* in English is fairly clear; the rest is Japanese, spoken in short, energetic bursts. Although Harris cannot decipher the director's message and feels certain the translation he's receiving is not verbatim, the emotion behind the words is obvious.

"Right side . . . and, uh, with intensity," the interpreter explains, hesitating for a moment.

"Is that everything?" Harris asks again. "I mean, it seemed like he said quite a bit more than that."

The director, exasperated, now uses even more Japanese. Only the English word *whiskey* is recognizable. Harris looks beseechingly toward his interpreter as the director seems to berate him.

"Like an old friend," Ms. Kawasaki calmly explains, "and into the camera."

As the director smiles and jabbers at Harris again, using a few English words and phrases, such as *whiskey, it's Suntory time,* and *okay,* it dawns on Harris that he may just have to wing it.

* * *

For most of us working in health care, winging it is not an option; there's simply too much on the line if we can't understand what our patients are telling us. In fact, health care providers who serve a multicultural patient population probably find Harris's predicament eerily familiar—and not because the scene is funny (though it *is* that).

Imagine, for example, a first-time meeting between an English-speaking provider and a patient who knows no English. The provider asks the patient a few health-related questions through an interpreter. The interpreter turns to the patient, and the two get into a lengthy discussion in their native tongue as the provider waits, basically left out. Finally the interpreter turns and says, "She said no." When the provider asks the interpreter to elaborate, the interpreter just smiles and says, "Oh, it doesn't matter. She means no."

Like Bob Harris in the scene above, the provider who hears this may be dumbfounded by such a response. What more did the patient say that the provider needs to know? Was it small talk? Has the interpreter excised information, determining that some of what the patient said simply wasn't important enough to translate? And who decides what's important enough to translate?

HEALTH CARE IN MULTICULTURAL AMERICA

Answers to such questions matter more all the time. As we saw in chapter 5, Factoring Culture Into the Care Process, the United States is becoming increasingly diverse, both culturally and linguistically. More than 31 million foreign-born people live in the United States, and 18% of those report speaking a language other than English at home (Herndon & Joyce, 2004). Roughly 46 million Americans do not speak English as their primary language. Though more than 215 million Americans do speak English, the number of Spanish speakers is a staggering 28 million. Around 78% of Latinos in the United States speak a language other than English. In California alone, 224 different languages are spoken, but some experts estimate that Spanish-speaking Latinos will ultimately provide 60% of new growth in the state's population between 1990 and 2010 (California Healthcare Interpreters Association, 2002, p. 16).

After Spanish comes Chinese, with more than 2 million speakers in the United States, followed by French (1.6 million) and German (1.3 million). Tagalog has 1.2 million speakers, Vietnamese and Italian have roughly 1 million each, and Korean and Russian round out the top 10 U.S. languages with roughly 900,000 and 700,000 speakers, respectively (Shin & Bruno, 2003).

The bottom line is that clinicians must serve a significant number of non-English-speaking patients. In addition, bear in mind that some who claim to speak English well actually have trouble with the language. According to the 2000 U.S. Census, 21 million Americans consider their ability to speak English as "less than very well" (Shin & Bruno, 2003; U.S. Census Bureau, 2000). A study by the U.S. Agency for Health Care Research and Quality put the number of Americans with little or no understanding of English at 10 million (Shedden, 2006).

How do these statistics affect patient care? Beginning with the obvious, they affect communication in the patient–provider clinical encounter. We know that miscommunication is common between people who speak the same language, so interactions between those who speak different languages are likely compromised that much more. And because providers cannot reasonably be expected to speak every language their patients do, use of trained translators and interpreters is vital and necessary for achieving good patient outcomes.

Transparency: An Essential Ingredient

Studies show that language barriers in the health care setting contribute to health disparities, negatively affecting patients' access, satisfaction, and quality of care (Mullins, Blatt, Gbarayor, Yang, & Baquet, 2005). In some cases these barriers result in increased expenditures by patients, as when patients treated inadequately must return for a second or third visit to receive additional care (Shedden, 2006). Clinicians in various settings, from hospitals to community health centers to private practices, often duplicate their efforts when they cannot communicate effectively in their patients' primary language, wasting time and money and putting their patients' health at risk.

Lacking in exchanges like the one between Bob Harris and the Japanese director in *Lost in Translation* and between the provider and the patient whose interpreter offered only "she means no" is *transparency,* the principle that everything said by any party in an interpreted conversation "should be rendered in the other language, so that everything said can be heard and understood by everyone present" (Bancroft, 2005, p. 36). In fact, any time an interpreter enters into the conversation by talking directly to either party in either language, he or she is obligated to interpret both his or her speech and that of the party spoken to. Failure to do so is not only discourteous but also arguably compromises the clarity and integrity of the exchange.

Lack of transparency does not go unnoticed by non-English-speaking patients. In a study examining factors that contribute to quality of care among Chinese and Vietnamese American patients, for example, complaints about the quality of interpreter services were common. One Chinese patient with diabetes remarked rather tellingly, "The doctor speaks so much, but the translator says only a few words" (Ngo-Metzger et al., 2003, p. 48). In clinical interactions that require the services of an interpreter, good patient–provider communication relies on the mutual trust transparency helps create.

LOW HEALTH LITERACY AND THE NEED FOR INTERPRETERS

Not surprisingly, patients with low health literacy are disproportionately affected by language barriers. Most clinicians seem to understand this, even if they do not conceive of their patients' problems strictly in terms of literacy. In a study by Hatton and Webb (1993), nurses identified patients' characteristics they considered relevant to interactions that involved interpretation. These included acculturation, education, age, and complexity of health-related problems.

All of these factors are correlated with low health literacy, as we've seen. In fact, in this context the word *acculturation* is probably equivalent to *low health literate.* Nurses in the study described patients as not having familiarity with clinical topics discussed, noting that there were some who "[didn't] understand the calendar" and others who had trouble making and keeping appointments (Hatton & Webb, 1993, p. 144).

Patients with low health literacy face similar obstacles in their pursuit of quality health care. Even if limited English proficiency (LEP) is not precisely equivalent to limited health literacy (e.g., many LEP patients are proficient in their own language, have some medical training, and are familiar with clinical terms and concepts), many barriers faced by LEP patients are remarkably similar to those faced by low-health-literate patients. And therein lies the critical importance of effective interpretation and translation in the health care field.

"In no other time in history," writes David Galbis-Reig, MD, "has the art of providing culturally competent translation and interpretation services been more important than at the current time. In no other field (except perhaps in international politics) do translators and interpreters play such a crucial role as they do within the health care profession" (Galbis-Reig, 2000). Some research findings bear out Galbis-Reig's assertion. In one study performed by Bernstein and colleagues (2002), use of trained health care interpreters was associated with increased intensity of emergency department (ED) services, reduced return rate, increased clinic use, and lower 30-day charges, with no corresponding increase in length of ED stay or cost of visit.

DIFFERENCE BETWEEN INTERPRETING AND TRANSLATING

In what follows we distinguish between a *translator* and an *interpreter*. Though the two are similar, some differences are important to understand. In general, as the American Translators Association (ATA) states, "Translation is written, whereas interpretation is spoken" (Aparicio & Durbin, 2003). Both require a thorough understanding of the source language of the speaker or text, as well as the language into which the translator or interpreter transforms the original utterance or written material.

The following definitions, taken from the *Glossary of Interpreting Terminology* prepared by the National Council on Interpreting in Health Care (NCIHC), elaborate somewhat on the ATA's simple distinction, but note the similarities:

> **Interpreter:** A person who renders a message spoken in one language into a second language, and who abides by a code of professional ethics
>
> **Translator:** A person who translates written texts, especially one who does so professionally (Bancroft, 2005, pp. 35, 36).

According to the NCIHC, interpreting is the "process of understanding and analyzing a spoken or signed message and re-expressing that message faithfully, accurately and objectively in another language, taking the culture and social context into account." The purpose of interpreting is to "enable communication between two or more individuals who do not speak each other's languages" (Bancroft, 2005, p. 36).

It would be wrong, however, to suggest that interpreters abide by a code of ethics, whereas translators do not. The ATA has a Code of Professional Conduct and Business Practices (2006) that can be viewed at http://www.atanet.org// membership/code_of_professional_conduct.php. The code contains language targeted at translators themselves, as well as some language targeted at businesses that employ translators.

The primary goals of health care interpreting and translating are similar, of course. Both activities are concerned with communicating a message from one language to another so that each party—the provider and the patient—can understand one another better. But the term *translator* has broader connotations than does the term *interpreter*. A translator is any person "who expresses or renders the meaning of a text and/or verbal material from the source language into a language different from that of the source language" (Galbis-Reig, 2000). What distinguishes an interpreter from a translator, then, is not so much the difference between oral and written messages, but whether the act of translation takes place in "real" time, as Galbis-Reig notes:

> An interpreter is a translator who accomplishes the same goal [that is, of expressing or rendering the meaning of a text and/or verbal material from the source language into a different language] in "real" time either through verbal or written means (e.g., a person translating for a live speaker or an individual transcribing for a live speaker into a different target language at a conference or seminar).

In this chapter, our focus is on health care interpreters as opposed to translators. (For a discussion of translation as it relates to the needs of low-literate patients, see chapter 8, Principles of Writing for Low Literacy.) And because quality interpreting is so critically important for low-literate and LEP patients, in this chapter we take a broad view of interpreting as a field, considering the contexts in which it takes place, ideas about the proper role of the interpreter in the clinical encounter, and some of the most effective interpretive methods and technologies for patients who speak little or no English.

INTERPRETING IN NONCLINICAL CONTEXTS

Interpreters make valuable contributions in many fields other than medicine, and different kinds of interpreting are used in different circumstances for different reasons. Simultaneous interpretation is the method used at the United Nations, for example, where interpreters translate while a speaker is talking (Hwa-Froelich & Westby, 2003). Accurate interpretation requires care and patience; even with simultaneous interpreting there can be a short delay to give the interpreter time to catch up.

A famous example of this delay occurred in the tense exchange between U.S. Ambassador Adlai Stevenson and Soviet Ambassador Valerian Zorin during the Cuban Missile Crisis. On October 25, 1962, at an emergency session of the UN Security Council, Stevenson tried to force an answer from Zorin as to the existence of Soviet nuclear weapons in Cuba, demanding, "Don't wait for the translation! Yes or no?" When Zorin didn't answer, Stevenson produced photos taken by U.S. surveillance clearly showing the missile installations *(Foreign Relations of the Unites States,* 1996). One hopes that the stakes in the average interpreting exchange, high as they are, are not so grim.

In contrast to simultaneous interpretation there is consecutive interpretation, during which speakers pause to allow the interpreter or signer to convert their message into the other language. This kind of interpreting is common in all contexts.

Although professional interpreters were once employed primarily for diplomatic interpretation and translation (as in the example above), in international justice efforts, and at international conferences, increasingly they are used in medical, educational, and community settings, often in collaboration with speech-language pathologists (Hwa-Froelich & Westby, 2003).

INTERPRETING IN CLINICAL CONTEXTS

Health care interpreting is a distinct and specialized area of practice, as the NCIHC notes in its *National Standards of Practice for Interpreters in Health Care* (2005). Under Title VI of the Civil Rights Act of 1964 and Executive Order 13166, issued in August 2000 by President Clinton, patients with LEP have the right to a trained interpreter (Herndon & Joyce, 2004). Studies have shown that LEP patients are less likely to have a regular source of primary care and less likely to receive preventive care. They also are less satisfied with care they do receive and more likely to report overall problems with care (Green et al., 2005).

What's more, LEP and low health-literate patients are at increased risk for medical errors (Jacobs, Shepard, Suaya, & Stone, 2004). One way to avoid mistakes is to avoid making assumptions about patients' educational levels (Bernadett, 2005; Roat, 2005). It is incumbent on health care providers to understand their patients' needs and to seek help accordingly. Recognizing the need for an interpreter is important. Failure to use interpreters for LEP patients has been shown to lead to higher hospital admission rates, increased use of testing, poorer patient comprehension of diagnosis and treatment, and misdiagnosis and improper treatment (Herndon & Joyce, 2004).

Health care interpreters range from professionals employed by hospitals and other institutions to ad hoc, untrained individuals, such as family members (including children), the patient's friends, and nonclinical hospital employees—even strangers from the waiting room (Flores et al., 2003). As Phelan and Parkman (1995) note, the best option for most patients is a fluently bilingual health care worker; that is, a clinician who is fluent in both English and the patient's language. A certified interpreter who is trained in cross-cultural communication and is an experienced clinician would be ideal, of course, but individuals with such broad-based training are rare.

Often nonclinical bilingual assistants lack the appropriate training in cross-cultural communication, making the use of such ad hoc interpreters risky. As the following passage makes clear, the California Healthcare Interpreters Association (CHIA) strongly opposes the use of untrained bilingual interpreters:

> Fundamental ethical aspects of healthcare between providers and patients are compromised when people who have not received healthcare interpreter training are asked to interpret. These include . . . the loss of confidentiality, potential misdiagnosis, and potential invalid informed consent. . . . There is a misconception that bilingual individuals without training can provide adequate interpreting. Unfortunately, the parties most affected by the interpreting lack the skills to judge its quality. They assume the person providing the interpreting is doing an adequate job. This may create a misplaced sense of security that effective communication is taking place (CHIA, 2002, p. 9).

Others agree that using ad hoc interpreters can have negative clinical consequences (Flores et al., 2003; Marcos, 1979; Vasquez & Javier, 1991).

In some contexts, however, such as in smaller practices that cannot afford to hire full-time professional interpreters or in crowded EDs where the rushed pace of care may prevent interpreting in the context of brief clinical encounters, ad hoc interpreting is likely to continue. One medical center in Southern California simply asks prospective employees during their interview about their foreign-language skills, regardless of what position they are ultimately hired to fill—from surgeons to receptionists to nurses to janitors. Other medical centers doubtless have similar practices. Those interviewees who report having foreign-language skills, if hired, are usually expected to serve as ad hoc interpreters during their regular shifts (S. Knight, personal communication, November 2005).

Efforts to certify health care interpreters and to further professionalize the field should be applauded. Nevertheless, the practice of using ad hoc interpreters will likely continue for the foreseeable future. As Sevilla Mátir and Willis (2004) note, bilingual staff members can serve as effective interpreters, but only if they have been specifically trained to fill such a role. In this spirit, Sevilla Mátir and Willis offer the following eight rules that bilingual staff members with no formal training should follow when interpreting for patients:

1. Use the universal form of the language whenever possible.
2. Refrain from assuming the role of interviewer or decision maker.
3. Let the patient lead the discussion.
4. Translate everything.
5. Be aware of culturally significant issues that affect patient care, and translate in a way that conveys the cultural framework.
6. Meet the patient prior to the medical encounter.
7. Develop interpreter-physician work plans for each patient.
8. Seek continuing education.

Knowing how to speak another language does not make someone an interpreter. The work of interpreting is complex, as Hatton (1992) learned during 8 months of participant observation and engaging in conversations of varying length with interpreters, patients, health care providers, and ancillary staff in various community health settings. The interpreters she observed were not conduits who took one language and simply turned it into another; instead they performed "information processing," a multifaceted activity.

"The work of the translators in these bilingual, bicultural settings was, indeed, interpretation (i.e., a very complex clarification and explanation of ideas from one language to another and from one individual to another)," Hatton explains.

> This process involved judgment and decision about the circumstances under which [translators] sent information back and forth.... The translators were ... interpreters who had the power to vary the quantity as well as the quality of the information sent between client and provider and vice versa (Hatton, 1992, p. 55).

Later in this chapter we discuss other challenges and benefits to using untrained interpreters. For now, let's turn to the question of the interpreter's role in the health care arena.

ROLES INTERPRETERS PLAY: SOME CONCEPTUAL MODELS

There is no consensus about the precise role an interpreter should play in the clinical environment, though the basic function of an oral language interpreter is not in dispute. His or her goal should be to provide "a linguistic conversion of a message spoken in one language into another" (Beltrán Avery, 2001, pp. 2–3).

Despite this basic agreement, however, there remains what Maria-Paz Beltrán Avery, PhD, calls "creative tension" among professionals about such issues as the scope of the interpreter's role, the extent of patient advocacy he or she can appropriately engage in, the extent of the interpreter–patient relationship, and even the nature of interpretation itself (Beltrán Avery, 2001). Should an interpreter be seen as a genuine member of the health care team, for example, or as a tool to aid the provider in carrying out his or her function? This much is certain: the patient's health and well-being should be a mutual first priority for all parties involved.

The field of health care interpreting is always evolving, so perceptions about interpreter roles tend to be in flux. In *The Role of the Health Care Interpreter: An Evolving Dialogue* (2001), Beltrán Avery describes the "early dichotomy" that once existed between neutral, uninvolved, *passive* interpreting (i.e., message passing) and *active* interpreting, in which there is recognition of an interpreter's obligation to help both parties—patients and providers—explore and negotiate whatever impediments to understanding arise. Although these polar extremes continue to "tug at each other," says Beltrán Avery, the dichotomy has given way to a range or continuum, with the notion of the "neutral interpreter" softening into that of the "interpreter as conduit." She cites four perspectives that she says "continue to inform practice in the field [of interpreting] today." These four perspectives are summarized below:

1. The interpreter as conduit, which is a step up from pure neutrality because it recognizes that accurate message transmission must be based on equivalencies of concepts. Serving as a conduit also requires knowledge of the cultural context and familiarity with the background of the patient and the medical culture.

2. The interpreter as manager of cross-cultural and cross-language encounter, in which he or she not only provides the appropriate linguistic conversion from one language to another but also actively assists to overcome barriers to communication embedded in cultural, class, religious, and other social differences.

3. The incremental intervention model, which recognizes the need for the interpreter to stay in the background supporting communication while allowing the interpreter a legitimate way to intervene if he or she perceives that a misunderstanding is taking place.

4. The interpreter as embedded in his or her cultural-linguistic community, which recognizes that the core function of the interpreter is to transmit messages from one language to another, but assumes that the person performing this function is there as a whole person embedded in the social fabric of his or her community. This social fabric cannot be separated from who the interpreter is, how the interpreter relates to the patient, what the nature of his or her relationship is to the provider and the institution of medicine, and what the historical and political context of that community is in the United States (Beltrán Avery, 2001, p. 6).

Passive and Active Interpreting

The ideal of the neutral interpreter who merely passes messages back and forth from one person to another has gradually given way, both on pragmatic and on moral grounds. Interpreters serving only as conduits may theoretically be neutral, but that kind of interpretation is not realistic in real-life clinical encounters.

Active interpreters, by contrast, can negotiate between cultures and establish ties of trust and respect (Hwa-Froelich & Westby, 2003). In fact, those who advocate the incremental intervention model described above see disengaged neutrality, even in the face of obviously ineffective communication, as "unacceptable," "morally and legally irresponsible," "detrimental to advancing the goal of the encounter," and "not serving anyone's interests" (Beltrán Avery, 2001, p. 9).

Most interpreters fall somewhere along a passive–active continuum. In other words, it's not so much an either-or choice between a passive or active interpreter as an "evolving dialogue" between advocates who emphasize either end of a single spectrum. Beltrán Avery explains,

> Both polarities are critical. The conduit perspective keeps the field grounded in the central function of the interpreter—the linguistic conversion that allows communication between a patient and provider who do not speak the same language. The embeddedness perspective challenges the profession to consider its place in a holistic view of the patient's well-being—a wholeness of heart, mind, and spirit. One without the other is incomplete (Beltrán Avery, 2001, p. 14).

The active mode is popular among small, closely knit communities and among those who interpret for communities in which "relational ties form the foundation of trust and credibility" (Beltrán Avery, 2001, p. 4). Trust and respect are extremely important for ensuring fair and accurate interpreting. Interpreters embedded within the community often are personally involved in the process, actively influencing its direction.

In their analysis of 50 semi-structured interviews, Edwards, Temple, and Alexander (2005) determined that the issue of trust in people's understandings and experiences of needing and using interpreters was a recurrent theme, regardless of the person's ethnic affiliation, gender, or age; what kinds of services he or she needed; and the type of interpreter used.

Other Models of Interpreting

Other models of interpreting are equally valid, of course. One cited by Hwa-Froelich and Westby (2003, p. 82) conceives of the interpreter's role as that of listener, speaker, gatekeeper, interviewer, social agent, or conversationalist. These researchers note that interpreters and employers of interpreters need extensive training so that the desired role for an interpreter is defined and he or she can choose to operate within it or negotiate a different role.

Whatever role or roles an interpreter assumes, what matters is that he or she "may define his or her role differently than the other involved persons" (Hwa-Froelich & Westby, 2003, p. 82). If a clinician sees an interpreter's role one way while the interpreter sees it another, problems and miscommunication—even destructive power struggles—can result. Again, communication is key.

Clinicians and interpreters should agree about the interpreter's role, engaging in a dialogue about their expectations well before the patient enters the picture.

CHIA has its own guidelines about interpreter roles and interventions designed specifically to address barriers to cross-cultural communication, such as language differences, language complexity, and differences in cultural norms (CHIA, 2002, p. 40). In *California Standards for Healthcare Interpreters: Ethical Principles, Protocols, and Guidance on Roles & Intervention* (2002), the authors describe the most frequent roles of the health care interpreter—in order of increasing complexity and controversy—as those of *message converter, message clarifier, cultural clarifier,* and *patient advocate.* Though each role is discussed at length in the CHIA document, here is a summary explaining what each role entails:

- *Message converter.* In this role, interpreters listen, observe body language, and convert the meaning of all messages from one language to another without unnecessary additions, deletions, or changes in meaning.
- *Message clarifier.* In this role, interpreters are alert for possible words or concepts that might lead to misunderstanding and identify and assist in clarifying possible sources of confusion for the patient, provider, or interpreter.
- *Cultural clarifier.* The cultural clarifier role goes beyond message clarification to include a range of actions that typically relate to an interpreter's ultimate purpose of facilitating communication between parties that do not share a common culture. Interpreters are alert to cultural words or concepts that might lead to misunderstanding and act to assist parties to clarify culturally specific ideas.
- *Patient advocate.* In this role, interpreters actively support change in the interest of patient health and well-being. Interpreters require a clear rationale for the need to advocate on behalf of patients.

Interpreters move in and out of each of these four roles, notes Bernadett (2005), as they work to overcome linguistic, register, cultural, and systematic barriers to patient–provider communication. *(Register* refers to the varieties of language a speaker or writer uses in a particular social context. An informal register, used with friends, might include slang or swearing; a formal register is preferable for speaking or writing that takes place in a professional or academic environment.)

The extent to which interpreters should act as patient advocates is a matter of some controversy. One risk is that the health care provider may resent the interpreter's efforts toward patient advocacy, thereby diminishing the quality of care or access for the patient. If an interpreter does choose to act as a patient advocate, some suggest that the advocacy should be limited in scope. The NCIHC's *National Standards for Practice for Interpreters in Health Care* (2005) includes both impartiality and advocacy as expected standards of practice.

On the one hand, interpreters should not allow personal judgments or cultural values to influence their objectivity, and they should disclose potential conflicts of interest, withdrawing from assignments if necessary. The example given by NCIHC is that interpreters should avoid interpreting for a family member or a close friend. Avoiding such situations is considered being impartial. On the other hand, interpreters are advised to "speak out to protect an individual from serious harm" and to "advocate on behalf of a party or group to correct mistreatment and abuse" (NCIHC, 2005, p. 10). That is considered acceptable advocacy.

Just short of outright patient advocacy—though clearly a form of "active" interpreting—is what Beltrán Avery, the Massachusetts Medical Interpreters Association (MMIA), and other professionals in the field have described as "the interpreter as manager of a cross-cultural/cross-language mediated clinical encounter." To imagine what this might look like, think of an

> Asian interpreter . . . [who uses] a more respectful approach when speaking to an older Asian man or a highly educated person but use[s] a more equal-power communication style with someone who is the same gender, age, and/or education level. [Such an] [interpreter] focus[es] on the communication between the involved parties, considering conversational flow and pace to benefit communication and understanding. It does not mean the interpreter becomes an advocate for either party. This role model works best when service providers have received training on working with an interpreter and see interpreters as part of their team (Hwa-Froelich & Westby, 2003, p. 81).

Such an approach is consistent with NCIHC standards of practice, according to which interpreters should strive to understand cultures associated with languages they interpret, including the biomedical culture (NCIHC, 2005, p. 7). Cultural awareness is related to the ethical principle that interpreters "strive to develop awareness of cultures encountered in the performance of interpreting duties."

The interpreter's role as a member of the health care team is one focus of a study by Hatton and Webb (1993). The authors conducted interviews with 22 registered nurses, 15 of whom were interpreters themselves. Sixty to 90% of patients in the study spoke a language other than English.

Data analysis revealed three types of interactions among nurses, interpreters, and patients: (1) the interpreter as voice box, (2) the interpreter as excluder, and (3) the interpreter as collaborator. Only three nurses advocated use of the voice box approach under all circumstances. Voice box is a passive approach in which the interpreter translates word for word what is said, but does not intervene in the discussion, much like the way in which translation is performed at the United Nations. In the excluder role, by contrast, the interpreter takes over, as in the earlier example in which the interpreter said to the provider, "She means no."

Well-trained interpreters ideally convert the meanings of messages from one language to another without unnecessary additions, deletions, or changes in meaning and without injecting their own opinions (Herndon & Joyce, 2004). The following excerpt, in contrast, offers an example of the excluder role in action. Even a well-meaning interpreter can let personal bias cloud his or her judgment. Although prejudices among family members may be a concern when clinicians allow family members to interpret, this British child psychiatrist warns,

It can also be important when [other] interpreters are used, as I found when interviewing a young widow from an Asian culture.

I first met the family when I saw both parents about their son's behavioural problems at primary school. The father was much older than his wife, and it was clear that he thought that his son was perfect and that the mother was supposed to serve the boy, whatever issue was involved.

When the father died of a sudden heart attack we heard reports of the mother's grief and of the boy's intense distress. Because the mother was supposed to speak little English (the father's good knowledge of English had meant that this was not a factor in earlier meetings), we organised the services of an interpreter for a meeting with her and her son.

After considerable discussion of the widow's feelings, and after we had asked the son to leave the room, I felt justified in verbalising my impression that the widow was experiencing not only pain but also relief at her husband's death. When I asked the interpreter to convey this to the mother he laughed and told me that my idea was plainly wrong. After some discussion he said something to the mother, but her facial expression suggested that she had not been told my views, and I had to argue this further with the interpreter. Finally, he said something to the widow that must have been closer to my interpretation, since she smiled, nodded vigorously, and said—in English—that perhaps it was wrong that she should harbour such feelings but that she certainly did so (Brafman, 1995, p. 1439).

Sometimes, however, "taking over" by the interpreter is essential, as a few of Hatton and Webb's interviewees made clear in their study, "especially when the interpreter and nurse [have] been unable to contact the [patient] because the family did not have a phone. . . . On these visits, the nurse and interpreter found themselves at the [patient's] front door negotiating entrée, and the interpreter relied on his or her own linguistic and interpersonal skills to enter the [patient's] home" (1993, p. 142).

A synthesis of the voice box and excluder roles results in the interpreter as collaborator, which is an especially effective approach that may occur more commonly when an interpreter has worked with a particular clinician or at a particular institution over an extended period of time. In the study by Hatton and Webb, a community health nurse described a case in which she had to teach a client how to use an apnea monitor. "The turn of a knob was critical. By collaborating, the [nurse] and interpreter acknowledged the situation's difficulties and managed them as a team" (1993, p. 144). Hatton and Webb also emphasize the importance of the interpreter "striking accord" with the patient to become a "cultural connector" between patient and provider (1993, p. 145).

CHOOSING THE RIGHT KIND OF INTERPRETER

Earlier we mentioned that bilingual clinicians could act as ideal health care interpreters, but this assumes they are truly fluent in the language and understand the patient's cultural and economic circumstances. Even the most gifted polyglot cannot be versed in every language encountered in the course of clinical practice;

the U.S. 2000 Census prepared language codes for 380 categories of single language or language families (Shin & Bruno, 2003).

Roat (2005, p. 10) describes the pros and cons of using bilingual physicians and bilingual staff and discusses four categories of "dedicated interpreters": staff interpreters, contracted interpreters, agency interpreters, and volunteer interpreters. "Dedicated interpreters," she writes, "are those whose only reason for being at your practice is to interpret" (2005, p. 11). Such interpreters can be contracted for in three ways (Roat, 2005, p. 12):

1. Agency interpreters are contracted by a language agency that usually provides on-site and telephonic interpreting for a fee. A good agency has highly qualified professional interpreters and provides recruiting, screening, contracting, and dispatching interpreters as part of its service. This option can be expensive, but it is a good idea to know which agencies are available in case of an emergency.

2. Contracted interpreters are independent business people who can be called directly when they are needed. Usually paid hourly, they tend to be highly experienced in the more common languages, but in the case of walk-in patients the clinician must wait for them to arrive.

3. Staff interpreters are employed by your practice just to do interpreting. Often these are the best and most experienced interpreters, though they do represent a significant financial investment. They are usually justified only if you have a high enough LEP population in the language or languages in which such interpreters are fluent to keep them busy all day, every day.

Among interpreters there are generalists and specialists. Many interpreters specialize with complementary language pairs, such as Spanish-to-English, or vice versa. Native speakers of a language often can decipher subtle nuances and have greater cultural competence than do generalists, who have either received formal training or whose experience, though it may be extensive, probably isn't focused within a specific area of specialization (Galbis-Reig, 2000).

INTERPRETING AND TECHNOLOGY

Now that we've considered the various roles that interpreters can play, as well as various types of interpreters, let's turn to the physical context in which interpreting takes place. Most often, patient–provider–interpreter encounters occur face-to-face in real time. The provider and the patient engage in a clinical dialogue with the help of an interpreter standing close by, usually off to one side so the provider can address his or her questions directly to the patient. But other scenarios are equally common, such as interpreting over a telephone line.

Telephonic Interpreting

Telephonic interpreting can be conducted using a speakerphone, but should never take place within earshot of other patients; using a private room away from busy waiting areas is preferable. Finding a private space may be difficult in public environments, such as the ED, but to maintain HIPAA (Health Insurance Portability and Accountability Act of 1996) compliance, providers should make every effort to safeguard their patients' privacy (Moskop, Marko, Larkin, Geiderman, & Derse, 2005). (For more about the effects of HIPAA on health care interpreters, see the section later in this chapter titled "HIPAA and the Patient's Privacy.") Telephonic interpreting is less likely to be used when there are delays in contacting an interpreter or when it is difficult to use a telephone at the patient's bedside (Kazzi & Cooper, 2003). However, as technology improves and cell phones become more widely available, such obstacles should gradually be overcome.

Because telephonic interpreting is costly, health care providers should use the time wisely. On-site interpreters usually charge by the hour, whereas telephonic interpreting is assessed on a per-minute basis. Providers should closely assess their needs to determine the most cost-effective approach. For example, if you must pay $40 per hour for an on-site interpreter and $2.50 per minute for a telephonic interpreter, you will save money if you use a telephonic service for calls lasting less than 16 minutes (Roat, 2005, p. 19). After 16 minutes, the hourly rate would be less expensive.

Telephonic interpreting compares favorably with ad hoc interpreting among Spanish-speaking patients. Lee, Batal, Maselli, and Kutner (2002) surveyed adult English-speaking and Spanish-speaking patients in an urban, university-affiliated walk-in clinic to examine the effect of interpreting method on their satisfaction with care. Spanish-speaking patients using a telephonic interpreting service were as satisfied with their care as those who saw language-concordant providers (that is, Spanish-speaking patients seen by Spanish-speaking providers), whereas patients using family or ad hoc interpreters were less satisfied. The researchers concluded that clinics serving large Spanish-speaking populations could enhance patients' satisfaction by avoiding the use of untrained and ad hoc interpreters, such as family members.

Many telephonic interpreting companies offer a wide variety of languages to choose from—some as many as 160. Yet the disadvantages of telephonic interpreting are similar to those mentioned in chapter 6, Improving Patient–Provider Communication, with respect to telephone medicine. Telephonic interpreters do not have a chance to consider nonverbal cues in the exchange (Herndon & Joyce, 2004). Social scientists tell us that more than 70% of a message can be read in the nonverbal language accompanying the spoken word, all of which is lost to a telephonic interpreter (Roat, 2005, p. 14).

As Cynthia E. Roat, MPH, recommends in her report, *Addressing Language Access Issues in Your Practice* (2005), use of face-to-face interpreters is preferable when patients have any degree of hearing loss, are from very traditional cultures that rarely use the telephone, are afraid or distraught, will be receiving bad news, or are visiting a provider for the first time. In addition, conversations involving more than two participants, visits involving teaching (especially when visual aids are used), psychiatry or mental health encounters, and sight translations should take place in person. However, telephonic interpreting is advisable in the following circumstances:

- for conversations that will be conducted over the phone anyway
- when the content to be discussed is relatively simple
- for determining what language a patient speaks
- when you need immediate access to an interpreter in emergencies
- when you cannot get or there will be an unacceptably long wait for a trained on-site interpreter
- when privacy and confidentiality are issues, especially if the patient's community is small and close-knit
- when health and hygiene are issues, such as the case in highly communicable diseases
- for quick questions to inpatients
- for doctors' rounds with inpatients (Roat, 2005, pp. 21–22)

Another option is the dual-handset telephone, which looks like a regular telephone but has two handsets attached to the base rather than one. Clinical staff can use one handset to dial an off-site language translation service while the non-English-speaking patient uses the other handset to hear the dialogue in translation. Unlike speakerphones, dual-handset phones can assure confidentiality in an open area or in an exam room with thin walls. According to Language Line Services (2005), additional advantages to using a dual-handset phone include better hygiene (the phones safeguard against spreading disease through a single handset), simplicity (because interpreter service numbers can be programmed into the phone), and speed (that is, there's no need to pass the phone back and forth between the provider and the patient). Other companies such as CyraCom also offer dual-handset telephone services; theirs is called the CyraPhone®(CyraCom, 2006).

One disadvantage of dual handsets is that they tether the health care provider and patient to the telephone base and can be awkward for family members who accompany the patient because they will be unable to hear the interpretation (Roat, 2005).

Alternative Interpreting Technologies

Remote simultaneous interpretation is relatively new. In this model, both the patient and the health care provider are supplied with headsets, which in turn are linked to an interpreter in a remote office. As the physician speaks, the interpreter interprets at the same time, just as UN and conference interpreters do. The listener hears the message at the same time the speaker is speaking (Roat, 2005, p. 14). One drawback of this method is that it is difficult to find and train enough interpreters who are competent in the simultaneous mode and who are willing to work for the relatively low rates paid to health care interpreters.

In its research on remote simultaneous interpreting, the Cambridge Health Alliance found that this technology takes out the "middle man," potentially allowing for a more direct patient–provider relationship; speeds up communication during the appointment (especially for longer ones); and increases patient privacy. However, remote simultaneous interpreting lacks visual cues, exposes the provider to technical problems, is awkward, fails to block out sounds with disposable headsets that are nonetheless costly, feels isolating for some patients, and limits the number of participants to one provider and one patient at a time (Saint-Louis, Friedman, Chiasson, Quessa, & Novaes, 2003, p. 47).

Software developed by Spoken Translation, called HealthComm, is a combination of voice recognition and machine translation software. The program types a written version of the message it believes the health care provider has voiced. The provider can correct any errors, at which point the computer produces a written translation into the other language and a back-translation into English. After additional corrections are made, the computer "speaks" the message to the patient. Though the technology shows promise, at present it is too slow and cumbersome for clinical use, as Roat (2005, p. 15) suggests.

The Phraselator, a one-way, voice-activated handheld device, matches English spoken phrases to prerecorded phrases in another language. (In the section "Front Office and Other Clinical Staff," we discuss a manual approach called FAST, which uses cue cards. The Phraselator is similar to FAST, but with a technological twist.) It is useful for giving basic information and for asking simple questions that call for a yes or no answer, but complex medical interviews or questions calling for narrative answers are not adapted so easily to this device (Roat, 2005, p. 15).

As use of the Internet continues to grow, patients and providers will use its resources with increasing frequency to obtain information regarding available health care services and resources, including medical translation and interpreting services. The worldwide, high-speed connectivity available through the Internet has served to blur the boundaries between cultures and nations (Galbis-Reig, 2000). In fact, video interpreting using a Web cam and software to allow the interpreter, the health care provider, and the patient to see one another from remote sites around the world is now available from some telephonic interpreting agencies, though it remains expensive for private practices. Of course, the price will likely decrease as the technology becomes more common (Roat, 2005).

SKILLS NEEDED BY INTERPRETERS

An excellent source describing the qualifications of a health care interpreter and detailing an assessment process is the NCIHC's *Guide to Initial Assessment of Interpreter Qualifications* (Beltrán Avery et al., 2001). "When assessment precedes training," note the authors,

> its purpose may be simply to provide a standard for accepting applicants. But, it may be used diagnostically to determine what knowledge, language skills and interpreting skills the candidate needs to further develop, and whether the person is ready for training and what training is needed" (Beltrán Avery et al., 2001, p. 1).

Six components comprise the NCIHC's process for initial interpreter assessment:

1. basic language skills
2. ethical case study
3. cultural issues
4. health care terminology
5. integrated interpreting skills
6. translation of simple instructions (Beltrán Avery et al., 2001)

Although we do not describe each of these areas in detail here, interested readers—especially those charged with recruiting and hiring health care interpreters—may wish to consult the original NCIHC document at http://www.ncihc.org/workingpapers.htm.

Providers and interpreters should understand basic interpreting etiquette and maintain good communication practices before, during, and after encounters with non-English-speaking patients. Some basics involve body language, eye contact, and seating arrangement. Health care providers should do what they can to create a warm, friendly environment, beginning with a smile and a handshake as well as an introduction of the interpreter. Greet the patient first, not the interpreter (Roat, 2005, p. 11). If you must address the interpreter about some issue of communication or culture, let the patient know you will be doing so first (Roat, 2005, p. 11).

Some recommend that the interpreter, patient, and provider form a triangle, with the patient and provider facing one another and the interpreter off to the side (Bernadett, 2005; Phelan & Parkman, 1995). Others note that the provider should refrain from saying "tell him" or "tell her" and instead should speak directly to the patient while maintaining eye contact if it is culturally appropriate to do so. Similarly, interpreters should be trained to use "I" language and to "exercise discretion in switching to the 'third person' when the first person form causes confusion or is culturally inappropriate for either or both parties" (CHIA, 2002, p. 36).

Providers also should remember that the interpreter is a professional and should respect his or her role in the clinical encounter. Other protocols for effective provider–interpreter communication before, during, and after encounters with patients are described in some detail in the CHIA document *Ethical Principles, Protocols, and Guidance on Roles & Intervention* (2002).

STANDARDIZED INTERPRETING PROTOCOLS: MAXIMIZING GOOD COMMUNICATION

As Bernadett (2005) notes, standardizing interpreting protocols offers several benefits. It provides a framework that guides the interaction among interpreters, patients, and health care providers. For those patients and providers unfamiliar with how best to use the services of an interpreter, formal standards inform them about the interpreter's role as well as how to proceed and what to expect during a typical clinical session. Standards allow interpreters to set the stage for a smooth experience and enable them to focus on their interpreting task.

Most prominent among national organizations trying to standardize interpreter protocols is the National Council on Interpreting in Health Care, or NCIHC, but other groups such as CHIA and MMIA have an interest in advancing certification efforts in their respective states. (It's a step-by-step process. A first step, well before that of certification, is the standardization of practice from state to state.) Only Washington and Oklahoma currently offer certification for interpreters working in health care (Cynthia E. Roat, personal communication, February 2006), but two reports have documented various training programs in California (Roat, 2003) and throughout the United States and Canada (Roat & Okahara, 1998) that teach a variety of techniques and practices. Issues discussed in these reports include course design and administration, protocols, testing, instructors, and advice for course planners. Funded by the California Endowment, the survey of California programs (Roat, 2003) analyzes trends in training and acts as a resource compendium for those seeking to be trained as health care interpreters.

Unfortunately, though awareness of our need for trained medical interpreters continues to grow, there has been "a lack of clarity and consistency on the national level in defining the characteristics and competencies of a qualified health care interpreter, leaving interpreters and health care facilities, as well as other stakeholders, with little or no guidance in identifying the performance requirements of the interpreter role" (NCIHC, 2005).

In 2004, however, the NCIHC published its *National Code of Ethics for Interpreters in Health Care* following an extensive period of gathering input and counsel from working interpreters and their colleagues. Once this code was in place, the NCIHC built on the work of the MMIA and CHIA to create a set of national standards of practice for interpreters working in health care settings. First, an environmental scan was conducted to analyze standards of practice in the United States and around the world. A total of 145 documents in 11 languages from 25 countries were analyzed (Bancroft, 2005). It became clear as a result of the scan that unified standards of practice were necessary:

> The scan uncovered a number of contradictions among certain standards of practice, both within and across different sectors of interpreting. For example: whether the interpreter should remain alone with a client; be completely impartial or support and advocate the client; always interpret completely or sometimes summarize; restrict the interpreter's role to interpreting or include other roles (such as information and referral or mediation); interpret offensive language or offer the speaker a chance to rephrase. . . . While standards of practice both across and within sectors contradict each other, they also affirm basic principles and practices common to nearly all professional interpreters (Bancroft, 2005, p. viii).

The NCIHC used the information gathered in the scan along with feedback from focus groups, stakeholders, and conferences across the United States to draft national standards for practice for health care during 2004 and 2005. The standards are designed to correct for the uneven and inconsistent quality of health care interpreting that has characterized practice until now (Bidar-Sielaff & Ruschke, 2005). They are intended to guide the practice of all interpreters and to acquaint noninterpreters with the standards recognized within the interpreting profession (NCIHC, 2005).

Nine overall standards are discussed in the document (see below), each of which is related to one or more ethical principles already established by the NCIHC (i.e., the document spells out the relationship between the ethical principles and the nine overall standards). In turn, several *individual* standards are enumerated under the umbrella of each of the nine overall standards; a total of 32 individual standards are therefore listed in the document (e.g., the interpreter renders all messages accurately and completely, without adding, omitting, or substituting; the interpreter advises parties that everything said will be interpreted; the interpreter is prepared for all assignments). As mentioned, the 32 standards are categorized under the following nine major headings:

1. accuracy
2. confidentiality
3. impartiality
4. respect
5. cultural awareness
6. role boundaries
7. professionalism
8. professional development
9. advocacy

"While each standard has merit and can stand on its own," note the authors, "the full implication of each standard is best understood when seen in its connection and interdependence with the other standards" (NCIHC, 2005, p. 3). The full document may be viewed on or downloaded from the NCIHC's Web site, http://www.ncihc.org/NCIHC_PDF/National_Standards_of_Practice_for_Interpreters_in_Health_Care.pdf.

Federal and State Regulations

The public sector also advocates on behalf of non-English-speaking patients, basing many of its activities on language in the Civil Rights Act of 1964. In fact, several other federal laws recognize the need for language assistance, among them the Voting Rights Act, the Food Stamp Act, the Older Americans Act, and the Substance Abuse and Mental Health Administration Reorganization Act (Office for Civil Rights, 2001). Federal funds are available to provide language services to low-income individuals through the Medicare, Medicaid, and State Children's Health Insurance Program. Many states also have laws about health care interpreting (ACORN, 2004).

The Joint Committee on Accreditation of Healthcare Organizations (JCAHO), which accredits hospitals and other health care institutions, requires language assistance in a number of situations. For example, its accreditation manual for hospitals provides that written notice of patients' rights be appropriate to the patient's age, understanding, and language. The National Committee for Quality Assurance (NCQA), which provides accreditation for managed care organizations, requires language assistance in several settings. As part of its evaluation process, the NCQA assesses managed care member materials to determine whether they are available in languages other than English that are spoken by major population groups (ACORN, 2004).

In August 2000, President Clinton signed Executive Order 13166, which required all federal agencies to provide guidance to recipients of their funds on how to comply with Title VI and to produce a plan on how to provide language access to their own services. Although there have been congressional efforts to have the order revoked, none have succeeded thus far.

After President Clinton left office, the American Medical Association wrote to Secretary of Health and Human Services Tommy Thompson complaining that providing interpreter services was too expensive and that the Office for Civil Rights (OCR) should not implement the order. The OCR responded that the regulations governing access had been in place since 1964 and that Congress would have to rescind the entire 1964 Civil Rights Act to cease implementing the guidance (NCIHC, 2003–2004).

In response to concerns about the cost of interpreter services, Congress requested that the Office of Management and Budget (OMB) investigate the cost of implementing the order (NCIHC, 2003–2004). The OMB concluded that the cost of implementing the executive order "could be substantial," particularly to the health care sector, but said this was "tempered by the fact that many government agencies and private entities that serve a significant LEP population have already taken steps to provide language services" (Office of Management and Budget, 2002, p. 4). The report catalogued many benefits of offering language services, but concluded that "the ultimate benefits and costs of [Executive Order 13166] will depend on how it is implemented" (OMB, 2002, p. 5).

Some researchers have sought to estimate the cost of providing interpreting services in the health care environment. Jacobs and colleagues (2004) assessed the impact of interpreter services on the cost and use of health care services among patients with LEP enrolled in a health maintenance organization (HMO). In their study, the estimated cost of providing the services was $279 per person per year.

There were limitations in the study: a small sample size, data abstracted for a period of only 1 year following implementation of the interpreter services, and a sample limited to enrollees who were continually insured for an average of 3 years. In addition, the researchers based their assessment on interpreter services that were higher than the average cost in the market at the time ($79 in the study compared to the estimated average of $35 per interpretation) and did not measure all of the potential benefits of the services, such as improved communication and quality of care (Jacobs et al., 2004).

However, because the use of interpretation increased patients' use of preventive and primary care services (such as follow-up visits and medications), and because annual Medicaid expenditures for patients with mood disorder, diabetes, and heart disease were $1,957, $1,563, and $2,328, respectively, at the time of the study, the researchers concluded that the estimated cost of the interpreter services seemed reasonable (Jacobs et al., 2004).

Another federal effort associated with the provision of interpreter services is the development of 14 national standards for Culturally and Linguistically Appropriate Services (CLAS). Produced by the Office of Minority Health in 2001, CLAS standards are designed to improve access to health and social services by minority populations who encounter barriers to care. Basically, they aim to help eliminate racial and ethnic health disparities and to improve health care for all Americans. The 14 standards are grouped under three themes: culturally competent care, language access services, and organizational supports for cultural competence (Putsch, SenGupta, Sampson, & Tervalon, 2003).

According to the U.S. Office for Civil Rights, at least 26 states and the District of Columbia have enacted legislation requiring language assistance, such as the use of interpreters and/or translated forms and other written materials for LEP persons. However, a report by the National Health Law Program claims that "states, health care providers and managed care organizations are largely unfamiliar with the numerous federal and state civil rights laws that protect limited English speakers against discrimination in the delivery of health care" (Perkins, Youdelman, & Wong, 2003).

States that require language assistance include California, which mandates that intermediate care facilities use interpreters and other methods to ensure adequate communication between staff and patients; New Jersey, which provides that drug and alcohol treatment facilities offer interpreter services if their patient population is non-English-speaking; Pennsylvania, which provides that a patient who does not speak English should have access, where possible, to an interpreter; and Massachusetts, which in April 2000 enacted legislation requiring acute care hospitals to offer competent interpreter services to LEP patients in connection with all state ED services (Office for Civil Rights, 2001).

In Minnesota, the Bilingual Services Act of 1995 affirms the following:

> Every state agency that is directly involved in furnishing information or rendering services to the public and that serves a substantial number of non-English speaking people shall employ enough qualified bilingual persons in public contact positions, or enough interpreters to assist those in these positions to ensure provision of information and service *(Minnesota Refugee Health Provider Guide,* 2004).

Similarly, Rhode Island requires hospitals to provide interpreters as a condition of continued licensure and requires posting this availability in conspicuous places in at least three widely used languages other than English (ACORN, 2004). The Massachusetts Emergency Services Interpreter Law of 2001 mandates that all acute care facilities offering ED services provide interpreter services for all patients (ACORN, 2004).

Laws governing the use of health care interpreters—including who is qualified to do interpreting (Sevilla Mátir & Willis, 2004)—vary by state. Those interested should contact health officials in their own state to learn about applicable laws.

WORKING WITH CERTIFIED AND NONCERTIFIED INTERPRETERS

The benefits of using trained interpreters are well recognized in facilitating history taking, reducing unnecessary diagnostic tests, and assisting a patient's education regarding disease, treatment, and prevention (Kazzi & Cooper, 2003). Training can take place in multiple contexts, from hands-on experience interpreting in a hospital to courses offered at institutes or in colleges and universities.

But certification is a different story. As Beltrán Avery and colleagues (2001) explain, certification calls for formal assessment by a certifying body using an instrument tested for its validity and reliability. Apart from a few private programs, only a handful of formal certifications in interpreting exist in the United States, among which are federal court interpreter certification, the state court certification, and certifications offered by the Registry of Interpreters for the Deaf (Beltrán Avery et al., 2001).

Use of certified interpreters might be desirable, but presently few foreign-language interpreters are certified. As of February 2006, Washington and Oklahoma were the only two states that certified interpreters (Cynthia E. Roat, personal communication, February 2006), though two commercial telephonic interpreting companies—Language Line Services and NetworkOmni—also have a certification process in place. Prospective employers should therefore be wary about any interpreter who boasts of being "certified" on his or her resumé. Completion of a few hours of training by a referral agency without formal testing does not constitute certification (Beltrán Avery et al., 2001).

Meanwhile, the NCIHC continues to explore certification on the national level. Interpreters legitimately certified through a national program might be more serious about advancing in and making contributions to their chosen field. Whether those individuals would necessarily be "better" interpreters than their noncertified peers, however, remains open to debate.

On the state level, MMIA in Massachusetts and other regional groups also are pursuing certification efforts. CHIA, the California public charity mentioned earlier, is developing a skills summary for interpreters until certification is available. This will make it easier to "compare interpreter A with interpreter B to determine who is more qualified" (Cynthia E. Roat, personal communication, February 2006). As of February 2006, the following states were pursuing certification efforts: Oklahoma, Oregon, Indiana, Iowa, Georgia, Massachusetts, and North Carolina.

"California has no real effort under way to certify clinical interpreters," says Cynthia E. Roat, chair of the NCIHC advisory committee and a consultant and prolific writer in the field of health care interpreting. "The California State Personnel Board does offer a medical interpreters test, but it's designed to test the skills of interpreters serving in workers compensation cases, not in clinical contexts" (personal communication, February 2006).

Although certification remains a long-term goal in California, CHIA Executive Director Don Schinske points to a set of regulations that went through the California legislature and were signed into law by Governor Gray Davis in 2003.

The bill, SB 853, focused on cultural and linguistic requirements for commercial HMOs in the state, requiring all commercial health plans to develop standards for language assistance. Specifically, the law was designed to ensure that enrollees in managed care organizations and other insurance plans in California are provided with language assistance on a par with that provided by Medi-Cal and other public health programs (California Update, 2003). Although the law falls short of requiring certification, it might be seen as an initial step along that path (D. Schinske, personal communication, January 2006).

In addition to federal standards such as CLAS and requirements by national accrediting bodies like JCAHO, states play an important role in helping eliminate barriers between LEP patients and high-quality health care.

> The hospitals are the first adopters of standards for their own provision of language services. State regulations add another prong: they make health plans responsible. But services must be provided for all downstream contractors. It's challenging enough for a hospital, but at the office level, that's where the rubber hits the road. Should there be acknowledgment of the need for language services in health care contracting? Is that another negotiable item in the contract? (D. Schinske, personal communication, January 2006)

More data are needed before national certification becomes available. Schinske continues,

> In terms of certification the biggest hurdle in California, Massachusetts, and elsewhere around the country are the costs involved. Also, what does a good certification exam look like? Standards are important; there is no fundamental disagreement between CHIA and NCIHC about what constitutes professional health care interpreting. But when it comes to developing tests and assessing them, it would take at least $1 million to get it done. There isn't a big pot of money out there to develop a certification test (D. Schinske, personal communication, January 2006).

Still, groups like CHIA periodically talk about partnering with other groups to achieve a national certification test because the point, says Schinske, is not who does it, but to have it in place.

Cynthia Roat has this to say about certification:

> The first thing that's important to understand about certification is that it's just part of a quality assurance program. In lieu of national or state certification, it is important to find interpreters who have had their language skills screened and who have been trained. Many people who end up working as interpreters got into the field because they wanted to be of service to their community. Often they were the only ones around who spoke another language, but many are "heritage speakers" who grew up in the United States speaking a language other than English at home. In many cases their language skills simply are not up to interpreting, which is why language screening is important (Cynthia Roat, personal communication, February 2006).

Interpreting is a learned skill that requires training, she notes. "Certification is only one part of the puzzle; good recruiting and language screening and training ought to precede assessment, which ought to be followed by careful monitoring and continuing education efforts. If you can't get certification, you can still work toward quality" (Cynthia E. Roat, personal communication, February 2006).

Front Office and Other Clinical Staff

Earlier we discussed the use of dedicated interpreters, briefly mentioning the advantages and disadvantages of hiring them. When health care providers can speak other languages fluently, LEP patients appreciate their efforts and feel more comfortable in their care. Another resource on which providers might draw is the use of office staff with foreign-language skills. Because office staff members are usually the first people to interact with patients, they are uniquely positioned to establish rapport, determine the patient's needs, and extract information.

Some things to consider when relying on bilingual staff, however, are (1) that doing so may disrupt the operation of the office (if the employee is interpreting instead of processing patients), (2) that it has hidden costs because the employee is potentially less productive, and (3) that there is a possibility staff members do not have the linguistic competence, education, or capacity to serve as qualified interpreters (Roat, 2005).

In some environments, such as acute care, use of interpreters for every clinical encounter is neither possible nor practical. However, clinical staff still must communicate basic instructions to patients, even when they have no understanding of the patient's language. For this reason, researchers at the University of Kentucky Medical Center developed what they call the Focused Accessible Spanish Translator (FAST) to deal with their patient population, a majority of whom speak Spanish (Bernard et al., 2005). The FAST is simply a cue card small enough to fit in the clinician's pocket (Figure 10.1). On the card are phrases that intensive care nurses (on one side) and surgeons (on the other side) can use in their daily practice, such as "Can you breathe?," "Are you in pain?," "We are going to bathe you," "You had surgery," and "Do you need us to contact [your] family/friend?" Each phrase is accompanied by a translation into basic Spanish on the same line. Words and phrases in FAST are divided into general/greetings, commands, and (for surgeons) rounds.

A survey on how FAST was used (Bernard et al., 2005) found that 94% of nurses and 88% of physicians at the hospital still had their cards 7 months after a formal training session. Among physicians, lack of intent to use the card was directly correlated with their ability to speak Spanish. Most respondents found the FAST easy to use and portable and said that it met their needs at the bedside, but still acknowledged the effectiveness of on-site interpreters. As the researchers make clear,

> The FAST was not designed to be all inclusive and did not supplant interpreters because the quality of communication obtained with interpreters is considered the reference standard. Professional interpretation is important for in-depth discussion such as detailed history taking, discussing complex treatment options, preoperative planning for surgery, discussing prognosis, addressing social issues, ensuring

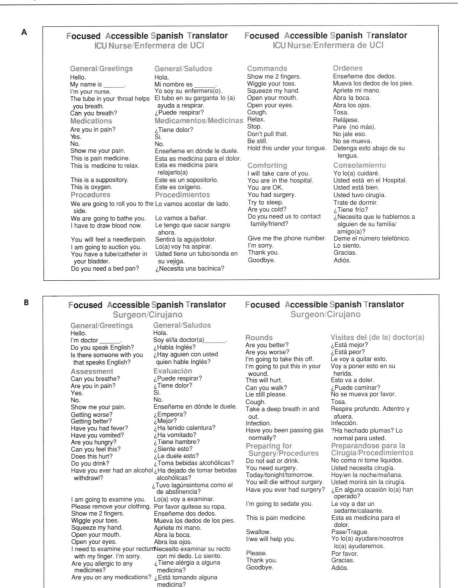

FIGURE 10.1 Focused Accessible Spanish Translator (FAST). Most critical care nurses and physicians surveyed at the University of Kentucky Medical Center in Lexington, KY, where the FAST card is used, said they found it helpful. Health care providers, especially nurses, said they experienced decreased stress levels when using the translator, which is a simple 128 mm × 77 mm card kept in the provider's pocket. *Source*: Bernard, A. C., Summers, A., Thomas, J., et al. (2005). Novel Spanish translators for acute care nurses and physicians: Usefulness and effect on practitioners' stress. *American Journal of Critical Care, 14*(6), 545–550. © 2003 Andrew C. Bernard, MD. Reprinted with permission.

informed consent, and so on. The FAST provides essential information for routine acute care practice environments when interpreters cannot be continually present and interrupting care to refer to a conventional translation tool is impractical (Bernard et al., 2005, p. 546).

Although the study did not address low health literacy, the phrases are simple enough that they could help when communicating with low-health-literate patients. And whereas the FAST is geared toward English-to-Spanish translation, it could be adapted to languages spoken in any institution's catchment area.

Family Members

Most clinicians agree that using family members for medical interpreting is not a good idea. Family members often lack knowledge about clinical services and procedures, for example. Unlike trained interpreters, they generally do not understand terms used by medical specialists and may become embarrassed about conveying personal information.

And then there are privacy concerns: because family members know the patient, they may inadvertently share information with mutual acquaintances or other members of the patient's family whom the patient may not wish to have that information (Boyar, 2005; Edwards et al., 2005). Often family members unconsciously screen what they hear and give a summarized interpretation to the patient. Doing so decreases the accuracy of the interpretation and could weaken the patient–provider relationship. As Phelan and Parkman (1995) note, violent spouses could try to hide the true cause of a patient's injuries, and incidents of child or sexual abuse might remain secret if family members are permitted to interpret.

Of course, there also are some advantages to having family members do the interpreting. Generally speaking, patients trust members of their own family to work in their best interests. Family members are readily available and have a shared history of understanding and obligations with the patient. They are morally committed to carrying out medical instructions and can help with everyday matters and with transportation. And presumably family members work for free; they do not require payment (Edwards et al., 2005, p. 88).

Still, in light of the potentially serious ethical drawbacks mentioned above, when trained interpreters are not available it is probably better to use bilingual staff members (if properly trained) than to use family or friends (Herndon & Joyce, 2004). For billing purposes, if a patient insists on using a family member, clinicians should document that it was by choice (i.e., "per patient request"). Providers cannot bill the patient for the actual service provided by the interpreter, but a prolonged service code (99354–99357) may be acceptable in addition to the appropriate evaluation and management code (Herndon & Joyce, 2004; Sophocles, 2003).

Children, on the other hand, should never be used for health care interpreting, according to Sevilla Mátir and Willis (2004), unless there is no alternative. Children often substitute the wrong terms or filter information to try to protect their parents. Consider the following exchange between a pediatrician and a Spanish-speaking woman who brought her 2-year-old child in to see her pediatrician for vomiting and dehydration. The interpreter was the child's 11-year-old sister:

Pediatrician: So [he vomited] five times between 1:00 and 3:00? And after that he hasn't thrown up?

Interpreter: Que si desde eso él no ha vomitado? [That if since that (time) he has not vomited?]

Mother: No. Ahora tiene como dolor de oido y eso. [No. Now he has like pain in the ear and so on.]

Interpreter: Yes, he havin' pain.

Mother: Dile que él tiene algo en la boca. Dile. [Tell her (the pediatrician) that he has something on his mouth. Tell her.]

[SILENCE]

Pediatrician: How old is he now?

Interpreter: Three (Flores et al., 2003, p. 9).

In this exchange the pediatrician does not receive a response about how many times the child had vomited before the visit. Also, note that the interpreter omits the mother's statements about the child's ear pain and oral lesion (and gets the child's age wrong as well). Adults must think of the children here: it is not fair to put that kind of burden on young people who are neither emotionally nor intellectually mature enough to deal with the consequences of failing in such a critical task.

ERRORS IN CLINICAL INTERPRETING

Use of children to perform the complex job of health care interpreting raises the issue of medical errors. Because of the inherent communicative uncertainties in any language, all clinical encounters that involve interpreting are prone to error. Nevertheless, use of nonprofessional interpreters only increases the risk.

During a 7-month period, Flores and colleagues (2003) audiotaped and transcribed 13 clinical encounters in a hospital outpatient clinic in which a Spanish interpreter was used. Six encounters involved professional hospital interpreters; the others used ad hoc interpreters, such as nurses and social workers and even an 11-year-old sibling. (An excerpt from the transcription of that clinical encounter appears in the section above.) A total of 396 errors were recorded, with a mean of 31 per encounter. Most common was omission (52%), followed by false fluency (16%), substitution (13%), editorialization (10%), and addition (8%). Sixty-three percent of the errors had potential clinical consequences, with a mean of 19 errors per encounter.

Although there was no significant difference between hospital and ad hoc interpreters in the mean number of errors committed per clinical encounter, errors committed by ad hoc interpreters were significantly more likely to have clinical consequences than were errors committed by hospital interpreters (Flores et al., 2003). Most alarming, perhaps, is the statistic that more than half of the errors made by hospital interpreters had potential clinical consequences, suggesting that most hospital interpreters receive inadequate training at their institution (Flores et al., 2003; Ginsberg, Martin, Andrulis, Shaw-Taylor, & McGregor, 1995).

Other studies have found that clinically relevant interpreter-related distortions could lead to the misevaluation of patients' mental status (Marcos, 1979; Vasquez & Javier, 1991). Citing such evidence as lawsuits over misinterpreted words in the ED and a report of children placed in state custody for mistaken child abuse because of a misinterpreted word (and the associated failure of clinicians to call for an interpreter when one was needed), Flores and colleagues (2003) argue that third-party reimbursement for trained medical interpreter services is necessary. They note that such reimbursement would prevent physicians from having to cover the costs of complying with the OCR's guidance memorandum, which states that denial or delay of medical care for LEP patients because of language barriers is a form of discrimination.

A decade ago, according to Ginsberg and colleagues (1995), only 14% of U.S. hospitals offered training for volunteer interpreters, and in half of these the training was not mandatory. Often interpreter training is limited to short orientation sessions or to shadowing more experienced interpreters, which potentially increases the risk for miscommunication and medical errors. As we saw in chapter 4, errors in clinical practice can have dire consequences for patients of all kinds, but they are particularly hazardous for those with low health literacy and LEP.

Elderkin-Thompson, Silver, and Waitzkin (2001) recorded 21 medical encounters involving Spanish-speaking patients who required a nurse-interpreter to communicate with physicians. In successful interpretations where misunderstandings did not develop, nurses translated the patients' comments as accurately as possible and physicians extracted clinically relevant information.

Roughly half of the recorded encounters contained serious miscommunication problems that affected either the physician's understanding of the symptoms or the credibility of the patients' concerns. In those encounters containing errors, one or more of the following occurred: physicians resisted reconceptualizing the problem when contradictory information was mentioned; nurses provided information consistent with clinical expectations but not with patients' comments; nurses slanted interpretations, reflecting unfavorably on patients and undermining patients' credibility; and patients explained symptoms using a cultural metaphor not compatible with Western disease classification (Elderkin-Thompson et al., 2001).

Death, serious illness, adverse reactions, and other poor outcomes can result when patients receive substandard interpreter services (or, for that matter, no interpreter at all). Each of the following real-life stories helps illustrate this point:

Albuquerque, NM: Abusive husband causes preterm labor, then serves as interpreter. A young Vietnamese woman who spoke no English came to the ED in preterm labor (37 weeks), crying and very upset. Her husband was used to interpret for the delivery. The patient cried through the whole delivery. Weeks later, she was interviewed by a Vietnamese-speaking resident who discovered that the reason she was in tears was that her husband had beaten her up, and this had caused her preterm labor. The lack of an interpreter made her dependent on her abuser for care.

Philadelphia, PA: Relative misinterprets for patient, which leads to unnecessary surgery. A relative, trying to interpret for a patient who could not speak English, did so inaccurately. Based on this misinterpretation, the doctor scheduled the patient for surgery. On the morning of the procedure, a trained interpreter conveyed information that showed the surgery was not only unnecessary but also likely to be harmful to the patient.

Oregon: Patient loses sight due to lack of third-party translation. A Mexican laborer was hit in the eye with a nail gun while on the job. He went to a nearby clinic and was treated by a physician who only spoke English. The clinic provided an interpreter by phone, but the patient never spoke directly to the interpreter and therefore could not communicate the exact nature of his injury. The patient had been to the clinic previously after being hit in the eye by a wood chip, so the doctor assumed he was there for the same injury and treated him accordingly. The lack of interpretation meant the doctor never realized the laborer had been hit by metal. The patient's condition worsened and by the next morning he was back at the clinic. He was sent to a nearby hospital, where surgery was performed to remove the metal. Three subsequent surgeries were performed, but none of them succeeded. The laborer's sight remained impaired. The man sued. At the trial an expert testified that if the surgery had been performed earlier, the man's sight could have been saved. The jury agreed (Roat, Alvarado-Little, & Jacobs, 2003).

In each of these cases, better communication and the provision of a trained interpreter might have led to a better outcome for the patient. Much like patients with low health literacy, LEP patients often are at the mercy of the health care system. What they don't know can harm them unless someone familiar with their plight is available to advocate for them.

Sometimes interpreters simply are not called when patients need them. In a cross-sectional survey of 467 native Spanish-speaking and 63 English-speaking Latino patients presenting with nonurgent medical problems, Baker, Parker, Williams, Coates, and Pitkin (1996) found that when the patient's English and the examiner's Spanish were poor, an interpreter was not called 34% of the time. Eighty-seven percent of the patients who did not have an interpreter thought that one should have been used. Professional interpreters were used for only 12% of the patients, with nurses and physicians interpreting most frequently (49% of the time). The investigators concluded that interpreters are often not used despite a perceived need by patients and that the interpreters who were used usually lacked formal training.

CULTURAL ISSUES IN CLINICAL INTERPRETING

Messages that are translated from one language into another also make a shift from one cultural context to another, meaning that translations must be phrased in such a way as to be responsive to the cultural needs of the foreign-language-speaking population (Boyar, 2005). Some clinicians see interpreters as "culture brokers" because they also must bear in mind social gestures and other culture-specific behaviors (Hatton & Webb, 1993, p. 143).

Although most consider the interpreter as "collaborator" to be the most effective type of interaction, Beltrán Avery (2001, pp. 6–7) warns against cultural brokering, or the shared exchange of cultural information on the part of the interpreter, saying it can be dangerous on two levels. First, it may offer cultural information only as the interpreter views it, not as the patient views it. Second, it may be seen as a quick fix that covers up the shortcomings of the institution. In other words, if the interpreter is skilled as a culture broker, the provider needn't do any better in terms of achieving cultural competence. Then, if one day that interpreter is no longer available, the provider will have to begin again from scratch (Beltrán Avery, 2001).

Then there are problems of different dialects within ethnic subcultures. Consider the following remarks by Maroof Khan, a Bangladeshi man interviewed by Edwards and colleagues:

> I think most people who do interpreting speak Dhaka dialect. This can cause problems for a Sylheti-speaking person. I think Sylheti-speaking interpreters should be provided for Sylheti people. Another example, say a person is from the Chittagong area. If you have a Sylheti-speaking interpreter then this person won't understand the Sylheti dialect. For them, there should be someone from Chittagong doing the interpreting (Edwards et al., 2005, p. 84).

Census data in 2001 indicated that Bangladeshis were 6% of the minority population in Great Britain. At the time, the country's 283,000 Bangladeshis were concentrated in London and, to a lesser extent, in Birmingham (Lupton & Power, 2004). Although such numbers may or may not support the hiring of multiple Bangladeshi interpreters in any one clinic or hospital, through telephonic interpreting Mr. Khan's wish could be granted. Either way, his point that interpreters ought to speak the dialect of the patient for whom they interpret is difficult to dispute.

Unfortunately, training programs often do not provide instruction in awareness of multiple cultures and/or training in how to translate and interact in culturally appropriate ways during interpreting interactions (Hwa-Froelich & Westby, 2003). In some cultures, language itself is proscribed by custom. A Navajo woman who attended one of the formative working group meetings of the NCIHC in Seattle in 1998 captured this idea well. Here she describes some of the culturally imposed limitations she must undergo in performing her work as an interpreter:

> There is a clan system. There are certain things I can't interpret if it's for my husband's clan . . . or for my father's clan, especially if it is about certain sensitive things, like the male parts of the body. There are certain things that I, as an interpreter, cannot interpret if the person I am interpreting for is older than me. I can't say certain things to a male that I can say to a female. There are certain things a young female interpreter can't say to a young man. There are certain things a male interpreter can't say to a woman.

And, then there is spirituality. There are certain things I can't interpret to anybody because of the spiritual part of it. In our culture, there are some things you don't say. So, I have two worlds that I have to take the patient through—Western medicine that is separate from our lives and the Indian way of life where we're at all the time. By knowing both sides, I bring those two forces together. I show the patient—this is what is over there. I show the provider—that is what is over there (Beltrán Avery, 2001, pp. 10–11).

Cross-cultural communication calls for wisdom and experience. Health care interpreters ought to translate messages carefully so that they convey the cultural framework in which care takes place. Take, for example, a patient from a matriarchal culture. Imagine that this patient does not want to take a certain medicine because it will be costly and would not please his or her mother. Rather than assume that the health care provider understands the cultural context, the interpreter should translate that concern in such a way that the provider understands why the mother is such an important figure in the patient's life (Sevilla Mátir & Willis, 2004, p. 35).

Whether a health care interpreter is professionally trained, part of the clinical staff, or simply called in for a particular interpreting task, culturally aware interpreting can help build trust and rapport with non-English-speaking patients, potentially improving health care outcomes. Unfortunately, highly skilled interpreters who are well versed in the cultures of their patients' population are rare. As Beltrán Avery suggests,

> People who possess the skills to bridge the cultural and linguistic gaps are few and in great demand. Those who possess these skills often have training in more than one job role. Thus, it is the nurse, the social worker or the case manager who also serves as the interpreter. In these situations, as in the incremental intervention approach, transparency is again of utmost importance in order to maintain trust among the members of the triad (Beltrán Avery, 2001, p. 11).

WORKING WITH INTERPRETERS: HOW PROVIDERS CAN HELP

Family physicians and other health care providers can take several important steps to facilitate the interpreting process, such as asking for an interpreter of the same gender as the patient. Often patients feel more comfortable when discussing personal issues with a member of the same sex (Herndon & Joyce, 2004). Because interpretation may take longer than anticipated, clinicians should allow extra time when scheduling consultations with LEP patients. As Herndon and Joyce (2004, p. 38) advise,

> When interacting with LEP patients, keep your sentences brief and pause often to allow time for interpreting. Avoid highly technical medical jargon and idiomatic expressions that may be difficult for the interpreter to convey and the patient to comprehend. Use diagrams and pictures to facilitate better understanding.
>
> It's also important to listen without interrupting and to make it a point to confirm that the patient understands by asking him or her to repeat important

instructions back to you. Pause at several points during the conversation to ask whether the patient has any questions. Many cultures see questioning physicians as a sign of disrespect and may be hesitant to respond initially.

Phelan and Parkman (1995) offer similar advice, listing the following "key points when interviewing with an interpreter":

- Address the patient in the second person.
- Talk directly to the patient.
- Keep control of the consultation.
- Pause frequently.
- Appear attentive when the patient responds.
- Respond to the patient's nonverbal cues.
- Check the patient's understanding.
- Make use of written material.

In *Addressing Language Access Issues in Your Practice,* Roat (2005, p. 7) advises providers to develop a language access strategy. The first steps in this process include asking patients about their language preference, tracking their language preferences, and determining the current and future demands of the patient population. "If you and your patient don't speak the same language," says Roat, "and if you are committed to communicating clearly, you basically have three choices": (1) the patient learns English, (2) you learn the patient's language, or (3) you use the services of an interpreter. "Having patients learn English is a worthwhile goal and one that every immigrant and refugee needs to consider," she points out (Roat, 2005, p. 8).

In fact, many non-English-speaking patients are trying to learn English, according to a California Media telephone survey conducted in June 2003. For those clinicians serious about communicating with patients in another language, Roat recommends having language fluency assessed through proficiency testing. Language Testing International, Language Line Services, and other entities offer such testing (Roat, 2005).

HOW TO FIND INTERPRETERS

After you've determined what kind of interpreters you'll need for your practice, the next step is finding them. National associations such as NCIHC and state groups such as CHIA and MMIA may be good places to start. (For a list of health care interpreter associations throughout the United States, visit the NCIHC Web site at http://www.ncihc.org and click on the link to "Health Care Interpreter Associations in the U.S.") Clinicians with large non-English-speaking patient populations may wish to consider contracting with one or more of the outside interpreter services mentioned earlier in this chapter. Here is a partial list of companies along with their Web addresses:

- 1-800-Translate: http://www.1-800-translate.com/Medical.html
- CyraCom International: http://www.cyracom.net
- Global LT: http://www.languatutor.com

- Language Line Services: http://www.languageline.com
- MultiLingual Solutions: http://www.mlsolutions.com
- NetworkOmni: http://www.networkomni.com
- Telelanguage: http://www.telelanguage.com

Contacting health care interpreters in your local area can be a challenging task. However, the American Translators Association (ATA) offers a database of more than 3,700 professional translators and interpreters on its Web site, http://www.atanet.org. The database lists ATA members throughout the country and the world and can be accessed by clicking "services directories" on the home page. Two directories are available: one for individuals (called "Directory of Translation and Interpreting Services") and one for companies (called "Directory of Language Services Companies"). The advanced search option enables users to narrow down a search to a particular state or city, with an option to select a specific mile radius (ATA, 2006).

A potential drawback is that ATA membership dues are fairly high. As of January 2006, an associate membership was $145, though student membership (limited to 4 years) was $80. Institutional membership with the ATA was $180 and corporate membership was $300. This means that some professionals on the database may charge a premium for their services that smaller hospitals or practices couldn't afford.

Using ATA's online database, a quick search for individual Spanish-language interpreters within a 50-mile radius of the zip code 90005 (in downtown Los Angeles) brings up a list of 71 interpreters. Expanding the search to a 100-mile radius results in 89 names. The database may have a few serious gaps, however. No records are found, for example, for Vietnamese interpreters within 100 miles of Los Angeles, meaning that those searching the directory for interpreters in Westminster or Garden Grove, CA—where the Vietnamese American population is highly concentrated, constituting roughly 30.7% and 21.4% of their residents, respectively (U.S. Census Bureau, 2000)—would have little luck finding them using ATA, at least as of January 2006, when this particular database search was performed.

Using the local Yellow Pages to determine whether there are interpreters or translators working in your area, either as individual contractors or as members of businesses, is yet another option, though it may take time and patience to sift through the listings to find what you need.

In fact, some smaller, local organizations keep databases of their own— smaller versions, perhaps, of ATA's national directories. When health care providers call and ask for a translator or interpreter, typically these businesses ask a series of questions to determine the specific needs of the job and then consult their own local contacts and lists to find a candidate whose qualifications match. For example, Milla Ismailova, managing director of the California English Language Center in Lake Forest, CA, notes that her organization keeps a database of 2,000 translators and interpreters.

"I usually look at the background of the interpreter or translator first," she says, "to see if they are right for the job. We have nurses who come to this country who are bilingual and know English very well; often they have training in their own countries. We establish good relationships with interpreters and translators throughout the United States."

Although continuing education and certification signal professional advancement in most fields, experience goes a long way, too. Consider Ismailova, an immigrant from Russia who has lived in both Azerbaijan and Siberia. She earned a master's degree from the Azerbaijan Institute of Foreign Languages, where she specialized in English as a foreign language, before settling in the United States. She has training both in interpreting and translating, having completed postgraduate course work and certification in Azerbaijan. She also has 20 years' experience doing Russian-to-English and English-to-Russian interpreting and translating (M. Ismailova, personal communication, February 2006).

Ismailova looks for others like herself to fill the most challenging jobs. In fact, many companies that offer interpretation and translation services have developed their own procedures for "qualifying" their professionals. Still, even as these agencies provide verification of their employees' training and certification, caveats mentioned earlier about the nature of certification should be kept in mind.

Trained interpreters are costly, but can save time and resources in the long run by decreasing the number of callbacks, misdiagnoses, and unnecessary tests and increasing patients' comprehension, compliance, and satisfaction (Herndon & Joyce, 2004). How costly these professionals are depends on the needs of the regions in which they work, such as the numbers of people speaking languages they interpret and the cost of living.

Rates at the International Institute of New Jersey (IINJ), for example, which contracts with roughly 120 freelance interpreters, are on the low side: around $60 per hour with a 2-hour minimum for health care interpreting. IINJ provides translating and interpreting services for courts, hospitals, youth and family services, boards of education, the Social Security Administration, and social services in Jersey City and across the northern part of the state (J. Dee, personal communication, February 2006).

The law of supply and demand determines rates. Because Chinese-language interpreters are harder to find, interpreting to and from Chinese costs a little more than other languages. National averages vary from $100 to $125 per hour, with interpreters in ethnically diverse, highly populated areas such as New York and California commanding the highest fees.

Occasionally, charges for health care interpreting are reimbursable. As of July 2003, nine states offered direct reimbursement for the costs of language interpreters: Idaho, Hawaii, Maine, Massachusetts, Minnesota, Montana, New Hampshire, Utah, and Washington (Language Services Action Kit, 2003). These states have set up their own reimbursement systems, with some contracting with language agencies, others reimbursing providers who screen and hire interpreters, still others reimbursing interpreters directly, and one enrolling the interpreters as Medicaid providers. Reimbursement rates vary from $7 to $50 per hour (Carter-Pokras et al., 2004; Language Services Action Kit, 2003). Those facilities that serve a high number of LEP patients might be able to receive funding if they are considered "disproportionate share hospitals" (i.e., hospitals that serve a dispro-portionate share of Medicaid or uninsured patients; Carter-Pokras et al., 2004).

HIPAA AND THE PATIENT'S PRIVACY

Interpreters who work in health care settings should understand how HIPAA privacy requirements affect their work. HIPAA, which took effect in April 2003, provides a minimum set of national standards limiting the way health plans, pharmacies, hospitals, clinicians, and others (called "covered entities") can use personal medical information. The act regulates the conduct of three types of entities: a "member of the workforce" of a covered entity, a "business associate" of a covered entity, and a person approved by the patient. Because HIPAA also binds those who are controlled by covered entities, such as volunteers, and those with whom covered entities contract, interpreters who work as employees, in-dependent contractors, and volunteers generally are required to uphold HIPAA privacy regulations (National Health Law Program, 2005).

There are exceptions, however, to this privacy requirement. If a patient con-sents to an ad hoc interpreter who is not a member of the workforce or a business associate of the covered entity (such as another patient or a person in the health care facility), that interpreter may not be bound by the HIPAA privacy rule. Be-cause this distinction can be difficult to determine, health care facilities hoping to minimize their exposure to lawsuits should ensure that everyone working as an interpreter does everything within his or her power to maintain the patient's confidentiality. Even disclosure of a person's primary language (if, say, there are a relatively small number of foreign-language speakers in a particular commu-nity) could be a violation of privacy and would be prohibited under HIPAA. A good primer is the National Health Law Program's *HIPAA and Language Ser-vices in Health Care* (2005), available on the organization's Web site at http://www.healthlaw.org.

Generally speaking, any interpreter who is a member of a covered entity's workforce or a business associate of the covered entity must abide by the privacy rule and not disclose information about the patient, whether that information is in electronic, paper, or oral form (National Health Law Program, 2005). Different institutions have different requirements about when information can be disclosed and by whom. Information must be disclosed when patients or their personal representatives request access to their health information or when the Department of Health and Human Services is undertaking a compliance investigation, review, or enforcement action.

If an interpreter learns about child or elder abuse or hears threats of violence during the encounter, he or she is obligated to interpret the information, at which point the provider may address the situation and be required to report the information based on mandatory reporting laws. In some states, interpreters also may be considered mandated reporters (National Health Law Program, 2005).

Before any office visit that is going to involve interpreting, health care providers should give the necessary background information to the interpreter. They should remind the interpreter that everything that is interpreted must be kept confidential. They should also reassure the patient that everything said in the exchange will be kept confidential (Herndon & Joyce, 2004). If a speakerphone is going to be used, it should not be placed in any area such as a lobby or an open emergency room where other patients can overhear the conversation (Roat, 2005, p. 20).

In addition to the legal obligations that medical institutions have with respect to confidentiality, patients simply appreciate it when their privacy is taken into consideration, as Edwards and colleagues (2005, p. 87) learned in their research. "There are people who only interpret so that they can gossip about people," said Mrs. Topolska, a Polish woman interviewed in the Edwards study. "[The professional interpreter I used] never said anything she shouldn't have. . . . It is better to use someone who is neutral, and that he interprets honestly. So that he does not take sides."

In chapter 4 we mentioned the disconnect between the reading level of the typical HIPAA Notice of Privacy Practices and that of average patients, many of whom have low health literacy. Such documents pose a considerable challenge to health care interpreters, who often are expected to sight translate them, regardless of how long the forms are or whether they are written in understandable English as opposed to legalese.

"Interpreters cannot simplify or explain texts that we are asked to sight translate," says Cynthia Roat. "Sight translations should be done in the same register in which the document is written. If the form is grade 16, it should be translated into the same level in the target language" (Cynthia Roat, personal communication, February 2006). Incomprehensible English is replaced by an equally incomprehensible interpretation, and with the same result: the patient cannot understand.

There is a limit to what an interpreter can sight translate in the course of a medical visit. According to Roat, anything more than a page or page and a half is too much. "Ideally, the provider should orally summarize what's in the document first so the interpreter can interpret the provider's speech. With consent forms, it's better if the provider sits and explains the form and then has the patient sign it" (Cynthia E. Roat, personal communication, February 2006).

It is questionable whether simply providing an English privacy notice to an LEP patient constitutes a "good faith" effort to obtain informed consent (National Health Law Program, 2005). Having this notice interpreted at the same level would do little to increase the patient's understanding, as mentioned. Fortunately, new JCAHO standards require that the physician or other health care provider remain present during consent to give the patient time to ask questions and to get additional information (Cynthia E. Roat, personal communication, February 2006).

IMPROVING PATIENT ACCESS

Ultimately, LEP patients who are offered competent interpreting services benefit from increased access to quality care—the goal of all ongoing efforts to accommodate patients with low health literacy. However, as we've seen, barriers to the use of trained interpreters remain and include poor identification of the need for an interpreter by clinical staff, an acceptance of ad hoc interpreters, lack of awareness about access to health care interpreting services, and a desire by some patients to undertake the consultation in English without assistance (Kazzi & Cooper, 2003).

Studies have shown that LEP patients themselves experience barriers to access as a direct result of their limited language skills. Sometimes they experience delays in accessing interpreters and limited access after hours, for example (Kazzi & Cooper, 2003). Some LEP patients complain that it is difficult for them to obtain a professional interpreter unless they already can speak English. As Edwards and colleagues (2005) observed, LEP patients cannot always communicate clearly with receptionists or when they are trying to book a telephonist. Questions of access must be addressed before anything else.

Like so many issues in health care, however, language access is part of a complex system that involves issues of reimbursement, education and training, quality control, and even political will. Patients with limited literacy skills—many of whom cannot speak English—report poorer overall health, are less likely to make use of medical screenings, seek medical care after they have reached later stages of disease, are more likely to be hospitalized, have poorer understanding of their treatments, and have lower adherence to medical regimens (Berkman et al., 2004; Rudd, 2002). Ideally, those who need interpreting services would receive such services, either for free as a public benefit or as an expense reimbursable through private insurance.

But quality health care interpreters are in short supply, and their services often come at a high price. Average working Americans increasingly shoulder the burden of expanding health care costs, so the current health care system may be in no position to absorb the additional expenses associated with wider access to translators or interpreters. In an article in *The New England Journal of Medicine,* Paul G. Ginsburg, PhD, shares statistics that may have particular relevance to the general question of health literacy and the more specific question of language access:

> Between 1999 and 2003, the per capita spending for services covered by private health insurance increased by 39%. Given that the average hourly earnings of U.S. workers increased by only 14% during that period, affordability is an acute and growing concern. Unlike increased spending for most other goods and services, which often inspires a celebration of our economy's ability to shift resources rapidly to new products and services that consumers want, rapidly increasing health care spending is often viewed negatively—almost as a force of nature that lies outside consumers' control. The simple explanation for rapidly increasing health care costs is that people are getting more care, much of which is associated with new medical technologies. But many experts have doubts about the value of some of this care in relation to its cost. And when health care costs increase at a much faster rate than incomes, many people–especially those with low incomes—can no longer afford insurance coverage (Ginsburg, 2004, p. 1591).

Yet clear and effective communication is not like a new MRI machine or the latest procedure for balloon angioplasty. It is not so much a luxury whose use has the potential to prolong a patient's life as it is an essential ingredient in our daily lives and well-being; more like food or oxygen than, say, a treatment for depression. According to Hudelson (2005), health care interpreters believe that physicians and other providers need (1) more training in cultural competence to help raise their awareness about potential sources of misunderstanding and about the difficulties of health care translation, (2) additional background knowledge about patients' countries of origin, and (3) more flexibility adapting to patients' varied communication styles (Hudelson, 2005). If each member of the patient–provider–interpreter triad doubled his or her efforts toward effective communication, surely we could reduce errors and improve outcomes and patients' satisfaction.

But that impact remains to be seen. Conflicting data about basic questions with respect to LEP patients' needs have been found. Tocher and Larson (1999) compared physician time spent providing care for non-English-speaking patients with time spent providing care for English-speaking patients during 5 months in a general internal medicine clinic. Although a significant number of clinic physicians believed they spent more time during a visit with non-English-speaking patients (85.7%) and needed more time to address important issues during their visit (90.4%), no differences were actually found in time spent between the two groups. The researchers did not measure quality of care or patients' satisfaction, but they speculated that the physicians assumed they were spending more time with non-English-speaking patients because of the challenges of language and cultural barriers.

On the contrary, in a study examining the effect of language on visit time at general medicine and family practice clinics during 1996–1997, Kravitz, Helms, Azari, Antonius, and Melnikow (2000) found that Russian-speaking and Spanish-speaking patients averaged 9.1 and 5.6 additional minutes of physician time compared to English-speaking patients. They therefore concluded that additional reimbursement might be needed to ensure continued access and high-quality care for these populations.

Can politicians and administrators be convinced that low-cost interpreting is a necessity rather than a luxury? Only time will tell. Perhaps the best argument for such a shift in thinking is expressed as a long-term outcome: initial investments in language access services are balanced out by cost savings when those same LEP patients experience better health down the road.

REFERENCES

Aparicio, A., & Durban, C. (2003). *Translation: Getting it right: A guide to buying translations.* Alexandria, VA: American Translators Association. Retrieved January 3, 2006, from http://www.atanet.org/bin/view.pl/13761.html

Association of Community Organizations for Reform Now (ACORN). (2004, January). *Speaking the language of care: Language barriers to hospital access in America's cities.* Retrieved January 29, 2006, from http://acorn.org

Baker, D. W., Parker, R. M., Williams, M. V., Coates, W. C., & Pitkin, K. (1996). Use and effectiveness of interpreters in an emergency department [abstract]. *Journal of the American Medical Association, 275*(10), 783–788.

Bancroft, M. (2005, March). *The interpreter's world tour: An environmental scan of standards of practice for interpreters.* Retrieved January 13, 2006, from http://www.ncihc.org/NCIHCDocRep/Files/222224ff-6fc5-4bb7-86ad-7a699eebad09.pdf

Beltrán Avery, M.-P. (2001, April). The role of the health care interpreter: An evolving dialogue. *National Council on Interpreting in Health Care Working Paper Series.* Retrieved January 6, 2006, from http://www.ncihc.org/workingpapers.htm

Beltrán Avery, M.-P., Chun, A., Downing, B., Maynard, M., Ruschke, K. (2001, April). Guide to initial assessment of interpreter qualifications. *National Council on Interpreting in Health Care Working Papers Series.* Retrieved January 5, 2006, from http://www.ncihc.org/workingpapers.htm

Berkman, N. D., DeWalt, D. A., Pignone, M. P., Sheridan, S. L., Lohr, K. N., Lux, L., et al. (2004, January). *Literacy and health outcomes* (Evidence Report/Technology Assessment No. 87, AHRQ Publications No. 04-E007-2). Rockville, MD: Agency for Healthcare Research and Quality.

Bernadett, M. (2005, May). *Interpreters in a healthcare setting: Ethical principles, protocols, and guidance.* Paper presented at Culture, Language, and Clinical Issues: Operational Solutions to Low Health Literacy, Institute for Healthcare Advancement Fourth Annual Health Literacy Conference, Irvine, CA.

Bernard, A. C., Summers, A., Thomas, J., Ray, M., Rockich, A., Barnes, S., et al. (2005). Novel Spanish translators for acute care nurses and physicians: Usefulness and effect on practitioners' stress. *American Journal of Critical Care, 14*(6), 545–550.

Bernstein, J., Bernstein, E., Dave, A., Hardt, E., James, T., Linden, J., et al. (2002). Trained medical interpreters in the emergency department: Effects on services, subsequent charges, and follow-up [abstract]. *Journal of Immigrant Health, 4*(4), 171–176.

Bidar-Sielaff, S., & Ruschke, K. (2005, October 25). *National Council on Interpreting in Health Care develops national standards for interpreters* [press release]. Retrieved January 3, 2006, from http://www.cmwf.org/usr_doc/site_docs/pdfs/media/NationalStandardsofPractice_PressRelease.pdf#search='develops%20national%20standards%20for%20interpreters%20BidarSielaff'

Boyar, E. (2005). Found in translation. *ACTmagazine.com.* Retrieved January 7, 2006, from http://www.actmagazine.com/appliedclinicaltrials/article/articleDetail.jsp?id=168945

Brafman, A. H. (1995). Beware of the distorting interpreter [letter]. *British Medical Journal, 331,* 1439.

California Healthcare Interpreters Association (CHIA). (2002). *California standards for healthcare interpreters: Ethical principles, protocols, and guidance on roles & intervention.* Retrieved January 14, 2006, from http://chia.ws/documents/publications/CA_standards_healthcare_interpreters.pdf

California Update. (2003, October 21). In the last days of his administration, Governor Davis signs key bills affecting immigrants in California. *California Immigrant Welfare Collaborative.* Retrieved January 28, 2006, from http://www.nilc.org/ciwc/nwsltr/CAUPD5-03.pdf

Carter-Pokras, O., O'Neill, M. J. F., Cheanvechai, V., Menis, M., Fan, T., & Solera, A. (2004). Providing linguistically appropriate services to persons with limited English proficiency: A needs and resources investigation. *American Journal of Managed Care, 10*(10), 29–36.

Code of professional conduct and business practices. (2006). Retrieved January 2, 2006, from http://www.atanet.org//membership/code_of_professional_conduct.php

Coppola, S. (Writer/Director). (2003). *Lost in translation* [Motion picture]. United States: Focus Features, Universal Studios.

Edwards, R., Temple, B., & Alexander, C. (2005). Users' experiences of interpreters. *Interpreting, 7*(1), 77–95.

Elderkin-Thompson, V., Silver, R. C., & Waitzkin, H. (2001). When nurses double as interpreters: A study of Spanish-speaking patients in a US primary care setting [abstract]. *Social Science and Medicine, 52*(9), 1343–1358.

Flores, G., Laws, M. B., Mayo, S. J., Zuckerman, B., Abreu, M., Medina, L., et al. (2003). Errors in medical interpretation and their potential clinical consequences in pediatric encounters. *Pediatrics, 111*, 6–14.

Foreign relations of the United States, 1961–1963: Vol. XI: Cuban missile crisis and aftermath. (1996). Washington, DC: U.S. Department of State. Transcriptions of Records of NSC and EXCOMM Meetings, October 1962. Retrieved January 8, 2006, from http://www.cs.umb.edu/~rwhealan/jfk/cmc_excomm_meetings.html

Galbis-Reig, D. (2000). Assessing medical translation services on the Internet. *Internet Journal of Law and Health Ethics, 1*(1). Retrieved January 7, 2006, from http://www.ispub.com/ostia/index.php?xmlFilePath=journals/ijhca/vol1n1/trans.xml

Ginsberg, C., Martin, V., Andrulis, D., Shaw-Taylor, Y., & McGregor, C. (1995). *Interpretation and translation services in health care: A survey of US public and private teaching hospitals.* Washington, DC: National Public Health and Hospital Institute.

Ginsburg, P. B. (2004). Controlling health care costs. *New England Journal of Medicine, 351*(16), 1591–1593.

Green, A. R., Ngo-Metzger, Q., Legedza, A. T., Massagli, M. P., Phillips, R. S., & Iezzoni, L. I. (2005). Interpreter services, language concordance, and health care quality: Experiences of Asian Americans with limited English proficiency. *Journal of General Internal Medicine, 20*(11), 1050–1060.

Hatton, D. C. (1992). Information transmission in bilingual, bicultural contexts. *Journal of Community Health Nursing, 9*(1), 53–59.

Hatton, D. C., & Webb, T. (1993). Information transmission in bilingual, bicultural contexts: A field study of community health nurses and interpreters. *Journal of Community Health Nursing, 10*(3), 137–147.

Herndon, E., & Joyce, L. (2004, June). *Getting the most from language interpreters.* Retrieved January 7, 2006, from http://www.aafp.org/fpm/20040600/37gett.html

Hudelson, P. (2005). Improving patient-provider communication: Insights from interpreters [abstract]. *Family Practice, 22*(3), 311–316.

Hwa-Froelich, D. A., & Westby, C. E. (2003). Considerations when working with interpreters. *Community Disease Quarterly, 24*(2), 78–85.

Jacobs, E. A., Shepard, D. S., Suaya, J. A., & Stone, E.-L. (2004). Overcoming language barriers in health care: Costs and benefits of interpreter services. *American Journal of Public Health, 94*(5), 866–869.

Kazzi, G. B., & Cooper, C. (2003). Barriers to the use of interpreters in emergency room paediatric consultations. *Journal of Paediatrics and Child Health, 39*, 259–263.

Kravitz, R. L., Helms, L. J., Azari, R., Antonius, D., & Melnikow, J. (2000). Comparing the use of physician time and health care resources among patients speaking English, Spanish, and Russian. *Medical Care, 38*(7), 728–738.

Language Services Action Kit. (2003). *Interpreter services in health care settings for people with limited English proficiency.* Boston: National Health Law Program and The Access Project.

Lee, L. J., Batal, H. A., Maselli, J. H., & Kutner, J. S. (2002). Effect of Spanish interpretation method on patient satisfaction in an urban walk-in clinic [abstract]. *Journal of General Internal Medicine, 17*(8), 641–645.

Lupton, R., & Power, A. (2004, November). *Minority ethnic groups in Britain* (Centre for Analysis of Social Exclusion. CASE-Brookings Census Briefs. No. 2). London: London School of Economics.

Marcos, L. R. (1979). Effects of interpreters on the evaluation of psychopathology in non-English-speaking patients. *American Journal of Psychiatry, 2,* 171–174.

Minnesota Department of Health. (2004). Working with medical interpreters: Laws governing the use of medical interpreters. In *Minnesota refugee health provider guide.* Retrieved January 20, 2006, from http://www.health.state.mn.us/divs/idepc/refugee/guide/index.html

Moskop, J. C., Marko, C. A., Larkin, G. L., Geiderman, J. M., & Derse, A. R. (2005). From Hippocrates to HIPAA: Privacy and confidentiality in emergency medicine—Part II: Challenges in the emergency department. *Annals of Emergency Medicine, 45*(1), 60–67.

Mullins, C. D., Blatt, L., Gbarayor, C. M., Yang, H. W., & Baquet, C. (2005). Health disparities: A barrier to high-quality care. *American Journal of Health-System Pharmacy, 62*(18), 1873–1882.

National Council on Interpreting in Health Care (NCIHC). (2001). *Guide to initial assessment of interpreter qualifications.* Retrieved December 29, 2005, from http://www.ncihc.org

National Council on Interpreting in Health Care (NCIHC). (2005, September). *National standards of practice for interpreters in health care.* Retrieved January 12, 2006, from http://www.ncihc.org/NCIHC_PDF/National_Standards_of_Practice_for_Interpreters_in_Health_Care.pdf

National Health Law Program. (2005). *HIPAA and language services in health care.* Retrieved February 1, 2006, from http://www.healthlaw.org/search.cfm?q=HIPAA+and+Language+Services&fa=search&x=28&y=7

Ngo-Metzger, Q., Massagli, M. P., Clarridge, B. R., Manocchia, M., Davis, R. B., Iezzoni, L. I., et al. (2003). Linguistic and cultural barriers to care: Perspectives of Chinese and Vietnamese immigrants. *Journal of General Internal Medicine, 18,* 44–52.

Office for Civil Rights (OCR). (2001). Appendix B. Selected federal and state laws and regulations requiring language assistance. Retrieved Janaury 24, 2006, from http://www.hhs.gov/ocr/lep/appb.html

Office of Management and Budget (OMB). (2002, March 14). *Report to Congress. Assessment of the total benefits and costs of implementing Executive Order No. 13166: Improving Access to Services for Persons with Limited English Proficiency.* Retrieved January 26, 2006, from http://www.whitehouse.gov/omb/inforeg/lepfinal3-14.pdf#search='OMB%20Report%20to%20Congress%20tempered%20by%20the%20fact%20that%20many%20government%20agencies'

Perkins, J., Youdelman, M., & Wong, D. (2003, August). *Ensuring linguistic access in health care settings: Legal rights and responsibilities.* Washington, DC: National Health Law Program.

Phelan, M., & Parkman, S. (1995). How to do it: Work with an interpreter. *British Medical Journal, 311,* 555–557.

Putsch, R., SenGupta, I., Sampson, A., & Tervalon, M. (2003). *Reflections on the CLAS standards: Best practices, innovations and horizons.* Seattle: The Cross Cultural Health Care Program.

Roat, C. E. (2003, February). *Health care interpreter training in the state of California including an analysis of trends and a compendium of training programs.* Woodland Hills, CA: The California Endowment.

Roat, C. E. (2005). *Addressing language access issues in your practice: A toolkit for physicians and their staff members.* San Francisco: California Academy of Family Physicians.

Roat, C. E., Alvarado-Little, W., & Jacobs, E. A. (2003, November 23). *Letter to Deanna Jang, J.D., Senior Civil Rights Analyst, Office for Civil Rights. National Council on Interpreting in Health Care.* Retrieved January 24, 2006, from http://www.ncihc.org/NCIHC_PDF/ NCIHCcommentstoOCR2003final.pdf#search='deanna%20Jang%20jd%20we% 20are%20writing%20on%20behalf%20arizona'

Roat, C. E., & Okahara, L. (1998, May). *Survey of twenty-three medical interpreter training programs in the United States and Canada.* Seattle: The Cross Cultural Health Care Program.

Rudd, R. E. (2002). *Health literacy overview presentation.* Retrieved August 27, 2005, from the Harvard School of Public Health, Health Literacy Studies Web site: http:// www.hsph.harvard.edu/healthliteracy

Saint-Louis, L., Friedman, E., Chiasson, E., Quessa, A., & Novaes, F. (2003). *Testing new technologies in medical interpreting.* Somerville, MA: Cambridge Health Alliance.

Sevilla Mátir, J. F., & Willis, D. R. (2004). Using bilingual staff members as interpreters. Retrieved January 7, 2006, from http://www.aafp.org/fpm/20040700/34usin.html

Shedden, M. (2006, January 19). *More hospitals call on interpreters for help.* Retrieved December 20, 2006, from http://www.ncpa.org/sub/dpd/?page=article&Article_ID=2790

Shin, H. B., & Bruno, R. (2003). Language use and English-speaking ability: 2000. *Census 2000 Brief.* Retrieved January 3, 2006, from http://www.census.gov/prod/2003pubs/ c2kbr-29.pdf

Sophocles, A. (2003). *Time is of the essence: Coding on the basis of time for physician services.* Retrieved January 27, 2006, from http://www.aafp.org/fpm/20030600/27time.html

Tocher, T. M., & Larson, E. B. (1999). Do physicians spend more time with non-English-speaking patients [abstract]? *Journal of General Internal Medicine, 14*(5), 303–309.

U.S. Census Bureau. (2000). *United States Census 2000. Profile of general demographic characteristics.* Washington, DC: U.S. Census Bureau.

Vasquez, C., & Javier, R. A. (1991). The problem with interpreters: Communicating with Spanish-speaking patients. *Hospital and Community Psychiatry, 42*(2), 163–165.

AFTERWORD

Our emphasis throughout this book has been on the need for better patient–provider communication and for increased efforts to accommodate underserved patients who stumble when clinical language is written beyond their abilities, whether that language appears in the form of a sign in a hospital corridor or a package insert the patient receives with a prescription; whether the message takes written or spoken form; and whether it is conveyed in English, Spanish, Hmong, Russian, Urdu, or another language.

Awareness of blind spots in our health care system can help improve treatments for all patients, regardless of their reading or literacy level as measured by the National Assessment of Adult Literacy of 2003, the Test of English as a Foreign Language, or some other exam. Our hope is that *Health Literacy in Primary Care: A Clinician's Guide* can contribute to the national dialogue already under way about the effects of low health literacy on patient care. And we hope it goes further than that, raising awareness about the range of services and approaches available to improve the lives of those scores of millions of Americans who live with this serious but ultimately preventable condition.

INDEX

SPRINGER PUBLISHING COMPANY

Emerging Infectious Diseases
Trends and Issues, Second Edition

Felissa R. Lashley, RN, PhD
Jerry D. Durham, PhD, RN, FAAN, Editors

Emerging, reemerging, and antibiotic-resistant infectious diseases continue to increase at an alarming rate throughout the world. Written for a wide range of health professionals, particularly nurses, this revised edition provides a comprehensive and up-to-date overview of these diseases and their epidemiology, clinical manifestations, prevention, and treatment. Contributed by a multidisciplinary team of nurses, physicians, and infectious disease specialists, the book includes material on the most recent and important new EIDs, such as avian influenza and SARS; and special considerations, including bioterrorism, behavioral and cultural issues, infectious etiologies of chronic diseases, and travel and recreational exposure.

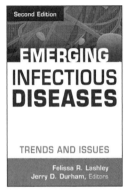

Table of Contents

May 2007 · 596pp · Hardcover · 978-0-8261-0250-8

11 West 42nd Street, New York, NY 10036-8002 • **Fax: 212-941-7842**
Order Toll-Free: 877-687-7476 • **Order Online: www.springerpub.com**

Dictionary of Health Insurance and Managed Care

David Edward Marcinko, MBA, CFP©, CMP©, Editor-in-Chief
Hope Rachel Hetico, RN, MSHA, CPHQ, CMP©, Managing Editor

"The Dictionary of Health Insurance and Managed Care *lifts the fog of confusion surrounding the most contentious topic in the health care industrial complex today. My suggestion therefore is to 'read it, refer to it, recommend it, and reap.'"*
—**Michael J. Stahl,** PhD, Physician Executive MBA Program, William B. Stokely Distinguished Professor of Business, The University of Tennessee, College of Business Administration

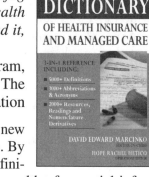

To keep up with the ever-changing field of health care, we must learn new and re-learn old terminology in order to correctly apply it to practice. By bringing together the most up-to-date abbreviations, acronyms, definitions, and terms in the health care industry, the Dictionary offers a wealth of essential information that will help you understand the ever-changing policies and practices in health insurance and managed care today.

Special Features

An Essential Tool for Every Health Care Industry Sector:
• Layman, purchaser, and benefits manager
• Physician, provider, and health care facility
• Payer, intermediary, and insurance professional

Key Benefits & Features Include:
• New terminology
• List for confusing terminology
• Expanded definitions of older terminology still in use today
• Simple examples
• Cross-references to research

Partial Contents:

• Foreword
• Preface
• Acknowledgments
• Dedication
• Instructions for Use

• Abbreviations and Acronyms
• Terminology: A-Z
• Appendix: Textbook References and Readings

2006 · 372pp · Softcover · 978-0-8261-4994-7

11 West 42nd Street, New York, NY 10036-8002 • **Fax: 212-941-7842**
Order Toll-Free: 877-687-7476 • **Order Online: www.springerpub.com**

SPRINGER PUBLISHING COMPANY

Modell's Essential Drugs in Current Use and New Drugs, 2006
52nd Edition

Milagros Fernandez, PharmD
Lydia Calix, BS Pharm, RPh, Editors

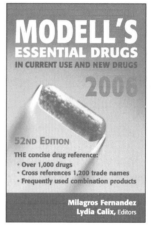

Now in its fifty-second year, this annually updated drug reference provides succinct information on the new drugs of this year and on medications in current use. It offers a concise and portable alternative to the mega drug reference volumes available elsewhere. The compact format contains essential information on nearly 1,100 generic drugs, with cross references to over 1,200 trade names. Highlights include a glossary listing the common side effects of the drugs. Special attention is given to the new drugs with expanded patient care implications for nurses and other allied health professionals.

Highlights to the 52nd Edition:

28 NEW drugs including:
- Telithromycin, from a new class of antibiotics known as ketolides
- Three new drugs for overactive bladders
- Five new agents for cancer
- Essential info on nearly 1,100 generic drugs
- Cross references to over 1,200 trade names
- List of most frequently used combination products
- Glossary listing common drug side effects

Table of Contents

Preface

Part I: New Drugs

Part II: Drugs in Current Use (an alphabetical listing)

Part III: Glossary of Side Effects

Part IV: References

2006 · 640pp · Softcover · 978-0-8261-7096-5

11 West 42nd Street, New York, NY 10036-8002 • Fax: 212-941-7842
Order Toll-Free: 877-687-7476 • Order Online: www.springerpub.com

SPRINGER PUBLISHING COMPANY

Teaching Cultural Competence in Nursing and Health Care

Inquiry, Action, and Innovation

Marianne R. Jeffreys, EdD, RN

Preparing nurses and other health professionals to provide quality health care amid the increasingly multicultural and global society of the 21st century requires a new, comprehensive approach that emphasizes cultural competence education throughout professional education and professional practice. Written in response to this need, *Teaching Cultural Competence in Nursing and Health Care* is intended as a primary resource for educators and graduate students in academic settings, health care institutions, and professional associations.

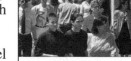

It is the only book that presents a research-supported conceptual model and a valid, reliable corresponding questionnaire to guide educational strategy design, implementation, and evaluation. *Teaching Cultural Competence in Nursing and Health Care* provides readers with valuable tools and strategies for cultural competence education that can easily be adapted by educators at all levels.

Unique features of this book include:
- A model to guide cultural competence education
- A questionnaire for measuring and evaluating learning
- A guide for identifying at-risk individuals and avoiding pitfalls
- Techniques for diverse learners
- Vignettes, case examples, illustrations, tables, and assessment tools

Table of Contents

June 2006 · 232pp · Softcover · 978-0-8261-7764-3

11 West 42nd Street, New York, NY 10036-8002 • Fax: 212-941-7842
Order Toll-Free: 877-687-7476 • Order Online: www.springerpub.com